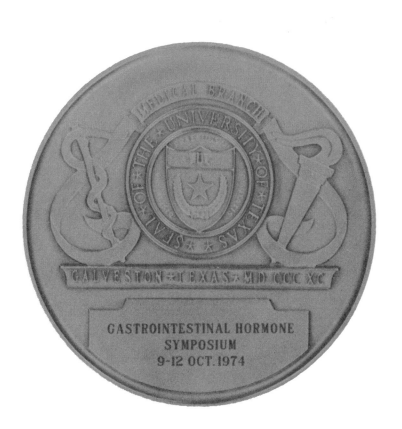

MEDICAL BRANCH
SEAL OF THE UNIVERSITY OF TEXAS
GALVESTON ★ TEXAS ★ MD CCC XC

GASTROINTESTINAL HORMONE
SYMPOSIUM
9-12 OCT. 1974

Gastrointestinal Hormones

GIH SYMPOSIUM Speakers

Front Row
Makhlouf, Track, Larsson, Grossman, Gregory, Thompson,
Bodansvky, Chey, Walsh, McGuigan, Cohen, Andersson

Second Row
Gardner, Solcia, Rayford, Adelson, Kelly, Lambert, Johnson,
Go, Hansky, Erspamer, Boden

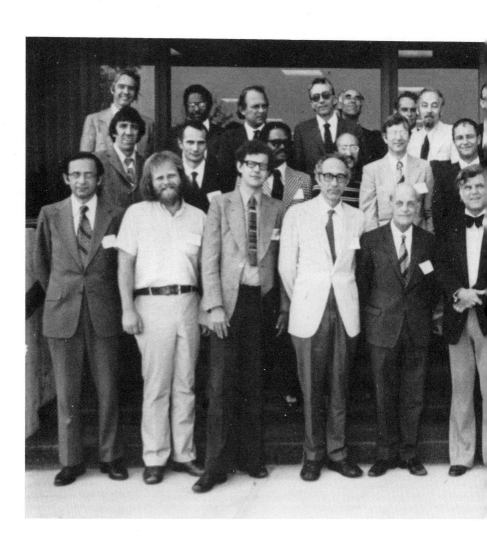

Third Row
Said, Debas, Unger, Creutzfeldt, Konturek, Barrowman,
Jacobson, Becker, Schofield, Dockray, Straus, Meyer,
Galardy, Brown, Olbe, Bloom, Rehfeld
Not pictured: Yalow.

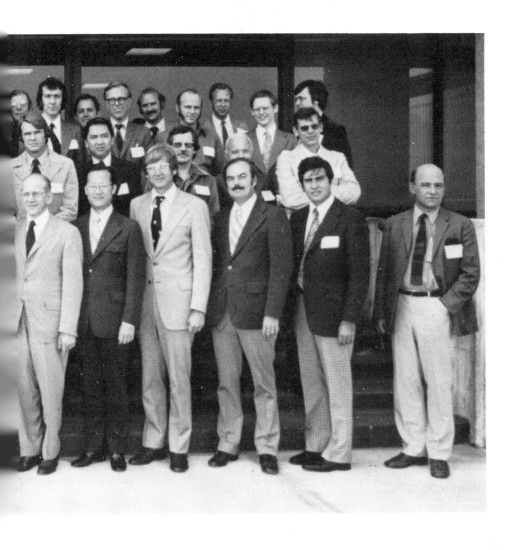

Technical Editor: Marilyn A. Thompson

Gastrointestinal Hormone Symposium, University of Texas Medical Branch at Galveston, 1971.

Gastrointestinal Hormones

A Symposium

Edited by James C. Thompson, M.D.

Foreword by Roderick A. Gregory, F.R.S.

Introduction by Morton I. Grossman, M.D.

University of Texas Press   Austin & London

For reasons of economy and speed this volume has
been printed from camera-ready copy furnished by
the editor. The individual authors assume full
responsibility for their contributions.

International Standard Book Number 0-292-72704-6
Library of Congress Catalog Card Number 75-3573
Printed in the United States of America

Second Printing, 1975

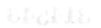

CONTENTS

ENDOCRINE CELLS

TROPHIC ACTIONS OF GI HORMONES

RELEASE OF GI HORMONES

FOREWORD

During the last 12 years there has taken place a
truly remarkable series of advances in our understanding of the physiology and biochemistry of the
gastrointestinal hormones, and on the occasion of
this Conference it is perhaps appropriate to consider
for a moment what has been accomplished in that short
period of time. At the outset, secretin - the first
hormone to be discovered - and gastrin - the second -
were isolated in a pure state and characterised as
basic and acidic peptides respectively after more than
half a century of endeavour and controversy. Within
a few years, both had become available in pure natural and synthetic forms and so for the first time
studies could be made in unequivocal terms of their
physiologic properties. These proved to be of unexpected range, involving virtually all of the muscu-
lar and glandular components of the digestive tract,
and even systems outside of it, relegating to history
the concept of 'one hormone, one action' which can be
seen upon reflection to have underlain much earlier
work.

A few years later, by the further efforts of the
late Erik Jorpes and Viktor Mutt - who was, alas,
prevented from attending on this occasion - there
was achieved a brilliant solution to the problem of
the nature of the duodenal hormones cholecystokinin
and pancreozymin by the demonstration that the actions
long attributed to these hormones were in fact prime
properties of a single peptide. Meanwhile gastrin
was shown to be the agent responsible for the Zollinger-Ellison syndrome, and in the last few years
'gastric inhibitory peptide', 'vasoactive intestinal
peptide' and 'motilin' have been added to the growing
family of peptides known to regulate the affairs of
the digestive tract. The first two of these have
been implicated in the Verner-Morrison syndrome of
watery diarrhoea, hypokalaemia and achlorhydria, and
the list of 'candidate hormones' is already an im-
pressive one. No crystal ball is needed to foresee

the many further advances that are to come from the continued study of what must now be recognised as certainly the largest and probably the most complex endocrine organ in the body - the gastrointestinal mucosa.

Perhaps the most important single consequence of the isolation and synthesis of so many hormones is that it has made possible the application of radio-immunoassay to their study, a great gift we owe to the late Solomon Berson and his colleague Rosalyn Yalow. This technique, one of the outstanding methodological advances of our time, has transformed every aspect of endocrinology, and something of its continuing impact can be seen in many of the contributions made to this meeting. A notable example is the discovery through the use of radioimmunoassay of the heterogeneity of circulating gastrin, which led to the recognition of 'big gastrin' and other circulating forms of the hormone. The scene is clearly set for similar advances in our understanding of the biosynthetic pathways and circulating forms of the other hormones.

At the very heart of that great afternoon's work in 1902, when Bayliss and Starling began it all with their discovery of secretin, was their recognition of the 'messenger' role of what later came to be called 'hormones', with its implication of the 'recognition' of the hormone molecule by a specific site on the surface of the 'target' cell. In this Conference were described the first assays in the study of the action of gastrointestinal hormones at their receptor sites in isolated cell systems: the shape indeed of things to come.

It was a timely moment for this Conference to bring together some two score of distinguished investigators from North America and Europe to discuss the present state of what Medawar has so aptly called "the art of the soluble" and to open exciting prospects of advances along new paths. It is safe to predict that every reader of this volume, the publication of which by the University of Texas Press has been so generously supported by the Moody Foundation, will find in it much that is new and important in his own sphere of interest, or if he is not already committed to work in this most active field, a unique introduction to some aspects of it which are presently engaging our interest.

For an occasion of this nature to be truly successful, not only must the time be ripe - as it was - but the participants and the program must be appropriately chosen. In this respect, full marks must surely go to Professor James Thompson and Dr. Morton Grossman, who organised the program. The University of Texas and its many generous benefactors made it all possible; and the Organising Committee, led by Professor Thompson and Dean Brandt, thought of everything - and a little more - that could possibly be conducive to a happy and smoothly flowing meeting. The result, deservedly, was a great success, crowned by a most gracious occasion at the end of the Conference when all participants dined by candlelight in the Hall of the Moody Medical Library to the music of a string quartet! An equally memorable event was the evening reception given in their home by Professor and Mrs. Thompson.

All those who were privileged to have attended this Conference must have come away very conscious of the burgeoning of this field of study, so long the 'Cinderella' of endocrinology, and wondering impatiently what new developments lie in store for the next occasion!

R.A. Gregory, FRS

PREFACE

A Symposium on Gastrointestinal Hormones was held
at The University of Texas Medical Branch, Galveston,
Texas on 9-12 October 1974; 41 scientists from 10
countries presented papers. The Symposium was nearly
four years in gestation; its eventual success was due
ultimately to these participants, whose works are
herein reported, and to the invited discussants.
The initial idea for the Symposium received enthu-
siastic support from Truman G. Blocker, Jr., M.D.,
then President of UTMB. A prospectus was prepared
for The Moody Foundation, whose Directors later acted
generously to grant funds to support publication of
these Proceedings.

The next step was to approach Dr. Morton I. Grossman
for advice and he graciously agreed to serve as Program Co-chairman. We selected topics to be covered
and who was best qualified to present them. Every
individual invited agreed to come (but one, and that
topic was deleted). The basic format for the meeting
was agreed upon in mid-1973, but fast-breaking new
discoveries resulted in additions to the program only
a few months before the meeting.

The Symposium was an extraordinarily happy affair.
I believe that everyone enjoyed it. Presentation
after presentation excelled expectations; discussions
were brisk and cordial and illuminating. A feast
was served to us: the structure of big gastrin was
revealed by Professor Gregory himself, exciting new
techniques were presented which allow close scrutiny
of hormone receptor sites, guideposts were provided
to the understanding of the physiologic significance
of molecular heterogeneity of peptide hormones,
elegant studies were presented on mechanisms of
release and actions of hormones, on new radioimmunoassays for secretin and cholecystokinin, on correlation of structure and function of GI endocrine cells.
At the end we had an extraordinary session on new
hormones.

An interesting outcome of the program was that
although most papers had a basic scientific orientation, several items of clinical interest were presented in addition to the role of gastrin in the
Zollinger-Ellison syndrome and VIP in the pancreatic
cholera syndrome (pp 635-642). It is clear that acid
secretion is suppressed by the entire secretin family
of hormones, and a clinical trial of GIP or VIP in
treatment of peptic ulcer disease might parallel or
follow the present trial with secretin. The property
of stimulation of intestinal motility shown by cholecystokinin (also by the octapeptide [OP-CCK] and
caerulein) might be worthy of a clinical trial of
treatment of postoperative ileus. Newer clinical
speculations involve the possible use of 1) VIP in
treating bronchospasm (pp 591-597), 2) CCK and
pentagastrin injections into the mesenteric arteries
in treating intestinal ischemia (pp 391-400), and
3) the use of CCK as a satiety factor in control of
obesity (pp 643-649). In all, the excellent quality
of the program was largely due to the prescience of
Morton Grossman.

The final Banquet ended with a beautifully
evocative and masterfully delivered talk by
Professor Gregory who gently illuminated all of
us. My thanks go to colleagues who made this
volume possible. I am sure that we all hope that
it will be of help to scientific and clinical
students of function of the gut.

James C. Thompson

Magnifications for photo- and electronmicrographs have been
recalculated to compensate for changes in size for final
printing; the magnifications given are correct.

Sequential amino acid formulas for gastrointestinal hormones
and related compounds are given in the Appendix, pp 651-654.

ACKNOWLEDGMENTS

We gratefully acknowledge help provided for the
Symposium on Gastrointestinal Hormones and for the
publication of this volume. Truman G. Blocker, Jr.,
M.D., President Emeritus, William C. Levin, M.D.,
President, and Edward N. Brandt, Jr., M.D., Ph.D.,
Dean of Medicine, of The University of Texas Medical
Branch, provided continued and unfailing assistance.
Local arrangements for the meeting were unusually
successful and that success was due to dedicated
efforts on the part of the Organizing Committee:
E.N. Brandt, Jr., M.D., Ph.D., Dean of Medicine,
Phillip L. Rayford, Ph.D., Assistant Professor of
Surgery, The Reverend W. Gammon Jarrell, Episcopal
Chaplain, UTMB, and Mr. Raymond M. Dunning, Jr.,
Assistant to the Chairman, Department of Surgery.
I would also like to thank my secretary, Mrs. Dorothy
LeFevers, and all of the members of the staff of the
Department of Surgery who made the participants
welcome.
Financial assistance was given generously by
Hoechst Pharmaceuticals, Inc., Lilly Research Labor-
atories, Mead Johnson Research Center, William H.
Rorer, Inc., E.R. Squibb and Sons, and The Upjohn
Company. Further help was provided by The University
of Texas Medical Branch and by a grant from the
Research and Development Fund of the Department of
Surgery, UTMB. We want to express our gratitude to
Mr. Glendon Johnson, President, American National
Insurance Company, and his colleagues for the use
of the splendid conference facilities in the ANICO
Building and for their cheerful help during the
Symposium.
We are grateful to Mr. Philip D. Jones, Director
of the University of Texas Press, and to his colleagues for their help and guidance in the publication of this volume. We are especially grateful
to Miss Julie Gips, Manuscript Typist, Department
of Surgery, for her excellent work in preparing
camera-ready copy for publication.

The elegant electronmicrographs of the G-cell and the S-cell which decorate the front and back of the dust jacket were provided by Dr. Juan Lechago and Dr. Enrico Solcia, respectively. Mr. Joseph Paderewski designed and engraved the Commemorative Medallion.

Costs of publication were underwritten by a grant from The Moody Foundation. We are most grateful to the Members of the Board and to Mr. Robert Baker and to Mr. Edward Protz of The Moody Foundation.

My greatest debt is to my wife, Marilyn A. Thompson, who has served expertly as Technical Editor for this volume.

JCT

SPEAKERS

Joel W. Adelson, Ph.D.	Department of Physiology, University of California School of Medicine, San Francisco, California 94143
Sven Andersson, M.D.	Department of Pharmacology, Karolinsa Institutet, 104 01 Stockholm 60, Sweden
James A. Barrowman, M.D.	Department of Physiology, The London Hospital Medical College, London E1 2AD, England
H. Dieter Becker, M.D.	Chirurgische Klinik Universität Göttingen, 34 Göttingen, Germany
Stephen Bloom, M.D.	The Royal Postgraduate Medical School, The Hammersmith Hospital, London W1P 7DE, England
Miklos Bodanszky, D.Sc.	Department of Chemistry, Case Western Reserve University, Cleveland, Ohio 44106
Guenther Boden, M.D.	Department of Medicine, Section of Metabolism and the General Clinical Research Center, Temple University Health Sciences Center, Philadelphia, Pennsylvania 19140
John C. Brown, Ph.D.	Department of Physiology, University of British Columbia, Vancouver 8, British Columbia, Canada
William Y. Chey, M.D.	Issac Gordon Center for Digestive Diseases, The University of Rochester School of Medicine and Dentistry, Rochester, New York 14607

Sidney Cohen, M.D.   Department of Medicine, Hospital
                                   of the University of Pennsylvania,
                                   Philadelphia, Pennsylvania 19104

Professor Werner Creutzfeldt   Medizinische Klinik Universität
                                   Göttingen, 34 Göttingen, Germany

Haile T. Debas, M.D.   Department of Surgery, University
                                   of British Columbia, Vancouver 9,
                                   British Columbia, Canada

Graham J. Dockray, Ph.D.   Department of Physiology, Univer-
                                   sity of Liverpool, Liverpool L69
                                   3BX, England

Professor Vittorio Erspamer   Instituto de Farmacologia Medica,
                                   Citta Universitaria, 001 00
                                   Rome, Italy

Richard E. Galardy, M.D.   Section of Cell Biology, Yale
                                   University School of Medicine,
                                   New Haven, Connecticut 06510

Jerry D. Gardner, M.D.   Section on Gastroenterology, Diges-
                                   tive Diseases Branch, National
                                   Institute of Arthritis, Metabolism,
                                   and Digestive Diseases, National
                                   Institutes of Health, Bethesda,
                                   Maryland 20014

Vay L.W. Go, M.D.   Gastroenterology Unit, Mayo Foun-
                                   dation, Rochester, Minnesota 55901

Professor R.A. Gregory   Physiological Laboratory, Uni-
                                   versity of Liverpool,Liverpool,
                                   L69 3BX, England

Morton I. Grossman, M.D.   VA Wadsworth Hospital Center and
                                   UCLA School of Medicine, Los
                                   Angeles, California 90073

Jack Hansky, M.D.   Monash University, Department of
                                   Medicine and Renal Unit, Prince
                                   Henry's Hospital, Melbourne,
                                   Australia 3004

Eugene D. Jacobson, M.D.	Program in Physiology, The University of Texas Medical School, Houston, Texas 77025
Leonard R. Johnson, Ph.D.	Program in Physiology, The University of Texas Medical School, Houston, Texas 77025
Keith A. Kelly, M.D.	Sections of Gastroenterologic and General Surgery and of Surgical Research, Mayo Clinic, Mayo Foundation, and Mayo Medical School, Rochester, Minnesota 55901
Stanisław J. Konturek, M.D.	Institute of Physiology, Medical Academy, Krakow, Poland
René Lambert, M.D.	Unité de Recherches de Physio-Pathologie Digestive, Hôpital Edouard-Herriot, 69374 Lyon, France
Lars-Inge Larsson, M.D.	Department of Histology, University of Lund, S-223 62 Lund, Sweden
Gabriel M. Makhlouf, M.D.	Department of Medicine, Medical College of Virginia, Richmond, Virginia 23298
James C. McGuigan, M.D.	Division of Gastroenterology, University of Florida College of Medicine, Gainesville, Florida 32610
James H. Meyer, M.D.	Veterans Administration Hospital and the University of California, San Francisco, California 94121
Lars Olbe, M.D.	Surgical Clinic II, Sahlgrenska Hospital, 413 45 Göteborg, Sweden
Phillip L. Rayford, Ph.D.	Department of Surgery, The University of Texas Medical Branch, Galveston, Texas 77550
Jens F. Rehfeld, M.D.	Department of Clinical Chemistry, Bispebjerg Hospital, DK-2400 Copenhagen, NV Denmark

Sami I. Said, M.D.	Departments of Internal Medicine and Pharmacology, University of Texas Southwestern Medical School and Veterans Administration Hospital, Dallas, Texas 75235
Brian Schofield, M.D.	Division of Medical Physiology, University of Calgary, Faculty of Medicine, Calgary, Alberta, Canada T2N 1N4
Enrico Solcia, M.D.	Instituto de Anatomia e Istologia Pathologica, Università de Pavia, 27100 Pavia, Italy
Eugene Straus, M.D.	Solomon A. Berson Research Laboratory, Bronx Veterans Administration Hospital, and Mt. Sinai School of Medicine, The City University of New York, New York 10468
James C. Thompson, M.D.,	Department of Surgery, The University of Texas Medical Branch, Galveston, Texas 77550
Norman S. Track, Ph.D.	Medizinische Klinik Universität Göttingen, 34 Göttingen, Germany
Roger H. Unger, M.D.	Veterans Administration Hospital and the University of Texas Southwestern Medical School, Dallas, Texas 75235
John H. Walsh, M.D.	Department of Medicine, University of California School of Medicine, Los Angeles, California 90024
Rosalyn S. Yalow, Ph.D.	Solomon A. Berson Research Laboratory, Bronx Veterans Administration Hospital, and Mt. Sinai School of Medicine, The City University of New York, New York 10468

INTRODUCTION

TRENDS IN GUT HORMONE RESEARCH

Morton I. Grossman

VA Wadsworth Hospital Center
and UCLA School of Medicine,
Los Angeles, California

HISTORICAL

When Bayliss and Starling[1] discovered secretin in
1902, they quickly saw its broad biologic implications. For them secretin was but one example of a
general mechanism, the coordination of body activity
by blood-borne chemical messengers. Here was a system
that, like the nervous system, allowed stimuli received at one part of the body to alter activity at a
distant part. To emphasize the generality of the concept, Starling[15] introduced the word hormone in 1905.

Although gastroenterology was clearly the mother of
endocrinology, the offspring quickly outdistanced the
parent. Chemical identification of the hormones is
the springboard from which rapid advances have occurred. Many peptide hormones were identified chemically long before the first determination of the structure of a gastrointestinal hormone, which was in 1964
when Gregory and associates[6] announced the amino acid
sequence of gastrin. Even though rapid progress has
been made in this first decade of the biochemical era
of gastrointestinal hormones, we still lag far behind
our colleagues studying other peptide hormones. It
is now time for the children to support the parent;
the principles garnered from the recent advances in
the study of other hormones should be applied to
hormones of the gut.

In what follows I offer some thoughts about aspects
of gastrointestinal hormone research that appear to
me to offer promise of important results in the near
future. I make no claims to powers of prophecy and I
fully recognize that the greatest advances are likely
to be the unpredictable ones.

HETEROGENEITY

It is now clear that many, perhaps all, peptide hormones occur in more than one molecular form. In at least six instances (gastrin,[7] insulin,[11] glucagon,[16] parathyroid hormone,[9] melanocyte-stimulating hormone,[2] and ACTH[18]), trypsin can transform a large form into a smaller form. In the first five of these, the structure of the point of cleavage is known and in each instance it contains at least two consecutive basic amino acids (Table 1). Steiner and associates[7] followed the transformation of proinsulin to insulin in isolated pancreatic islets and found that it involved trypsin-like cleavage followed by carboxypeptidase B-like action to remove the basic amino acids. The enzymes that perform the transformation are found in the secretion granules of the beta cell of the pancreatic islets.[12] It will be of great interest to determine whether the converting enzymes are the same in secretion granules of the various hormone-producing cells; for example, are the same enzymes found in the G-cell as in the beta cell of the pancreatic islets? Conversion from one molecular form to another is known to occur in the cell of origin. To date there is no evidence that it occurs in the circulation.

What biologic purpose is served by heterogeneity? In instances in which the precursor is essentially inactive and circulates in only small amounts, as with insulin, the main purpose is probably related to biosynthetic mechanisms. In the case of gastrin, however, the larger form predominates in the circulation and has definite biologic activity. The only obvious purpose served by the different gastrins is related to

Table 1.   Examples of hormones in which two consecutive basic amino acids are present at cleavage points

GASTRIN	-LYS-LYS-gastrin-17
INSULIN	B chain-ARG-ARG-connecting peptide-LYS-ARG-A chain
GLUCAGON	glucagon-LYS-ARG-
PARATHYROID	-LYS-ARG-parathyroid hormone
β-LIPOTROPIN	-LYS-LYS-β-MSH-LYS-ARG-

their different persistence of action because of their different half-lives.[17] A rapid burst of G-17 gets the targets going and a plateau of G-34 sustains that activity. An intriguing additional possibility is that the different molecular forms of gastrin might have different relative potencies on various targets; in this way they could function almost as though they were separate hormones. However, to date we have not found evidence for this kind of selectivity on various targets. For example, we found that the ratio of potency for acid secretion to potency for gallbladder contraction was the same for G-4, G-13, G-17, and G-34.

Although it has been known since 1968 that cholecystokinin exists in at least two molecular forms,[13] the second form has not yet been chemically characterized. Secretin has not yet been identified in heterogeneous forms.

Whatever its biologic meaning may prove to be, heterogeneity of circulating forms of a hormone can play havoc with attempts to relate total immunoreactivity to total bioactivity.

TROPHIC ACTION

One of the most intriguing - and perhaps one of the most important - actions of the gastrointestinal hormones, is their trophic action,[16] that is, their effect on the growth of cells. This has been studied most extensively for gastrin, but cholecystokinin also has trophic actions, and secretin counteracts the trophic actions of gastrin. The trophic effects are not nonspecific; they do not occur simply as a consequence of activation of the effector cell. Since the effector cells are not usually the proliferative cells, one must assume that separate receptors on the proliferative cells are involved in the trophic actions. The long lag between the time of exposure to hormone and the peak of the proliferative response indicates that a train of events is set in motion that continues even after the hormone has been metabolized. Since the epithelium of the digestive tract is among the most active tissues in the body in terms of replacement kinetics, it is not surprising that there are mechanisms regulating this replacement and that hormones are an important part of that regulatory mechanism.

The big swings in rate of mucosal growth that are associated with such physiologic states as weaning, starvation, and lactation, are correlated with changes in total food intake and are associated with corresponding changes in antral and serum gastrin (Lichtenberger, unpublished data). Similarly male-female differences in food intake are reflected in corresponding differences in antral and serum gastrin, and ovariectomy abolishes both the differences in food intake and in gastrin levels (Lichtenberger, unpublished data).

RECEPTORS

Until quite recently receptors were purely theoretical entities. Now we are beginning to get our first glimpses of the structure and properties of receptors. For the first time we are beginning to look at the binding of hormones to receptors rather than make deductions about such binding from the consequences that flow from the binding. In the past we deduced the kinetics of the reaction between hormone and receptor from the kinetics of a cellular response such as acid secretion. Now we can directly measure the binding of hormone to receptor and measure an immediate consequence of such binding, for example, formation of cyclic AMP.[14] It seems likely that within the next few years, the methods that have been used so successfully to study the receptor properties of cell membranes for other hormones will be applied to gastrointestinal hormones.

Receptors have been found on cells that do not respond to the hormone, for example, insulin receptors on lymphocytes.[5] A search for receptors for gastrointestinal hormones on such readily available cells should be made.

If a hormone or analog can be modified so that it attaches permanently to the receptor by covalent binding, the hormone can be labeled and act as a marker so the receptor can be isolated and its structure determined. The first steps in accomplishing this have already been taken[3] and we shall hear more about this exciting endeavor during this symposium.[4]

Receptors had been thought of as fixed objects, not subject to rapid changes. Recent studies on receptor binding have shown that the number of receptors is

Table 2. Classification of candidate gastrointestinal hormones

---

PURE PEPTIDES FROM INTESTINAL MUCOSA, HORMONAL STATUS UNCERTAIN

    Chymodenin
    Gastric inhibitory peptide (GIP)
    Motilin
    Vasoactive intestinal peptide (VIP)

PURE PEPTIDES WITH GASTROINTESTINAL ACTIONS, HORMONAL STATUS UNCERTAIN

    Pancreatic peptide
    Coherin
    Urogastrone

IMPURE SUBSTANCES WITH GASTROINTESTINAL ACTIONS, HORMONAL STATUS UNCERTAIN

    Gastrone

HORMONES POSTULATED ON PHYSIOLOGIC EVIDENCE, CHEMICAL EVIDENCE INCOMPLETE

    Bulbogastrone
    Duocrinin
    Enterocrinin
    Enterogastrone
    Enteroglucagon
    Incretin
    Villikinin

HORMONES POSTULATED ON PHYSIOLOGIC EVIDENCE, CHEMICAL EVIDENCE ABSENT

    Antral chalone
    Enterooxyntin
    Vagogastrone

---

remarkably labile.[5] The concentration of receptors
can quickly decrease in response to the presence of
the hormone. This provides an important mechanism
of autoregulation, which protects against overdoses
and enhances responsiveness when there is a deficiency.

CANDIDATES

In a recent review,[8] 18 candidate hormones from the
gut were listed (Table 2). The candidates include
both peptides seeking hormonal status and physiologic
events seeking peptide mimickers. Seven chemically
identified peptides are in candidate status, four
from intestinal mucosa (chymodenin, GIP, motilin,
and VIP) and three from extraintestinal sources (bovine or avian pancreatic peptide, coherin, and uro-
gastrone).

How does a candidate get admitted to the exclusive
ranks of the family of hormones? In essence, it must
be shown that the peptide in question is released in
amount and kind sufficient to account for the physiologic event under consideration. For example, we may
ask whether GIP is the enterogastrone (intestinally
derived inhibitor of acid secretion) that is released
by fat. Fat releases GIP and GIP inhibits histamine-
stimulated acid secretion. Can the effect of fat on
histamine-stimulated acid secretion be mimicked by
infusing GIP at a dose that gives a blood level of
GIP like that seen after fat ingestion? This is the
kind of evidence needed to move peptides out of the
candidate hormone category and into "full member"
status.

Acknowledgments

Supported by a Veterans Administration Senior Medical Inves-
tigatorship and by grant AM 17328 from the National Institute
of Arthritis, Metabolism, and Digestive Diseases to CURE, the
Center for Ulcer Research and Education.

References

1. Bayliss WM, Starling EH: The mechanism of pancreatic secretion. *J Physiol* 28:325-353, 1902.
2. Chretien M, Li CH: Isolation, purification, and character-ization of gamma-lipotropic hormone from sheep pituitary glands. *Canad J Biochem* 45:1163-1174, 1967.
3. Galardy RE, Craig LC, Jamieson JD, Printz MP: Photoaffinity labeling of peptide hormone binding sites. *J Biol Chem* 249:3510-3518, 1974.
4. Galardy RE, Jamieson JD: Photoaffinity labeling of secre-tagogue receptors in the pancreatic exocrine cell, in Thompson JC (ed), *Gastrointestinal Hormones,* Austin: University of Texas Press, 1975, pp 345-365.
5. Gavin JR III, Roth J, Neville DM Jr, De Meyts P, Buell DN: Insulin-dependent regulation of insulin receptor con-centrations: A direct demonstration in cell culture. *Proc Natl Acad Sci USA* 71:84-88, 1974.
6. Gregory H, Hardy PM, Jones DS, Kenner GW, Sheppard RC: The antral hormone gastrin: Structure of gastrin. *Nature* 204:931-933, 1964.
7. Gregory RA: The gastrointestinal hormones: A review of recent advances. (The Bayliss-Starling Lecture 1974). *J Physiol* 24:1-3, 1974.
8. Grossman MI and others: Candidate hormones of the gut. *Gastroenterology* 67:730-755, 1974.
9. Huang DWY, Chu LH, Cohn DV, Hamilton JW: N-terminal amino acid sequence of human proparathyroid hormone. *Fed Proc* 33:1512, 1974.
10. Johnson LR: Gut hormones on growth of gastrointestinal mucosa, in Chey WY, Brooks FP (eds), *Endocrinology of the Gut,* Thorofare, NJ: Charles B. Slack, 1974, pp 163-177.
11. Kemmler W, Peterson JD, Steiner DF: Studies on the con-version of proinsulin to insulin: I. Conversion *in vitro* with trypsin and carboxypeptidase B. *J Biol Chem* 246:6786-6791, 1971.
12. Kemmler W, Steiner DF, Borg J: Studies on the conversion of proinsulin to insulin: III. Studies *in vitro* with a crude secretion granule fraction isolated from rat islets of Langerhans. *J Biol Chem* 248:4544-4551, 1973.
13. Mutt V, Jorpes JE: Structure of porcine cholecystokinin-pancreozymin: 1. Cleavage with thrombin and with tryp-sin. *Eur J Biochem* 6:156-162, 1968.
14. Rodbell M, Birnbaumer L, Pohl SL, Sundby F: The reaction of glucagon with its receptor: Evidence for discrete regions of activity and binding in the glucagon mole-cule. *Proc Natl Acad Sci USA* 68:909-913, 1971.

15. Starling EH: On the chemical correlation of the functions
    of the body. *Lancet* 2:339-341, 1905.
16. Tager HS, Steiner DF: Isolation of a glucagon-containing
    peptide: Primary structure of a possible fragment of
    proglucagon. *Proc Natl Acad Sci USA* 70:2321-2325,
    1973.
17. Walsh JH, Debas HT, Grossman MI: Pure human big gastrin.
    Immunochemical properties, disappearance half time,
    and acid-stimulating action in dogs. *J Clin Invest*
    54:477-485, 1974.
18. Yalow RS, Berson SA: Characteristics of "big ACTH" in
    human plasma and pituitary extracts. *J Clin Endocr
    Metab* 36:415-423, 1973.

GASTRIN

THE CHEMISTRY OF THE GASTRINS: SOME RECENT ADVANCES

R.A. Gregory, H.J. Tracy

Physiological Laboratory, University
of Liverpool, Liverpool, England

It is now a little over ten years since the isolation of the hormone gastrin from porcine antral mucosa in the form of the heptadecapeptide was reported in detail.[8],[9] We had in fact obtained pure material early in 1962,[4] but it was not until later in the year that the quantitative amino-acid composition of it was established unequivocally by our colleague Professor Kenner and his group in Liverpool. The second member of the pair of heptadecapeptides was discovered in December 1962, but the fact that the only difference between them consisted of sulphation of the single tyrosine residue present was not realized until synthesis had been completed.[5]

Since those early days, much further knowledge has accrued concerning the various forms of the hormone that are to be found in antral mucosa of different species, in gastrinomas, and in the circulating plasma in both normal and pathologic conditions.[7] It may be of interest on this occasion to recount some of our more recent experiences with the isolation of those forms of the hormone with which we have been concerned, particularly "big" gastrin.

THE "LITTLE" GASTRINS (heptadecapeptides)

The original method of extraction of gastrin from antral mucosa,[9] which is suitable also for gastrinoma tissue and forms the basis for the method of isolation of the big gastrins, has been modified in a few respects over the years of its usage in our laboratory,

and some of the changes have recently been described.[6]
The initial steps are now essentially as follows:
1. Uptake of hormone from an aqueous extract
    with DEAE powder.
2. Isopropanol extraction at pH 9 in presence
    of salt.
3. Filtration on Sephadex G50.
4. Chromatography on aminoethylcellulose (AE).
   At this stage, the gastrins are clearly defined.
For completion of the purification of little gastrin
(and the minigastrins, see later) repetition of 4
above, column electrophoresis, and filtration on
Sephadex G25 are necessary. For isolation of big
gastrin, repeated chromatography on DEAE must be
added to these. In all column procedures, with the
exception of gel filtration, we now use as buffer
triethylamine-carbonate instead of ammonium bicarbonate. It is easily prepared by gassing a solution
of triethylamine with CO_2. It is readily volatile,
is free from traces of amino acids often present in
ammonium bicarbonate (an advantage when isolating
very small amounts of peptides for amino acid analysis), can be used at a lower pH, and gives residues
on lyophilisation of peptide solutions which are not
electrically charged. Column electrophoresis (for
which an apparatus is used that will be described in
detail elsewhere) is superior for preparative purposes to paper electrophoresis, particularly in isolation of the big gastrins, since these run badly
with the latter technique. Recovery is complete
(as shown by running picogram amounts of radiolabeled gastrin) and good resolution is obtained.[10]

Little Gastrins II A and II B

   During our first isolation of human big gastrins
from gastrinoma tissue[10] we observed that in addition
to the usual pair of little gastrins (sulphated and
unsulphated), having the expected amino acid composition, there was also present in the chromatographic
profile of these peptides on AE a third small peak.
Unfortunately the amino acid analysis of the small
amount of material present was not satisfactory, and
it could not be positively identified. In September
1972, thanks to the efforts of Drs. Edward Passaro
and Morton Grossman of Los Angeles, there came into

our hands a very large amount of gastrinoma tissue
(an hepatic metastasis) from a patient with the
Zollinger-Ellison syndrome. In preparing the various
forms of gastrin present in this material, we identified in the heptadecapeptide fraction not only the
usual little gastrins I and II, with the same amino
acid composition as previously described, but also
small amounts of two further peptides which we term
little gastrins II A and II B (Fig. 1). Amino acid
analysis shows that they have the same composition
as the heptadecapeptides, and both have sulphated
tyrosine. They both have the expected potency in
stimulating gastric acid secretion. The reason for
their greater polarity is obscure. The possibility
that these little gastrins may be artifacts cannot
be excluded until it can be shown either that they
are present in the circulation or that they can be
demonstrated in gastrinoma or antral tissue by the
use of a "cold" mild method of extraction.[11]

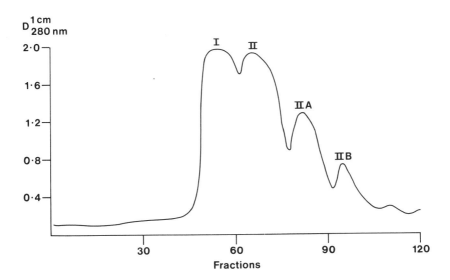

Figure 1. Gastrinoma extract. Chromatography of the heptadecapeptide fraction obtained by filtration on Sephadex G50
superfine. Gradient of pH and concentration on aminoethylcellulose column. Triethylamine-carbonate buffer. For explanation of I, II, IIA, IIB, see text.

THE "BIG" GASTRINS

We first became aware in 1968 that when extracts
of porcine antral mucosa were filtered on Sephadex
G50 columns there was detectable, in a region approximately halfway between the void volume protein and
the salt zone, a very small amount of gastrin-like
activity. It was obviously larger than the heptadecapeptide also present, which emerged in the vicinity of the salt zone. When injected subcutaneously into pouch dogs, this "bigger" gastrin gave a
response of much slower onset and more protracted
time-course than the heptadecapeptide given in the
same manner. It seemed to us that if this material
were not merely an artifact due to the binding of
some little gastrin to larger material, it might be
a precursor form of the hormone, and we set out to
try to isolate it. For a combination of reasons
the task proved extremely difficult.
In the first place, there was very little "big"
activity present in our extract compared with the
heptadecapeptide. When we improved the yield by
lowering the salt concentration in the isopropanol
extraction stage, this greatly increased contamination with a complex of pigment and acidic mucoprotein,
which was adsorbed on all types of columns and slowly
washed off during chromatography, thus obscuring the
normal profiles. Furthermore the "big" activity was
held on columns such as AE and DEAE partly by nonionic
forces, which gave a broad and 'tailing' type of elution profile. Finally there seemed to be more than
one "big" component present, so that gastrin activity
was often detectable over a wide range of fractions
and no useful 'cuts' could be taken. High-voltage
paper electrophoresis was useless and we could find
no suitable system of counter-current distribution.
However, we slowly made progress.
Early in 1970 we were afforded great encouragement
in our efforts by Drs. Yalow and Berson, who generously informed us, in advance of publication, of
their discovery that the form of immunoreactive gastrin usually predominant in serum was larger and less
acidic than heptadecapeptide. Their observations on
the behaviour of "big" gastrin (BG), as they named
the new serum component, proved of great value to us,[11]
and after further changes in our extraction procedure,
we finally succeeded early in 1972 in isolating from

porcine antral mucosa a pair of big gastrin peptides
(sulphated and unsulphated), which corresponded in
properties to the immunoreactive component Yalow and
Berson had discovered in serum. The porcine peptides
are now produced routinely in our laboratory. In our
hands the yield is no more than 1 mg of BG I and 2 mg
BG II from 20 kg of antral mucosa, obtained by dissection from about 600 antra. These amounts, at most,
are probably no more than half of the amounts originally present in the fresh mucosa, which we obtain
about 1 hour after killing. We would estimate the
total amount of BG in porcine antral mucosa to be
about 10% of the heptadecapeptide present.

At the same time as our isolation of the porcine
peptides, we extracted by a similar method an amount
of gastrinoma tissue that we had accumulated during
the previous four years, and from it isolated a few
milligrams of a pair of BG peptides that had an amino
acid composition closely similar to, and chromatographic and electrophoretic properties identical with
the porcine compounds and with immunoreactive BG in
serum.[10,11]

Yalow and Berson[16] had discovered that when serum BG
was digested with trypsin, it rapidly disappeared and
its place was taken by an equivalent amount of heptadecapeptide, or as they termed it "little" gastrin (LG).
From this they concluded that BG might consist of LG,
covalently linked through a lysine or arginine residue
to a further peptide chain of basic character. Experiments with the pure porcine and human BG peptides by
Kenner and his colleagues confirmed and clarified the
observations of Yalow and Berson. In each case the BG
molecule contained no arginine but two residues of lysine, which in sequence formed the link between the LG
portion and the rest. Depending upon the exact conditions of tryptic digestion, one or two "tryptic peptides" were liberated, together with free lysine and
LG, which at first had glutaminyl as the N-terminal
residue and was ninhydrin-positive. This spontaneously
changed to the pyroglutamyl form and the peptide became
ninhydrin-negative (Fig. 2). It was also established,
as had been anticipated, that the pair of BG peptides
in each species differed; in one the single tyrosine
residue (in the LG portion) was sulphated, whereas in
the other it was not, as in the free LG peptides. In
each species, the proportions of the types I and II
BG peptides were similar to those of the free LG peptides, namely, approximately 2:1 in favour of the un-

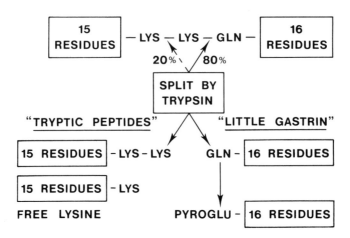

Figure 2. The structure of big gastrin. Cleavage by trypsin.

sulphated form in the human, and 2:1 in favour of the sulphated form in the hog.

At this stage, the amount of human material remaining was too small for any further structural studies, and there our progress would have come to a halt but for the arrival of the very large gastrinoma already mentioned. Our extraction of this material, which occupied more than a year, yielded several hundred milligrams of the free heptadecapeptides and about 15-20 mg of the BG peptides. A partial structure was deduced by Dr. Moira Barton from her studies of the enzymic degradation of the "tryptic peptide." The problem of sequencing human BG, however, was by no means solved, for the N-terminal residue (as in LG) was pyroglutamyl, which prevented the use of the classical Edman degradation.

A successful conclusion was reached by a fortunate combination of circumstances. First, Dr. Morton Grossman obtained for us from its discoverer, Professor R.F. Doolittle of the University of California, San Diego,[3] a supply of the enzyme pyrrolidonecarboxylyl peptidase, which specifically cleaves N-terminal pyroglutamyl from a peptide chain; and second, Professor Kenner secured the collaboration of Dr. Ieuan

Harris of the Molecular Biology Laboratory, Cambridge, England, whose outstanding expertise in the sequencing of peptides by micromethods is well known.

Using the Dansyl-Edman technique, Harris established the complete sequences of both human and porcine big gastrins. We are grateful to Dr. Harris and Professor Kenner for their permission to reproduce the sequences (Table 1) in advance of their account of the structural studies, which will be published in full elsewhere.

Table 1. Sequence of human and porcine big gastrins

HUMAN   Glp*-Leu-Gly-Pro-Gln-Gly-His-Pro-Ser-Leu-Val-Ala-

PORCINE   ——————————Leu———————————Pro————————

HUMAN   Asp-Pro-Ser-Lys-Lys-Gln-Gly-Pro-Trp-Leu-Glu-Glu-

PORCINE   ———Leu-Ala———————————————Met—————

HUMAN   Glu-Glu-Glu-Ala-Tyr-Gly-Trp-Met-Asp-Phe-NH$_2$

PORCINE   ————————————————————————————————

         * Pyroglutamyl

Meanwhile the synthesis of the human and porcine big gastrins is well advanced. For example, in the human peptide the sequences 1-12 and 13-19 have been prepared for coupling to the appropriate little gastrin. Completion of this and alternative routes of synthesis is going ahead on the basis of a collaborative effort between Kenner and his group in Liverpool and Professor Erich Wünsch in Munich.

Further Big Gastrins

During our recent studies with the gastrinoma tissue we have isolated from this source a third big gastrin, intermediate in polarity between BG I and BG II. It emerges when the BG II fraction, obtained by chromatography on AE of the BG 'cut' from Sephadex G50 filtration, is run on DEAE (Fig. 3). Harris has

established for us that the amino-acid composition
(acid hydrolysis) and end-groups of this variant are
the same as that of the other human BG peptides I
and II, and Dr. Barry Mason of Kenner's group has
shown that the tyrosine residue is not sulphated.

The peptide therefore belongs to type I and we propose to call it BG IA. Only 1.5 mg of it were obtained and it has not been sequenced. It seems likely
that there is some difference in amidation of the carboxyl groups in the molecule, compared with BG I or
II. In porcine antral extracts, from the corresponding BG fractions, we are in the process of purifying
small amounts of what appear to be two further BG

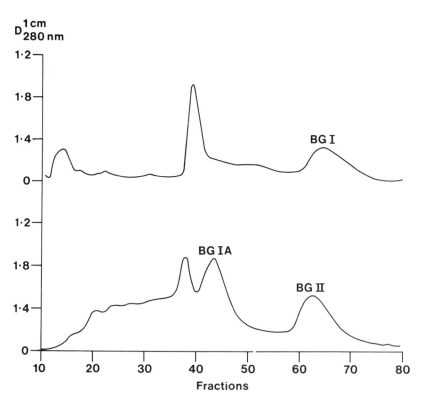

Figure 3. Chromatography of human big gastrins I, IA and II
on diethylaminoethylcellulose columns.

peptides, one less acidic than BG I and one intermediate in acidity between BG I and II. When the
chemical nature of these BG variants is firmly established, it will be necessary to determine whether
they are artifacts or whether they can be detected
in the circulation or in antral or gastrinoma extracts
made by the mildest possible means.

Finally, we must be reminded that although the BG
peptides isolated from gastrinoma tissue are termed
"human" BG (as indeed they are) it remains to be established whether or not they are identical with the
BG peptides produced in the antral mucosa, and this
will require the accumulation of sufficient human
antral mucosa from operation specimens to enable the
BG peptides to be isolated in adequate amounts for
sequencing.

THE "MINIGASTRINS" (tridecapeptides)

During our study of the various forms of gastrin
present in the very large gastrinoma already referred
to, we found in the heptadecapeptide fraction separated at the stage of Sephadex G50 filtration, a pair
of peptides (sulphated and unsulphated) that have an
amino acid composition corresponding to the C-terminal
tridecapeptide of little gastrin. These peptides
occur in the same proportions (2:1 in favour of the
unsulphated form) as do the little and big gastrins
in the same tissue and the little gastrins in human
antral mucosa. Only a few milligrams of each have
been isolated, compared with the hundreds of milligrams of the heptadecapeptides present in the tumour.
The isolation of these peptides[12] and their potency
and circulating half-lives[1] have been reported.

We were at first inclined to suppose that they
might be artifacts, but after their isolation, immunologic evidence was obtained by Dr. Rehfeld and his
associates that they can be found in the circulation
of patients with the Zollinger-Ellison syndrome and
in normal subjects after a meal.[14,15] We have not yet
detected minigastrins in hog antral extracts, but if
their proportionality with respect to LG is similar
to that found in the gastrinoma tissue, then only extremely small amounts are likely to be present.

OTHER GASTRIN COMPONENTS

The immunoreactive components described as "big big" gastrin and "Component I" are the subject of other reports in this symposium and so we shall not discuss them here, except to mention that in fractionation of gastrinoma or antral mucosal extracts by the methods we have described earlier, there can be found at the stage of Sephadex G50 filtration a) immunoreactive material in the void volume fraction,[17] and b) material similar to "Component I" which has some bio-logic activity and is immunoreactive.[15]

In 1967 we isolated from hog antral mucosa small amounts of a pair of inactive gastrin fragments cor-responding in amino acid composition to the N-terminal 1-13 portion of the heptadecapeptides, that is, they lacked the active C-terminal tetrapeptide. They were discovered when they separated as small peaks running ahead of the heptadecapeptides during final purifica-tion of large preparations of the latter on a long Sephadex G25 column; they were present in the same proportions (2:1 in favour of the sulphated form) as are the little and big gastrins in porcine antral mucosa. At the time, we made intensive but unsuccess-ful attempts to find the tetrapeptide and there the matter rested. However, an immunoreactive component which appears to correspond to the N-terminal 1-13 fragment of the heptadecapeptide has recently been identified in the serum of gastrinoma patients.[2] We have not yet detected this component in our extraction of gastrinoma tissue.

The discovery of BG and the clarification of its structural relationship to LG makes it likely that BG is a precursor of LG, the one being formed from the other by a process of trypsin-like cleavage at the -LYS-LYS- sequence. Support for this view is provided by the fact that in several other instances in which a larger precursor form of a hormone has been recognized, two consecutive basic amino acids are found at the cleavage point or points (Table 2).[13]

When proinsulin is converted to insulin, the C-pep-tide is released into the circulation. Clearly, it is likely that the "tryptic peptide" of BG may be similarly released and can be sought when an antibody to it can be raised. This should be possible when supplies of synthetic "tryptic peptide" become avail-able.

Table 2. Two consecutive basic amino acids at cleavage points

GASTRIN   -LYS-LYS-gastrin-17

INSULIN   B chain-ARG-ARG-connecting peptide-LYS-ARG-A chain

GLUCAGON   glucagon-LYS-ARG-

PARATHYROID   -LYS-ARG-parathyroid hormone

β-LIPOTROPIN   -LYS-LYS-β-MSH-LYS-ARG-

References

1. Debas HT, Walsh JH, Grossman MI: Pure human minigastrin: Secretory potency and disappearance rate. *Gut* 15: 686–689, 1974.
2. Dockray GJ, Walsh JH: Identification of an N-terminal fragment of heptadecapeptide gastrin in the serum of patients with Zollinger-Ellison syndrome (ZES). *Gastroenterology* 66:874, 1974.
3. Doolittle RF: Terminal pyrrolidonecarboxylic acid: Cleavage with enzymes, in Colowick SP, Kaplan NO (eds), *Methods in Enzymology*, New York: Academic Press, 25:231–244, 1972.
4. Gregory RA: Gastric secretion: A review of its chief nervous and hormonal mechanisms, in Smith AN (ed), *Surgical Physiology of the Gastrointestinal Tract*, (Symposium) Royal College of Surgeons Edinburgh, 1962, pp 57–70.
5. Gregory RA: Gastrin: The natural history of a peptide hormone. *The Harvey Lectures (1968–69)*, New York: Academic Press, 64:121–155, 1970.
6. Gregory RA: Gastrin, in Berson SA (ed), *Methods in Investigative and Diagnostic Endocrinology*, vol 2B, part 3, Amsterdam: North-Holland, 1973, pp 1029–1034.
7. Gregory RA: The gastrointestinal hormones: A review of recent advances. (The Bayliss-Starling Lecture 1973). *J Physiol* 241:1–32, 1974.
8. Gregory RA, Tracy HJ: Constitution and properties of two gastrins extracted from hog antral mucosa. *J Physiol* 169:18P–19P, 1963.

9. Gregory RA, Tracy HJ: The constitution and properties of
    two gastrins extracted from hog antral mucosa: I. The
    isolation of two gastrins from hog antral mucosa.
    II. The properties of two gastrins isolated from hog
    antral mucosa. *Gut* 5:103-117, 1964.
10. Gregory RA, Tracy HJ: Isolation of two 'big gastrins' from
    Zollinger-Ellison tumour tissue. *Lancet* 2:797-799,
    1972.
11. Gregory RA, Tracy HJ: Big gastrin. *Mt Sinai J Med*
    40:359-364, 1973.
12. Gregory RA, Tracy HJ: Isolation of two minigastrins from
    Zollinger-Ellison tumour tissue. *Gut* 15:683-685,1974.
13. Grossman MI: Trends in gut hormone research, in Thompson
    JC (ed), *Gastrointestinal Hormones*, Austin: University
    of Texas Press, 1975, pp 3-10.
14. Rehfeld JF, Stadil F: Gel filtration studies on immuno-
    reactive gastrin in serum from Zollinger-Ellison
    patients. *Gut* 14:369-373, 1973.
15. Rehfeld JF, Stadil F, Kilelsøe J: Immunoreactive gastrin
    components in human serum. *Gut* 15:102-111, 1974.
16. Yalow RS, Berson SA: Further studies on the nature of
    immunoreactive gastrin in human plasma. *Gastroenter-
    ology* 60:203-214, 1971.
17. Yalow RS, Wu N: Additional studies on the nature of big
    big gastrin. *Gastroenterology* 65:19-27, 1973.

HETEROGENEITY OF PEPTIDE HORMONES WITH RELATION TO GASTRIN

Rosalyn S. Yalow

Solomon A. Berson Research Laboratory,
Bronx Veterans Administration Hospital,
and Mt. Sinai School of Medicine, The
City University of New York, New York

In a Conference on Gastrin held just about a decade ago Gregory and Tracy[5] had the prescience to state, "We have termed the peptides we isolated Gastrins I and II, but we do not mean to imply by this that either is considered to be in the same form as the hormone is when released from antral mucosa. Clearly, there may be present in antral mucosa other gastrin composed of part of the peptides we have isolated, or indeed incorporating them, or the active parts, within a larger molecule. This consideration must apply also to the substance produced by Zollinger-Ellison tumors." A clear appreciation of the multiple forms of gastrin was not to develop, however, until almost six years later when we first demonstrated[11,12] using radioimmunoassay methods, that the predominant form of gastrin in the plasma of gastrin hypersecretors (patients with pernicious anemia or the Zollinger-Ellison syndrome) was a larger and more basic peptide than the heptadecapeptide gastrins I and II earlier purified by Gregory and Tracy.[4,8]

Our search for new forms of gastrin, which had been stimulated by our earlier studies[1] on the immunochemical heterogeneity of parathyroid hormone in plasma and by the discovery of proinsulin by Steiner and associates,[9] has led to studies in a number of laboratories, including our own, which suggest that many, if not all, peptidal hormones are found in more than one size in plasma and in glandular and other tissue extracts. These forms may or may not have biologic activity and may or may not be either precursor(s)

25

or metabolic product(s) of the well-known, well-characterized hormone.

TECHNIQUES FOR DETERMINING HETEROGENEITY

Before reviewing our studies on gastrin it is relevant to consider some general techniques for determining whether any hormone exists in heterogeneous
forms.

Immunochemical Heterogeneity

Measurement of hormone concentration by radioimmunoassay is performed simply by comparing the inhibition
of binding of labeled antigen to antibody that is observed in the unknown sample with the inhibition that
is produced by solutions containing known amounts of
unlabeled standard. A necessary condition for this
assay, which is also required for bioassay, is the
demonstration that the apparent hormonal concentration
is independent of dilution, that is, dilution curves
of unknown samples are superposable on the standard
curve. This condition is necessary but not sufficient
to assure identity of standards and unknowns. The
presence of heterogeneous forms may be suspected when
the apparent hormonal content of a specimen in terms
of a given standard, depends on the particular assay
system employed. Thus differences between unknown
and standard are suggested by discrepant results between bioassay and radioimmunoassay or by different
apparent concentrations when different antisera are
used for radioimmunoassay. Consideration should also
be given to the possibility of biologic heterogeneity
when discrepant results for hormonal concentration are
obtained when two or more different bioassay procedures
are employed.

Chemical Heterogeneity

Demonstration of the existence of chemical heterogeneity is dependent on fractionation in one or more
physicochemical systems. These may include, for
example: column fractionation using Sephadex gel,
Bio-rad gel, or ionic exchange resins; electrophoresis on starch gel, starch block or on paper; or

ultracentrifugation. Labeled or unlabeled marker molecules may be added to samples before fractionation and the position of the marker molecules may be determined by measurement of radioactivity or by specific radioimmunoassay. The size or charge of the various hormonal components can be compared to that of the known marker molecules, with the reservation that unlabeled and radioiodine-labeled marker molecules may not coincide because of changes in charge or molecular configuration that occur with the introduction of iodine into the molecule. Two other possible sources of error should be appreciated: on Sephadex gel, premature elution is observed with elongated molecules compared to globular molecules of the same weight, and delayed elution of basic peptides may occur with low ionic strength eluants.

Consideration must be given to the possibilities that larger molecular forms may arise from aggregation of hormone molecules or from nonspecific binding of hormone to tissue or plasma proteins, and that smaller molecular forms may be generated if the hormone is enzymatically degraded in tissue or plasma after removal of the sample from the body. Attempts should be made to dissociate larger molecular forms, perhaps complexed through noncovalent bonds, by changes in pH, by high concentrations of salt (6-8 M urea), or even by dilution. Failure to effect dissociation does not rule out the possibility that the larger molecular forms may arise from irreversible denaturation in some instances, or from dimerization that results perhaps from disulfide interchange. To diminish the possibility that molecular fragments arise from enzymatic conversion, it may be necessary on occasion to introduce bacteriostatic agents or enzyme inhibitors.

To characterize the various hormonal forms better, fractionation and refractionation in more than one system is generally preferable (for example, separation both on electrophoresis and on Sephadex gel filtration). Purification and sequencing are ultimately required to identify the possible precursor or metabolic forms of the peptide hormones. In advance of such definitive chemical characterization, however, the inference of distinct multiple forms is considerably strengthened by increasing the number of independent systems in which nonstandard forms can be demonstrated and the number of tests for their stability. Even when the smaller peptides can be demonstrated to have amino acid sequences identical with a portion of a larger

peptide, the possibility cannot be excluded that the
various hormonal forms could be synthesized independently on separate templates. Positive identification of precursor-product relationship, therefore,
requires biosynthetic studies in addition to demonstration of similar peptide structure.

GASTRIN

   In reviewing the multiple immunoreactive forms of
gastrin we have found in plasma and tissue, it must
be appreciated that the detection and quantitation
of the different immunoreactive hormonal components
depend on the characteristics of the antiserum(s)
employed. For instance, we have no evidence for
immunochemical heterogeneity of gastrin in nonfrac-
tionated plasma samples, since the apparent hormonal
concentrations in unknown plasma samples in terms

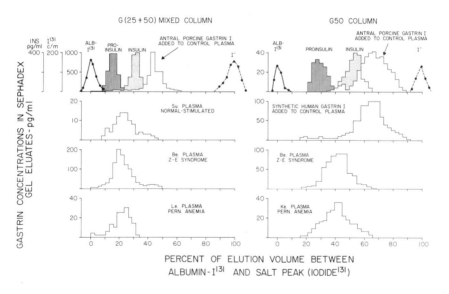

Figure 1. Distribution of immunoreactive gastrin in samples
of endogenous plasma or plasma-gastrin mixtures added to columns of Sephadex G50 (right) or mixtures of G50 and G25 (left)
for gel filtration (postmortem specimens). The zones of elution of the marker molecules are shown in the top frames.
(Reproduced, with permission of *Gastroenterology*.[11])

of a given heptadecapeptide gastrin standard, have
been the same with the several antisera we have produced in response to immunization with crude porcine
antral gastrin alone or coupled with carbodiimide to
rabbit albumin. Other investigators, perhaps because
of different immunization procedures, have described
the production of antisera with such specificities as
to preclude unique determination of hormonal content
in terms of the same heptadecapeptide gastrin standard.

Our early studies[11,12] were on plasma obtained primarily from patients who were gastrin hypersecretors,
that is, patients with Zollinger-Ellison syndrome
(ZE) or pernicious anemia (PA). Fractionation was
effected in a variety of physicochemical systems including Sephadex gel (Fig. 1), aminoethyl cellulose
columns (Fig. 2), starch block (Fig. 3), starch gel
(Fig. 4) and paper electrophoresis. From these studies we concluded that the major component of plasma
immunoreactive gastrin in the fasting state was, in
the patients studied, a new hormonal form that is a
larger and more basic peptide than heptadecapeptide
gastrin (HG), which we named big gastrin (BG). We
further demonstrated[2] that both BG and HG are present
in extracts of a Zollinger-Ellison pancreatic tumor
(Fig. 5) as well as in extracts of antrum and proximal small bowel (Fig. 6). In mucosal samples obtained more distally along the gastrointestinal tract,
BG becomes progressively more prominent in relation
to HG and the first part of the jejunum contains primarily BG, although at relatively low concentration (Fig. 6).

Big gastrin from plasma or from tissue is rapidly
converted to an HG-like peptide by tryptic digestion
with no significant change in immunoreactivity.[3,12]
This suggests that the antigenic site that reacts
with the antibodies in our antiserum is as fully
available when it is found in BG as it is when in HG.

We predicted on the basis of these studies[2,11,12]
that BG is composed of HG linked at its amino terminal end to a lysine or arginine residue of another
peptide, a prediction which has been confirmed by
the elegant chemical investigations of Gregory and
Tracy.[6,7]

More recently we have described another hormonal
form of gastrin.[13,14] This component which we have
called big-big gastrin (BBG) elutes in or just after

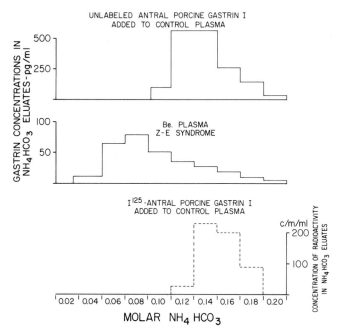

Figure 2. Discontinuous gradient elution from aminoethylcellulose (AE 41) in NH_4HCO_3 buffer. Distribution of immunoreactive gastrin components, on AE-cellulose column chromatography
in normal control plasma to which had been added porcine gastrin I (top), and in plasma of a patient (Be) with Zollinger-
Ellison syndrome (middle). Distribution of radioactive heptadecapeptide gastrin is shown at bottom. The slightly later
emergence of this preparation of iodogastrin than of unlabeled
gastrin is consistent with the increased negative charge frequently induced by iodination. (Reproduced, with permission
of *Gastroenterology*.[12])

Figure 3. Distribution
of immunoreactive gas-
trin components, on
starch block electro-
phoresis, in normal
control plasma to which
had been added porcine
gastrin I (top) and in
plasmas from two pa-
tients with Zollinger-
Ellison syndrome, Ro
(middle) and Be (bottom).
(Reproduced, with per-
mission of *Gastro-
enterology*.[12])

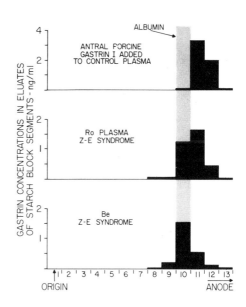

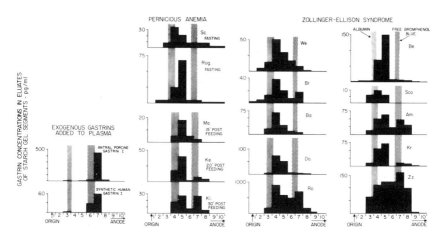

Figure 4. Distribution of immunoreactive gastrin components,
on starch gel electrophoresis, in plasmas from normal control
subjects to which had been added heptadecapeptide porcine
gastrin I or synthetic human gastrin I (left), and in plasmas
from patients with pernicious anemia (middle) and Zollinger-
Ellison syndrome (right). (Reproduced, with permission of
Gastroenterology.[12])

31

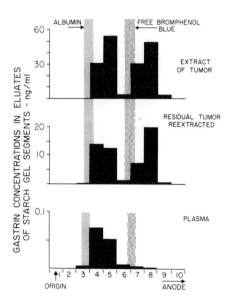

Figure 5. Distribution of immunoreactive gastrin on starch gel electrophoresis in extracts of a Zollinger-Ellison pancreatic tumor and in plasma obtained from same patient (Do). The concentration in the first crude extract was 44 µg/gm; concentration of gastrin in reextract of residual piece of tumor was 9 µg/gm. (Reproduced, with permission of *Gastroenterology*.[2])

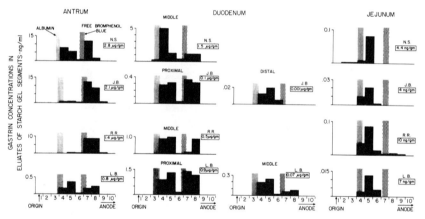

Figure 6. Distribution of immunoreactive gastrin, on starch gel electrophoresis, in extracts of antrum, duodenum, and proximal jejunum in postmortem material. The total concentration of gastrin (boxed values) in the crude extract for each sample is expressed as micrograms or nanograms gastrin per gram of mucosa. Since gel eluates from different gels were assayed at different dilutions, the absolute concentrations in the individual segments are to be ignored, since only the relative abundance of the components in each gel is of importance. (Reproduced, with permission of *Gastroenterology*.[2])

the albumin region on Sephadex G50 gel filtration. BBG is a prominent fraction of total plasma immuno- reactivity in fasting man, whether a normal subject or the usual duodenal ulcer patients (Fig. 7), or a fasting dog (Fig. 8), or pig (Fig. 9). It is gener- ally a very minor (<2%) or undetectable component in the plasma of PA and ZE patients[13],[14] (Fig. 10) and other patients who are gastrin hypersecretors (Fig. 7B).[13] BBG was the only component detectable in the plasma of an antrectomized patient, post-Billroth II (Ga, Fig. 7B), so that in this patient, at least, the antrum was not the source of BBG.

BBG is hardly detectable (<<1% of total immunoreac- tivity) in antral and duodenal extracts,[13],[14] although like BG it becomes relatively more prominent distally along the gastrointestinal tract, amounting to as much as 24% of some jejunal extracts.[13] It is only a minor component in extracts of a ZE tumor.[14]

Since the absolute concentration of BBG in plasma is generally considerably less than 50 pM/ml, we have not been able to characterize it readily in other physicochemical systems.

It should be noted, however, that plasma BBG is not as completely adsorbed to charcoal or to an anionic exchange resin as is BG or HG, so that plasma cannot necessarily be freed of immunoreactive gastrin by the use of materials which are specific adsorbents for BG or HG.[14]

Through the courtesy of Professor Gregory we have received material resembling plasma BBG which was extracted from a ZE tumor and which represented the void volume component following fractionation on a Sephadex G50 superfine column. On starch gel electro- phoresis BBG, like BG, migrates in the prealbumin re- gion on starch gel electrophoresis (Fig. 11).[14] From ultracentrifugal studies its molecular weight appears to be close to that of human growth hormone ($\sim$22,000 daltons).[14] Like BG, BBG is convertible by tryptic digestion to small forms with no loss in immunoreac- tivity (Fig. 12).[14] The failure to find significant BG as an intermediate in the conversion process is not surprising in view of the rapid conversion by trypsin of BG to HG.[3],[12]

A family of immunoreactive gastrins (BBG β), with an elution volume between BBG and BG, has been detec- ted as a minor component of a ZE tumor (Fig. 13) as well as of BBG following tryptic digestion.[14] These

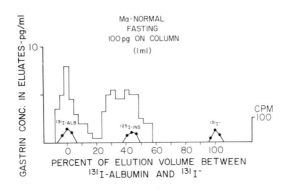

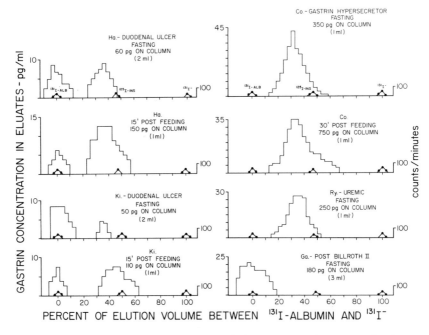

Figure 7. A & B – Distribution of immunoreactive gastrin in plasma of various human subjects on Sephadex G50 gel filtration. (Reproduced, with permission of *Gastroenterology*.[14])

different components maintain their integrity on refractionation (Fig. 13). Whether this family of gastrins is significant *in vivo*, however, or simply represents nonspecific degradation products of a larger hormonal form, has not been determined.

Gastrointestinal BG and HG are stimulated by feeding and are suppressed by antral acidification,[12],[14] but BBG is not.[14]

It should be appreciated that under steady state conditions, the relative plasma concentrations of each of the hormonal forms is determined not only by its secretion rate but also by its apparent space of distribution and its rate of degradation. In a recent study from our laboratory[10] we have shown that

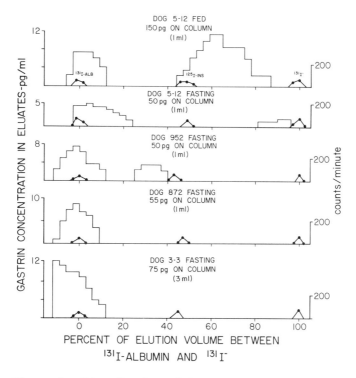

Figure 8. Distribution of immunoreactive gastrin in plasma from fasted or fed dogs on Sephadex G50 gel filtration. (Reproduced, with permission of *Gastroenterology.*[14])

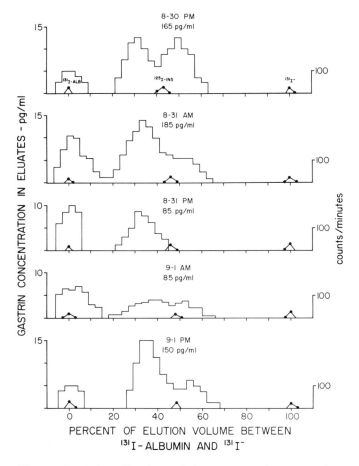

Figure 9. Distribution of immunoreactive gastrin in porcine plasma taken on three successive days on Sephadex G50 gel filtration. (Reproduced, with permission of *Gastroenterology*.[14])

36

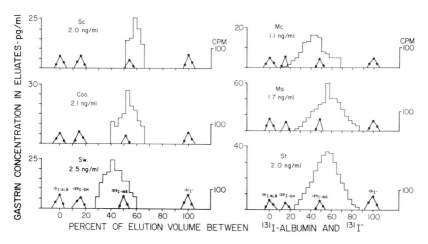

Figure 10. Distribution of immunoreactive gastrin on Sephadex G50 filtration of plasma from human subjects with Zollinger-Ellison syndrome (left) or pernicious anemia (right). (Reproduced, with permission of *Gastroenterology*.[14])

Figure 11. (Top) Gastrin concentration in eluates of starch gel segments. Upper panel, ^{125}I-porcine gastrin I added to hormone-free plasma. Lower panel, big-big gastrin (BBG) added to same plasma. (Bottom) Refractionation of pre-albumin segment 6 on Sephadex G50 gel filtration. (Reproduced, with permission of *Gastroenterology*.[14])

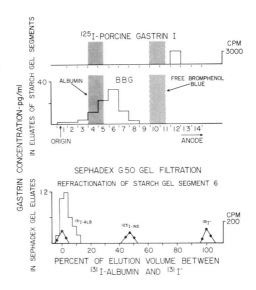

37

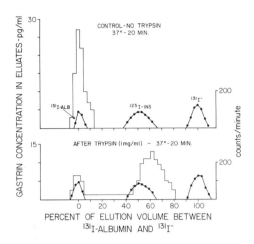

Figure 12. Refractionation of plasma "big-big" gastrin peak on Sephadex G50 filtration following incubation at 37C without (top) and with (bottom) trypsin (1 mg/ml). (Reproduced, with permission of *Biochemical and Biophysical Research Communications.*[13])

following a pulse injection in a dog the half-times for disappearance for HG, BG, and BBG were 3, 9 and 90 minutes respectively. Assuming the ultimate spaces of distribution to be the same, then endogenous secretion or exogenous administration of equimolar amounts of the three hormonal forms results in relative plasma concentrations approximately proportional to their turnover times; thus the relative concentrations of HG:BG:BBG would be about 3:9:90. This simplified calculation gives insight into the reason why BBG often predominates in the plasma of nonstimulated animals and man. Under nonequilibrium conditions the problem may be somewhat complicated by different rates of distribution for the different hormonal forms, but the same general principles obtain.

The fact that administration of *equimolar* amounts of different hormonal forms results in *different* plasma concentrations, poses an interesting question with respect to how to define biologic activity. Should the biologic response be measured in terms of the administered dose or in terms of the plasma concentration resulting from that dose?

An appreciation of the heterogeneity of peptide hormones leaves unanswered a host of other questions. Is the synthesis in a larger form essential only for proper storage or release or is another mechanism involved? What enzymes are involved in the conversion process? Are the converting enzymes hormone-specific? Are they species-specific? Are different enzymes involved when multiple hormonal forms are found? Is

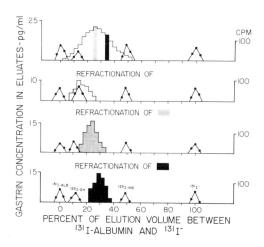

Figure 13. Top, distribution of immunoreactive gastrin in material (big-big gastrin 9β) supplied by Professor R.A. Gregory which consisted of the pooled eluates between the void volume and big gastrin regions of a Zollinger-Ellison tumor extract fractionated in Sephadex G50 superfine column eluated with 0.4% ammonium bicarbonate. Bottom three frames, refractionation of indicated eluates. (Reproduced, with permission of *Gastroenterology*.[14])

conversion effected in the secreting tissue or in the periphery or both? Which hormonal forms interact with the receptor(s)? These and related fundamental questions will continue to tantalize us for quite awhile.

SUMMARY

Many peptidal hormones are found in more than one size in plasma and in glandular and other tissue extracts. These forms may or may not have biologic activity and may or may not be either precursor(s) or metabolic product(s) of the well-known, well-characterized hormone. The presence of heterogeneous forms may be suspected when the apparent hormonal content of a specimen in terms of a given standard depends on the particular assay system employed. The demonstration of the existence of chemical heterogeneity is dependent on fractionation in one or more

physicochemical systems.   The detection and quantitation of the different hormonal components using
radioimmunoassay depends on the characteristics of
the antiserum(s) employed. Generally, the major component of plasma immunoreactive gastrin in the fasting
state of gastrin hypersecretors is big gastrin, and in
the fasting state of normal man, dog, or pig, or the
usual duodenal ulcer patient, is big-big gastrin.
Usually both big and heptadecapeptide gastrins are
stimulated by gastrin secretagogues. Heptadecapeptide
gastrin predominates in the antrum, but in mucosal
samples obtained more distally along the gastrointestinal tract, big gastrin becomes progressively more
prominent and predominates in the jejunum although
at low concentration. Both forms are found in extracts of Zollinger-Ellison tumors. Big-big gastrin
is virtually undetectable in tumor, antral, and duodenal extracts but accounts for 20% of immunoreactive
gastrin in some jejunal extracts.

References

1. Berson SA, Yalow RS: Immunochemical heterogeneity of para-
        thyroid hormone in plasma. *J Clin Endocr Metab* 28:
        1037-1047, 1968.
2. Berson SA, Yalow RS: Nature of immunoreactive gastrin ex-
        tracted from tissues of gastrointestinal tract.
        Gastroenterology 60:215-222, 1971.
3. Berson SA, Yalow RS: Heterogeneity of peptide hormones in
        plasma as revealed by radioimmunoassay, in *Les Adenomes
        Hypophysaires Secretants: Endocrinopathies et Immunolo-
        gie*, Paris: Masson et Cie, 1971, pp 239-269.
4. Gregory RA, Tracy HJ: The constitution and properties of
        two gastrins extracted from hog antral mucosa: I.   The
        isolation of two gastrins from hog antral mucosa.
        Gut 5:103-114, 1964.
5. Gregory RA, Tracy HJ: Studies on the chemistry of gastrins
        I and II, in Grossman MI (ed), *Gastrin*, Los Angeles:
        University of California Press, 1966, pp 9-26.
6. Gregory RA, Tracy HJ: Isolation of two "big gastrins"
        from Zollinger-Ellison tumour tissue. *Lancet* 2:797-
        799, 1972.
7. Gregory RA, Tracy HJ: Big gastrin. *Mt Sinai J Med* 40:
        359-364, 1973.
8. Gregory RA, Tracy HJ, Grossman MI: Isolation of two
        gastrins from human antral mucosa. *Nature* 209:583,
        1966.

9. Steiner DF, Cunningham D, Spigelman L, Aten B: Insulin
   biosynthesis: evidence for a precursor. *Science*
   157:697-700, 1967.
10. Straus E, Yalow RS: Studies on the distribution and degra-
    dation of heptadecapeptide, big, and big big gastrin.
    Gastroenterology 66:936-943, 1974.
11. Yalow RS, Berson SA: Size and charge distinctions between
    endogenous human plasma gastrin in peripheral blood
    and heptadecapeptide gastrins. *Gastroenterology* 58:
    609-615, 1970.
12. Yalow RS, Berson SA: Further studies on the nature of
    immunoreactive gastrin in human plasma. *Gastroenter-
    ology* 60:203-214, 1971.
13. Yalow RS, Berson SA: And now, "big, big" gastrin. *Biochem
    Biophys Res Commun* 48:391-395, 1972.
14. Yalow RS, Wu N: Additional studies on the nature of big
    big gastrin. *Gastroenterology* 65:19-27, 1973.

GASTRIN HETEROGENEITY IN SERUM
AND TISSUE: A PROGRESS REPORT

J.F. Rehfeld, F. Stadil, J. Malmstrøm,
M. Miyata

Department of Clinical Chemistry, Bispebjerg
Hospital, and Department of Gastroenterology C,
Rigshospitalet, Copenhagen, Denmark

In previous studies on the nature of gastrin in human serum we have described four components of different molecular size.[1,3,6] The smaller ones circulated in pairs. Component I apparently has the same molecular size as proinsulin, Component II corresponded to gastrin-34 (big gastrin), Component III to gastrin-17 (small gastrin), and Component IV to gastrin-13 (minigastrin).

With the fractionation techniques employed, we never observed big-big gastrin in serum.[3,6] During recent investigations on serum from normal subjects, we observed heterogeneity greater than earlier conceived. In order to define and separate the increasing number of gastrins, we have now optimized our gel filtration technique further and combined it with ion exchange chromatography and disc-gel electrophoresis.

At present, it looks as if characterization of all gastrins may be a lifetime work. This report, therefore, gives only a few new observations on the heterogeneity of gastrin in circulation and in tissue at our present stage of investigation.

MATERIALS

Sera were obtained from 14 normal subjects during fasting and after a protein-rich meal, 10 patients with pernicious anemia, eight patients with the Zollinger-Ellison syndrome, and six normal Danish pigs. The serum samples were treated as previously

43

described.[6] Biopsies of antral, duodenal, and jejunal mucosa were obtained from six healthy volunteers and 30 patients with duodenal ulcer (J Malmstrøm, unpublished technique).

METHODS

Synthetic human gastrin (SHG 1-17) was infused in a peripheral vein in six normal pigs (250 ng/kg/hr) for two hours. Blood was drawn from the aorta, the external jugular vein, the superior mesenteric vein, and a renal vein at the following intervals: -30, -20, -10, 0, 5, 10, 20, 30, 45, 60, 90, 120, 130, 140, 150, 165, 180, 195, 210, and 225 minutes.

Fractionation Procedures

Gel filtration was performed on Sephadex G50 super-fine columns with the following dimensions: 50x1 cm, 100x1.5 cm, 100x5 cm, 200x1.3 cm, 200x2.7 cm; 0.02 M Veronal buffer, pH 8.4 at 20C was used for elution on 50x1 and 100x1.5 cm columns. The remaining columns were eluted with 0.25 M ammonium bicarbonate, pH 8.1 at 4C. Anion exchange chromatography on AE-41 cellulose and disc-gel electrophoresis were performed as described in detail elsewhere.[6,10]

Gastrin Analysis

Gastrin concentrations were measured radioimmunochemically.[7,9] In the present study only antiserum 2604-8 was employed.[2] Monoiodinated ^{125}I-SHG was used as tracer[8] and anion exchange resin was used for separation of free and antibody-bound tracer.[4] An optimized assay with a detection limit $\leq$ 0.2 pg eqv SHG per ml sample, was used for gel filtration studies of serum and plasma from normal fasting subjects (Fig. 1). It could be shown, in accordance with previous studies[1,3,6] that all larger gastrin components were degraded by trypsin to gastrin-17, the same molecular form of gastrin as the assay standard. The gastrin concentration (expressed in equivalents of SHG) was similar before and after incubation with trypsin, both for isolated large molecular forms (Fig. 2) and for

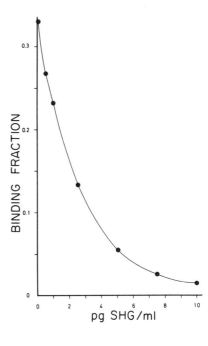

Figure 1. Optimized standard calibration curve for the radioimmunoassay of gastrin employing antiserum 2604-8. Detection limit ≤ 0.02 pg/ml.

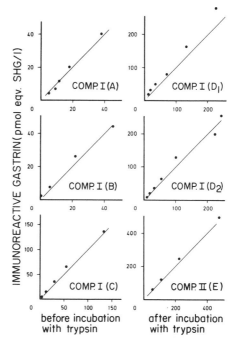

Figure 2. Effect of trypsinization on the immunoreactivity of five Component I's and one Component II at different dilutions. The antiserum used was 2604-8.

J.F. Rehfeld

all the gastrins in serum (Table 1). Since serial
dilution yielded straight-line curves before as well
as after trypsinization (Fig. 2), we assume that antiserum 2604-8 binds all gastrins larger than gastrin-13
with equimolar potency and that it is correct to express the concentration of the gastrins in molar
units.[5]

Table 1. Concentration of immunoreactive gastrin in serum
(pg eqv SHG/ml) before and after incubation with
0.2 mg trypsin per ml for 20 minutes at 20C. Inactivation by boiling for five minutes.

No.	Normal sera		Pernicious anemia sera		Zollinger-Ellison sera	
	Before	After	Before	After	Before	After
1	42	57	558	684	72000	79500
2	24	15	730	720	223000	234000
3	18	34	675	708	1080000	1016000
4	24	25	1026	972	288000	312000
5	42	42	1392	1206	21000	24000
6	21	9	498	528	6000	6000
7	54	36	639	684	4800	4080
8	39	36	732	588	6900	6300
9	42	38	384	480		
10	81	72	348	336		
11	24	33				
12	72	99				
13	72	72				
14	126	117				
Mean	48.6	48.9	698.2	690.6	212710	210230
2 p	> 0.9		> 0.8		> 0.9	

RESULTS AND COMMENTS

Gastrins in Serum

By copying the conditions under which big-big gastrin was found to be the dominating form of the circulating gastrins,[12] most gastrin immunoreactivity from plasma appeared in the void volume (Table 2). Increase of the ionic strength of the elution buffer, however, reduced the gastrin fraction eluted in the void volume significantly, and by subsequent incubation in 8 M urea and dialysis against a urea gradient, all gastrin in the void volume disappeared. The dialysis tube had an average pore radius of 2.4 nm, which allows even Component I with a Stokes' radius of 2.2 nm[1] to pass through the tube membrane. The results suggest that at least a significant part of gastrin described as big-big gastrin in *circulation* is due

Table 2. Big-big gastrin in 10 normal fasting subjects

	Material	Elution buffer*	Dialysis**	Fractions of Subjects	Immuno-reactivity
I	Plasma	0.02 M diemal pH 8.4	–	1.0	0.62
II	Serum	0.02 M diemal pH 8.4	–	1.0	0.39
III	Serum	0.1 M phosphate pH 7.4	–	0.3	0.04
IV	Serum	0.02 M diemal pH 8.4	Against elution buffer 20 hr, 4C	1.0	0.18
V	Serum	0.02 M diemal pH 8.4	Against elution buffer 8.0 M, 60 hr, 4C	0.0	0.00

* Elution on Sephadex G50 superfine columns (1 x 50 cm) at 20C.
** Dialysis in Visking tubes (mean pore radius 2.4 nm).

to nonspecific binding of smaller gastrins to plasma
proteins.

After preparative gel filtration of plasma from a
Zollinger-Ellison patient with high concentration of
gastrin (1.5 µmol/l), the fractions were pooled as
shown on Figure 3. After lyophilization and *three*
refiltrations on columns with a high resolution capacity (Fig. 4), Components I and II were each resolved into five well defined different peaks (Figs.
5 and 6). An ion exchange chromatography and disc-
gel electrophoresis have further disclosed that
Component I (C) and Component II (E$_2$) are paired.
Components III and IV are at present under similar
investigation.

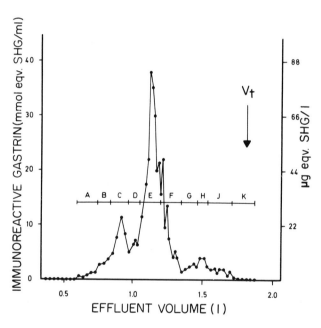

Figure 3. Elution diagram of immunoreactive
gastrin in a Zollinger-Ellison serum by gel filtration on Sephadex G50 superfine column
(100 x 5 cm) eluted at 20C with 0.25 M ammonium
bicarbonate, pH 8.1.

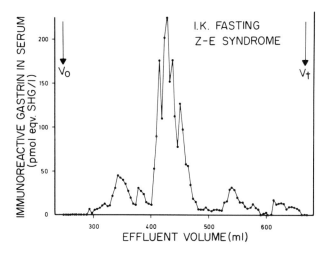

Figure 4. Calibration diagram of a Sephadex G50 superfine column (200 x 2.7 cm) eluted at 4C with 0.25 M ammonium bicarbonate, pH 8.1. A Zollinger-Ellison serum was used for the calibration.

Figure 5. Isolation of five different forms of Component I by three times refiltration on Sephadex G50 superfine columns (200 x 2.7 cm) eluted at 4C with 0.25 M ammonium bicarbonate, pH 8.1.

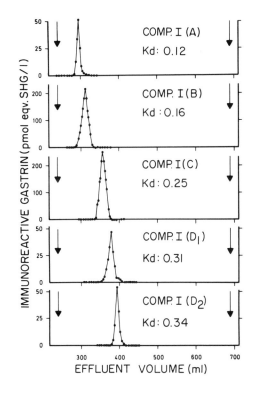

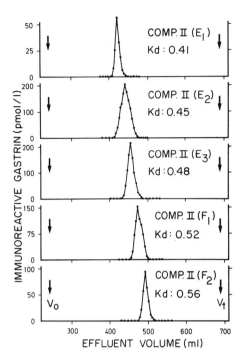

Figure 6. Isolation of five different forms of Component II by three times refiltration as described in Figure 5.

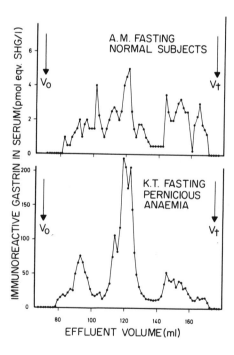

Figure 7. Elution diagram of immunoreactive gastrin in sera from a normal subject and a patient with pernicious anemia on Sephadex G50 superfine columns (200 x 1.3 cm).

50

In order to demonstrate that the high degree of heterogeneity found in the actual Zollinger-Ellison serum is a general phenomenon, sera from normal subjects and patients with pernicious anemia were gel filtrated and showed heterogeneity (Fig. 7) similar to that observed in Zollinger-Ellison sera.

Gastrins in Tissue

The concentration of gastrin in mucosa decreased dramatically from the antrum to the duodenal bulb, after which a further gradual decrease was observed (Fig. 8). The tissue gastrins have not yet been resolved corresponding to the serum gastrins, but gel filtration reveals that the predominating gastrins in the antrum are gastrin-17, constituting on an average 95% of total immunoreactivity (Fig. 9). In duodenum and jejunum the small gastrins constitute, on an average, half of gastrin in the eight biopsy specimens investigated so far. In some normal subjects, however, most duodenal and jejunal gastrin is composed of Components III and IV (Fig. 10).

Relationship Between Gastrins in Serum and Tissue

In serum the big gastrin molecules predominate in hypergastrinemic patients[1,3] as well as in normal subjects. Initially during meals the fraction of small gastrins increases, but in normal subjects Components I and II still constitute the majority of gastrin during the whole meal (JF Rehfeld and F Stadil, unpublished data). In tissue small gastrin molecules predominate because of the high concentration of Component III little or gastrin-17) in antrum.

The ratio in tissue between the amount of Component I and Component II on one hand and the amount of Component III and Component IV on the other, is roughly estimated to be 1:12 for the whole digestive tract. Considering a ratio of 1:5 for the metabolic clearance rate of big gastrin compared to little gastrin,[11] it can be calculated that big gastrin from tissue is to be secreted at a rate five times faster than that of small gastrin (on the assumption that all the circulating gastrins are derived from mucosa of the

Immunoreactive Gastrin

in mucosa biopsies from

antrum and duodenum.

(μg eqv. SHG/g mucosa)

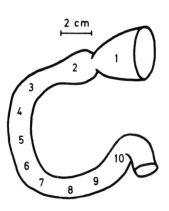

Healthy volunteers

1.   21.1 ± 4.7   (mean ± SEM, n =   6)

2.   1.8 ± 0.1   (———————, n =   6)

Ulcus duodeni patients

1.   27.1 ± 4.2   (mean ± SEM, n = 30)

2.   3.7 ± 0.7   (———————, n = 30)

3.   1.1 ± 0.2   (———————, n = 10)

4.   1.2 ± 0.2   (———————, n = 10)

5.   1.1 ± 0.3   (———————, n =   9)

6.   0.8 ± 0.2   (———————, n = 10)

7.   0.7 ± 0.1   (———————, n =   7)

8.   0.6 ± 0.3   (———————, n =   4)

9.   0.2 ± 0.1   (———————, n =   3)

10. 0.05   (n =   1)

Figure 8.   Total concentration of gastrin in antrum and duodenum in man.

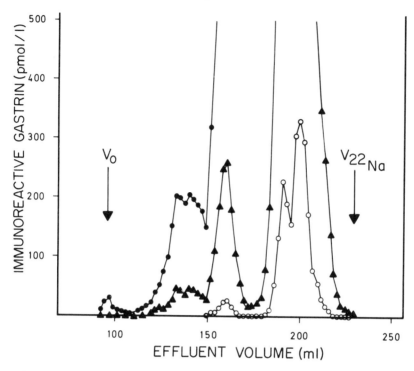

Figure 9. Elution diagram of immunoreactive gastrin in extract of human antral mucosa on Sephadex G50 superfine column eluted with 0.25 M ammonium bicarbonate, pH 8.1. V_O indicates void volume, $V_{22_{Na}}$ indicates total volume. The fractions were assayed in dilutions of 1:50 (•——•), 1:200 (▲——▲), and 1:1000 (o——o).

53

proximal gut). Such a high secretion rate is unlikely
and is not in accordance with the secretion pattern
in antral vein blood during stimulation (Stadil and
Rehfeld, unpublished data). The discrepancy may in
part be explained by conversion of secreted gastrin-
17 molecules to larger forms of gastrin. Such conversion has been observed in pigs during infusion of

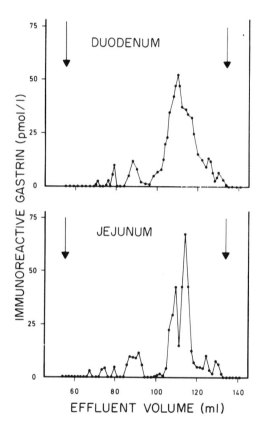

Figure 10. Elution diagram of immunoreactive gastrin in extract of human
duodenal and jejunal mucosa on Sephadex
G50 superfine column eluted with 0.25 M
ammonium bicarbonate, pH 8.1. Arrows
indicate V_o and V_t.

gastrin-17 (Fig. 11). Thirty minutes after start of
the infusion, small peaks corresponding in size to
Components I and II were found (Fig. 12), and after
150 minutes half of the gastrins in serum appeared
in the form of Components I and II (Fig. 13). The
observations were recently confirmed by infusion of
unlabeled or monoiodinated gastrins in man.

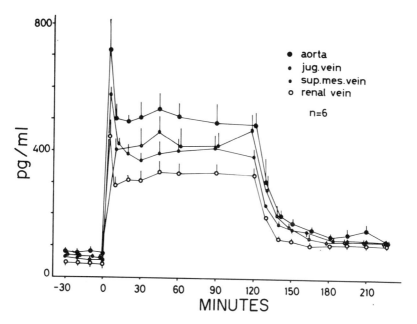

Figure 11. Mean + SEM concentration of immunoreactive gastrin
in serum in pigs during infusion of 250 ng SHG/kg/hour.

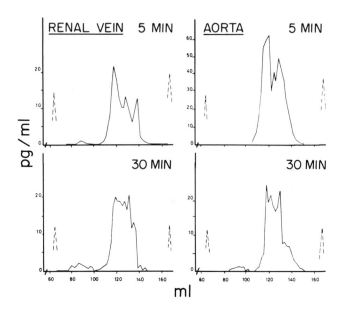

Figure 12. Elution diagram on Sephadex G50 superfine columns (100 x 1.5 cm) of immunoreactive gastrin in porcine serum from renal vein and aorta 5 and 30 minutes after beginning of SHG infusion.

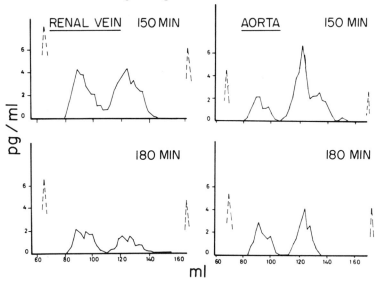

Figure 13. Elution diagram as in Fig. 12, 150 and 180 minutes after beginning of SHG infusion.

SUMMARY

Gastrin in human serum and tissue (antrum, duodenum, jejunum) was fractionated by gel filtration, ion exchange chromatography, and disc-gel electrophoresis. The fractions were assayed with an antiserum, which binds the components with equimolar potency. By gel filtration of plasma from normal fasting subjects, 62% of the gastrin immunoreactivity appeared in the void volume when elution buffer of low ionic strength was used. Increase of ionic strength decreased the percentage of gastrin in the void volume, and after incubation in 8 M urea and dialysis, no gastrin immunoreactivity was detectable in the void volume. Gel filtration with high resolution, subsequent ion exchange, and electrophoresis of serum, resolved both Component I and Component II (big gastrin) into six different gastrins each. Similar gastrins were found in antrum and duodenum.

The concentration of gastrin in human tissue varied from 12.9±2.0 (mean ± SEM) nmol/g mucosa in antrum, 1.8±0.3 nmol/g in the duodenal bulb to 0.1±0.05 nmol/g distal in duodenum. In the proximal jejunum 20 pmol/g mucosa were found. In the antrum 95% of the immunoreactivity in antrum was small gastrin, whereas half of the immunoreactivity in duodenum and jejunum was Components I and II (big gastrin). Preliminary infusion studies indicated that part of the discrepancy between the distribution of big and small gastrins in circulation and tissue may be explained by conversion of small gastrins (gastrin-17) to larger molecular forms outside the gut. The results suggest that in man:

    1) Big-big gastrin molecules are not normally present in circulation.

    2) Components I and II (big gastrin) consist of at least six different gastrins each.

    3) Antrum contains 5 to 10 times more gastrin than duodenum.

    4) Component III (little gastrin or gastrin-17) is the predominating tissue form of gastrin.

    5) Portions of Components I and II in circulation are conversion-products of Component III (little gastrin).

Acknowledgments

The skillful technical assistance of Jane Czuba, Annegrethe Pedersen, and Ulla Søegaard is gratefully acknowledged. The

studies were supported by grants from the Danish Medical
Research Council (j.nr. 512-2540, -3108, -3109, and -3954),
Den laegevidenskabelige Forskiningsfond for Storkøbenhavn,
Faerøerne og Grønland, Chr. X's Fond, and Landsforeningen til
Kraeftens Bekaempelse.

References

1. Rehfeld JF: Three components of gastrin in human serum: Gel
      filtration studies on the molecular size of immunoreac-
      tive serum gastrin. *Biochim Biophys Acta* 285:364-372, 1972.
2. Rehfeld JF, Stadil F, Rubin B: Production and evaluation
      of antibodies for the radioimmunoassay of gastrin. *Scand
      J Clin Lab Invest* 30:221-232, 1972.
3. Rehfeld JF, Stadil F: Gel filtration studies on immuno-
      reactive gastrin in serum from Zollinger-Ellison
      patients. *Gut* 14:369-373, 1973.
4. Rehfeld JF, Stadil F: (Letter) Radioimmunoassay for gastrin
      employing immunosorbent. *Scand J Clin Lab Invest*
      31:459-464, 1973.
5. Rehfeld JF, Stadil F: Units used to express the concen-
      tration of gastrin in biological fluids. *Gastroenter-
      ology* 65:859-860, 1973.
6. Rehfeld JF, Stadil F, Vikelsøe J: Immunoreactive gastrin
      components in human serum. *Gut* 15:102-111, 1974.
7. Stadil F, Rehfeld JF: Radioimmunoassay of human gastrin in
      human serum. *Scand J Gastroent* Suppl 9:61-65, 1971.
8. Stadil F, Rehfeld JF: Preparation of ^{125}I-labelled synthe-
      tic human gastrin I for radioimmunoanalysis. *Scand J
      Clin Lab Invest* 30:361-368, 1972.
9. Stadil F, Rehfeld JF: Determination of gastrin in serum:
      An evaluation of the reliability of a radioimmunoassay
      for gastrin. *Scand J Gastroent* 8:101-112, 1973.
10. Vikelsøe J, Rehfeld JF: Immunoreactive gastrin components
      in human antrum, in preparation.
11. Walsh JH, Debas HT, Grossman MI: Pure human big gastrin.
      Immunochemical properties, disappearance half time and
      acid-stimulating action in dogs. *J Clin Invest* 54:
      477-485, 1974.
12. Yalow RS, Wu N: Additional studies on the nature of big
      big gastrin. *Gastroenterology* 65:19-27, 1973.

PATTERNS OF SERUM GASTRIN AT REST AND AFTER STIMULATION IN MAN AND DOGS

Graham J. Dockray

VA Wadsworth Hospital Center,
Los Angeles, California

Gastrin, and other peptide hormones such as insulin, parathyroid hormone, and corticotrophin, exist in the blood and tissues in several different molecular forms.[11] The first suggestion of the molecular heterogeneity of gastrin came when Gregory and Tracy isolated heptadecapeptide (or "little") gastrin (G-17) from hog antral mucosa and showed it to exist in two forms, one unsulphated (G-17-I) and the other sulphated (G-17-II) at the tyrosine residue in position 6 from the C-terminus.[4] It is now known that gastrins of differing chain length also occur. Thus, the major form of gastrin in the circulation is larger and less acidic than G-17,[14] and is composed of 34 amino acid residues (G-34) of which the C-terminal 17 are identical to those in G-17.[5] As in G-17, the tyrosine residue at position 6 from the C-terminus of G-34 may be either unsulphated (G-34-I) or sulphated (G-34-II). Other molecular forms of gastrin have been described which correspond to the C-terminal tridecapeptide of G-17 (G-13),[6] and the N-terminal portion of G-17, possibly 1-13 of G-17.[2] In addition, two forms of gastrin which are larger than G-34 have been reported but not yet chemically and biologically characterized. These are Component I of Rehfeld and Stadil[9] and "bigbig gastrin" (BBG) of Yalow and Berson.[15,16]

The C-terminal tetrapeptide of G-17 is the minimal fragment of the molecule that possesses biologic activity,[8] so it is not surprising to find that the molecular forms known to share this tetrapeptide (G-17, G-34, and G-13) are all biologically active.[1,12] The properties of these peptides, however, are not identical. The clearance rate of G-34 was found

to be one-fifth that of G-17 and G-13; moreover, G-17
was found to be five times more potent than G-34 (with
potency expressed in terms of serum concentration
required for a given response) and twice as potent as
G-13 in stimulating acid secretion in the dog.[1,12]

Since the amino acid sequences of the C-terminal
portions of G-34, G-17 and G-13 are identical, it
seems reasonable to suggest that these molecules are
synthesized from the same gene and that G-34 represents
a biosynthetic precursor that yields G-17 and G-13 upon
cleavage. Because of the differences in biologic
activity of the different forms of gastrin, the factors
involved in regulating their relative rates of conversion and secretion are of particular biologic importance. As a first step towards understanding these
relationships, we studied the relative concentrations
of molecular forms in the serum and tissues of gastrinoma (Zollinger-Ellison syndrome) patients and in dogs
with antral pouches, both in the basal state and after
stimulation of gastrin secretion.

USE OF REGION-SPECIFIC ANTIBODIES TO GASTRIN

At the start of this study it was hoped that by
using antisera with specificity for different regions
of the gastrin molecule, it would be possible to
measure the molecular forms of gastrin in serum by
radioimmunoassay without prior fractionation. Thus,
an antibody with specificity for the C-terminus of
G-17 would estimate G-17 and G-34, whereas an antibody specific for the N-terminus of G-17 would measure
this molecular form alone. Appropriate antisera were
raised in rabbits immunized with G-17 conjugated to
bovine serum albumin. Figure 1 shows that for Ab 1296,
G-17-I and G-34-I inhibited binding of labeled [125]I
G-17, and that inhibition curves were parallel; other
peptides with the same C-terminal portion as G-17
(that is, 2-17 G-17 and G-13) also cross-reacted with
this antibody, but amino terminal fragments of G-17
(1-13 G-17 and desamido G-17) did not cross-react,
which indicated that Ab 1296 was specific for the C-
terminal part of G-17. In contrast, with Ab 1295,
binding of label was inhibited by G-17 and 1-13 G-17
but not by G-34; amino terminal fragments of G-17 such
as desamido G-17, also cross-reacted, but carboxyl
terminal fragments like 2-17 G-17 and G-13 did not,

so that this antibody was specific for the N-terminus
of G-17. With both antibodies, serum from a gastrinoma patient gave inhibition curves parallel to those
of G-17, which indicated that the antibodies were
suitable for use in estimating serum gastrin components.

The feasibility of using these two antibodies to
investigate concentrations of G-34 and G-17 in biologic samples was tested by applying them in the
radioimmunoassay of column eluates obtained when
serum from a gastrinoma patient was fractionated on

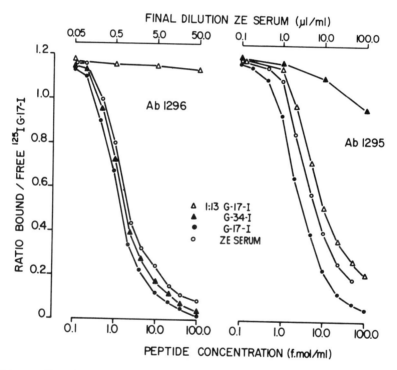

Figure 1. Competitive inhibition curves for G-17-I, G-34-I,
1-13 G-17-I and serum from patient with gastrinoma, with
Ab 1296 (final dilution 1:300,000) and Ab 1295 (final dilution
1:180,000). Trace was monoiodinated [125]I G-17-I. (Reproduced,
with permission of *Gastroenterology*.[2])

Sephadex G50. Figure 2 shows that Ab 1296 revealed
peaks of immunoreactivity in the eluates which emerged
in the same regions as standard G-34 and G-17. As
expected, Ab 1295 detected the G-17 peak but not the
G-34 peak. Unexpectedly, however, Ab 1295 also showed
a peak of immunoreactivity emerging between the G-34
and G-17 regions which had not been seen with Ab 1296.
The material in this peak had the pattern of immunoreactivity typical of an N-terminal fragment of G-17
and had the same elution volume as the 1-13 fragment
of G-17 (Fig. 2).

Amino terminal fragments of gastrin are not biologically active, but the possibility that 1-13 G-17
exists in serum and in antral extracts[3] is of particular interest, for when 1-13 sequence is removed from
G-17 the remaining portion is the C-terminal tetrapeptide which is the minimal fragment of the molecule
with biologic activity. Of course, one consequence
of the presence of N-terminal fragments of gastrin in
serum is that antibodies with specificity for the N-
terminus of G-17 cannot, by themselves, be used to
estimate G-17 concentrations in unfractionated samples.
In continuing studies on the relative concentrations
of the biologically active forms of gastrin in blood
and tissues, we have therefore used Ab 1296 and have
estimated concentrations of the molecular forms in
samples fractionated on columns (1 x 100 cm) of
Sephadex G50 run in veronal buffer, at 4C.

GASTRINOMA PATIENTS

Serum of 10 patients with gastrinomas was obtained
after an overnight fast and the molecular forms of
gastrin in the serum were separated on Sephadex G50.
In seven of the patients, samples of gastrinoma tissue
were obtained at surgery, extracted in boiling water,
and the extract chromatographed in the same way as
the serum samples. Biopsies of gastrinomas from
another three patients for which serum was not available were similarly studied.

Figure 3 shows a typical elution profile obtained
when serum and an extract of tumor from the same
patient were separated on Sephadex and immunoreactive
gastrin in eluates estimated with Ab 1296. In the
serum there was a major peak of immunoreactivity with
an elution volume (35%-45%) typical of G-34 and two

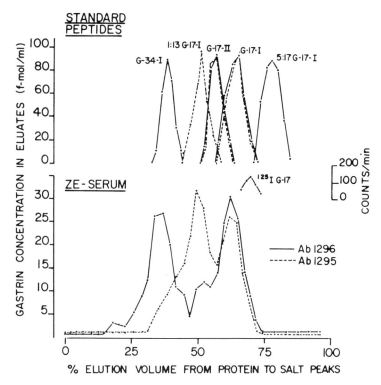

Figure 2. Upper trace. Record of five separate columns runs in which standard samples of G-34-I, 1-13 G-17-I, G-17-I, G-17-II and 5-17 G-17-I were applied to the same Sephadex column and eluted under conditions identical to those for gastrinoma serum shown in lower panel.

 Lower Trace. Elution pattern obtained when 0.5 ml serum of patient with gastrinoma was chromatographed on Sephadex G50 superfine (1 x 95 cm). Serum obtained at surgery.

 Flow: 6 ml/hr, fraction size 1.0 ml. All the tubes in the eluates were assayed with both Ab 1295 (---) and Ab 1296(——), and immunoreactivity is expressed in terms of a standard of G-17-I. Reproduced, with permission, *Gastroenterology*.[2])

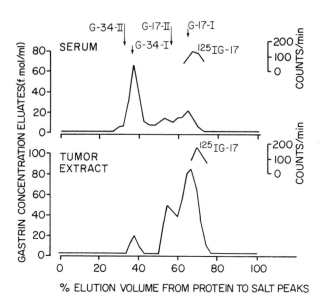

Figure 3. Elution profile of immunoreactive gastrin in a gastrinoma extract and in serum from the same patient taken preoperatively. Arrows indicate elution volumes of standard peptides on this column. Column conditions as in Figure 2.

minor peaks with elution volumes typical of G-17-II (55%-60%) and G-17-I (60%-65%). In the tumor extract, on the other hand, there was only a minor peak corresponding to G-34 but there were major peaks compatible with G-17-II and G-17-I. In the serum of three patients there was also a well-defined peak with an elution volume of 20%-30% corresponding to the Component I of Rehfeld,[9] and in two patients there was a peak of immunoreactivity in the column void volume corresponding to the BBG of Yalow;[15,16] in two other patients there were peaks of immunoreactivity with the gel filtration properties of G-13 (elution volume 80%-85%). The contributions to total immunoreactivity of serum by Component I, BBG, and G-13 together never exceeded 15% in any one serum.

There was a highly significant correlation between the concentration of G-34 and G-17 in both the serum (r=0.978, p <0.01) and in the tumor extracts (r=0.946, p <0.01) (Figs. 4a and 5a). There was no correlation, however, between ratio G-17/G-34 and the total immunoreactive gastrin in serum (Fig. 4b; r=0.296) and

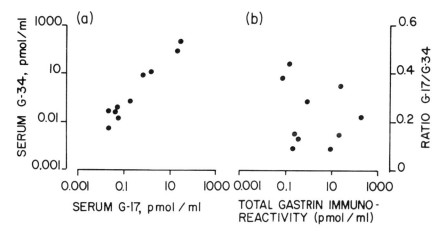

Figure 4. (a) G-17 concentration versus G-34 concentration in fasting serum of 10 ZE patients. The scales are logarithmic. Concentrations of G-17 and G-34 calculated from G50 elution profiles. Regression line: log y = 0.964 log x + 0.804; r = 0.978, *p* <0.01.

(b) Ratio of G-17/G-34 versus total gastrin immunoreactivity (on a log scale) in serum of same patients. Regression: y = 0.003 log x + 0.35; r = 0.296.

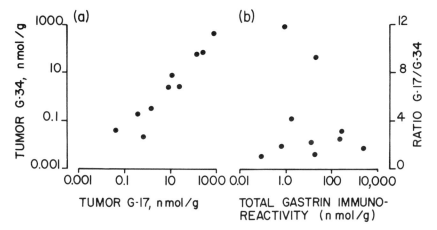

Figure 5. (a) As Fig. 2(a) but relative concentration of G-17 and G-34 in gastrinoma extracts of 10 patients. Note, seven patients were the same as those represented in Figure 2. Regression: log y = 1.0128 log x + 0.589; r = 0.946, *p* <0.01.

(b) As Fig. 2(b), but ratio of G-17/G-34 versus total gastrin immunoreactivity in gastrinoma extracts. Regression: y = 0.015 log x + 17.1; r = 0.19.

tumor (Fig. 5b; r=0.190). The mean relative abundances in serum of G-17 ($\frac{G-17}{G-17 + G-34}$) and G-34 ($\frac{G-34}{G-17 + G-34}$) were 0.18 and 0.82, respectively, compared to 0.73 and 0.27, respectively, in tumor extracts. Since the half-life of G-34 is 6-10 times greater than that of G-17 in man,[13] one would not expect to find equal ratios of G-17/G-34 in tissues and blood. Assuming that gastrinomas secrete G-17 and G-34 in the same ratio as they occur in extracts, then at a steady state condition, such as occurs in the basal fasting state, the ratio in blood can be predicted from the difference in half-lives:

$$\frac{G-17_g}{G-34_g} \quad \frac{G-17_{t\frac{1}{2}}}{G-34_{t\frac{1}{2}}} = \frac{G-17_s}{G-34_s}$$

where: g = concentration in gastrinoma
$t\frac{1}{2}$ = half-life in blood
s = concentration in serum.

The predicted relative abundance of G-17 in blood is 0.38 - 0.55, or about two to three times the observed value.

   Additional evidence that G-17 is the principal molecular form stored by gastrinoma tissue comes from stimulation experiments. Patients with gastrinomas respond to an intravenous injection of secretin with an increase in serum gastrin concentration, whereas in normal subjects secretin tends to depress serum gastrin levels.[7] Figure 6 shows that five minutes after the injection of secretin there is a pronounced increase in both serum G-17 and G-34 concentrations, although the G-17 response is proportionately greater than that of G-34. The concentration of G-17 returns to basal levels more rapidly than G-34, and this reflects the difference in half-lives of the two peptides. In a total of eight patients studied, six responded to secretin with an increase in serum gastrin. In these six the relative proportions of G-17 and G-34 in basal blood were 0.21 and 0.79, respectively, compared with 0.37 and 0.64 in serum taken five minutes after secretin. The relative increase in G-17 concentration was statistically significant ($p < 0.05$).

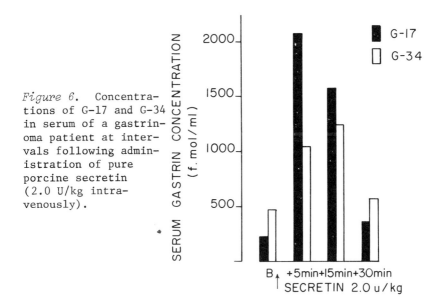

Figure 6. Concentrations of G-17 and G-34 in serum of a gastrinoma patient at intervals following administration of pure porcine secretin (2.0 U/kg intravenously).

ANTRAL POUCH DOGS

The secretion of the different molecular forms of gastrin was studied under physiologic circumstances in dogs with antral pouches. In three dogs with denervated antral pouches, serum samples were taken five minutes and three hours after instillation of 15% liver extract into the pouch (30-cm pressure). Suction biopsies of mucosa from the pouch were removed before and after the stimulation.

When serum taken five minutes after instillation of the liver extract was run on Sephadex G50, a peak of immunoreactive gastrin could be identified in eluates which had the elution volume (35%-45%) of G-34 (Fig. 7). In addition, minor peaks were identified which had elution volumes of 60%-65% and 70%-77%. The minor peaks probably correspond to G-17-II and G-17-I, respectively, although their elution volumes are about 10% greater than the corresponding peaks in eluates of ZE serum or pure human peptides. In the serum samples taken after three hours' stimulation of the antral pouch, the concentrations of G-17 were maintained while those of G-34 were approximately twice the values seen in the five-minute samples (Table 1). The shift in relative concentrations of G-17 and G-34 between five minutes' and three hours' stimulation may be accounted for by the longer

67

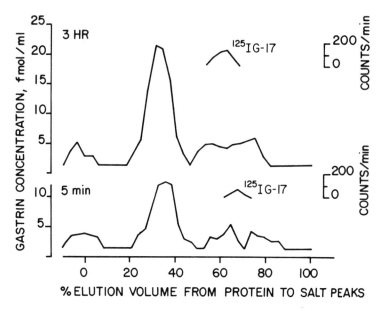

Figure 7. Sephadex G50 elution patterns of serum from a
dog with a denervated antral pouch taken 5 minutes and
3 hours after instillation of 15% liver extract into the
pouch at 30-cm pressure.

half-life of G-34 (15 min, in dogs) compared to G-17
(3 min) and thus the greater time taken to reach equilibrium in the blood after steady stimulation.

In many samples of dog serum that were run on
Sephadex G50 there was a peak of immunoreactivity in
the void volume of the column corresponding to
BBG.[15,16] In about 50% of samples of serum taken
from fasting unstimulated dogs, this was the only
peak of immunoreactivity; in approximately 25% of
studied dogs there were also small peaks corresponding to G-34 and G-17. Figure 7 shows that the concentration of BBG did not change throughout stimulation of the antral pouch. We have found that with
the antiserum (Ab 1296) used in this study, purified
bovine and human serum albumin, in concentrations
comparable to those of proteins in serum, inhibited
binding of label to antibody. Because of this we
ascribe at least some of the BBG seen in dog serum
to the action of serum proteins which elute in the
void volume of G50 columns and cause nonspecific
inhibition of antibody binding to label.

Table 1. Concentrations of G-34 and G-17 (fmol/ml) in serum of antral pouch dogs during stimulation by liver extract (6 experiments in 4 dogs)

| | Basal | Stimulated | |
		5 minutes	3 hours
Total gastrin immunoreactivity	15.0±3.0	110±12	164±18
Concentrations:			
G-17		38±7	46±7
G-34		58±13	102±15
Relative concentrations:			
G-17 observed		0.39	0.31
G-17 predicted*		-	0.64
G-34 observed		0.61	0.69
G-34 predicted*		-	0.36

* Predicted from antral ratio G-17/G-34 and half-lives of 3 minutes for G-17 and 15 minutes for G-34.

The principal molecular forms of gastrin in biopsies of antral mucosa had the same elution volumes on Sephadex G50 as the peaks identified as G-17-II and G-17-I in serum. The peak identified as G-34 in serum comprised only a minor proportion of the immunoreactivity in the antral biopsies. The relative concentrations of these molecular forms were not altered by stimulation of the pouch for up to three hours (Fig. 8). Also, the total gastrin immunoreactivity in the biopsies was not significantly changed after the period of stimulation (Table 2).

Table 2. Relative concentrations of G-17 and G-34 in biopsies of antral mucosa of antral pouch dogs before and three hours after stimulation with liver extract (6 experiments in 4 dogs)

	Before	After
Total gastrin immunoreactivity	10.6±2.7 nmol/g	8.4±2.2 nmol/g
Relative concentrations:		
G-17	0.89	0.90
G-34	0.11	0.10

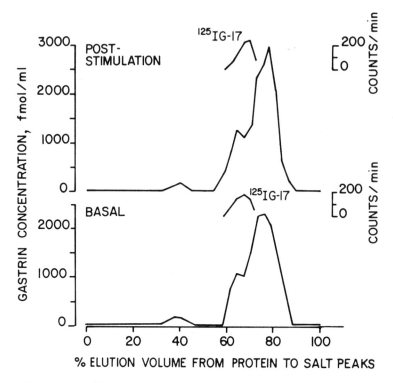

Figure 8. Elution patterns of extracts of biopsies of antral mucosa taken before and after instillation of liver extract into denervated antral pouch. Biopsies were boiled in water (5 minutes, 1 mg tissue/ml) and an aliquot of supernatant fluid applied to column.

Knowing the ratio of G-17/G-34 in antral mucosa and using the formula given in the previous section, the relative concentrations of G-17 and G-34 in serum following a steady stimulation of gastrin release can be predicted. Table 1 indicates that the predicted concentration of G-17 in serum is about twice the observed one.

Several factors may account for the discrepancy between the observed ratios of G-17 and G-34 in serum of gastrinoma patients and antral pouch dogs and the ratios predicted from tissue ratios and half-lives. First, there could be ultrarapid conversion of G-34 to G-17 during the extraction of tissues. We have observed, however, that [125]I G-34 added to tissue extracts can be recovered intact after passage of the

12. Walsh JH, Debas HT, Grossman MI: Pure human big gastrin:
    Immunochemical properties, disappearance half time,
    and acid-stimulating action in dogs. *J Clin Invest*
    54:477-485, 1974.
13. Walsh JH: Biologic activity and disappearance rates of
    big, little, and mini-gastrins in dog and man, in
    Thompson JC (ed), *Gastrointestinal Hormones*, Austin:
    University of Texas Press, 1975, pp 75-83.
14. Yalow RS, Berson SA: Size and charge distinctions between
    endogenous human plasma gastrin in peripheral blood
    and heptadecapeptide gastrins. *Gastroenterology*
    58:609-615, 1970.
15. Yalow RS, Berson SA: And now, "big, big" gastrin.
    Biochem Biophys Res Commun 48:391-395, 1972.
16. Yalow RS, Wu N: Additional studies on the nature of big
    big gastrin. *Gastroenterology* 65:19-27, 1973.

BIOLOGIC ACTIVITY AND DISAPPEARANCE RATES OF BIG, LITTLE, AND MINI-GASTRINS IN DOG AND MAN

John H. Walsh

Department of Medicine, University of California, Los Angeles, and VA Wadsworth Hospital Center, Los Angeles, California

The presence of multiple molecular forms of gastrin in the circulation and in gastrointestinal tissues is now well documented. In previous papers[3,4,6] it was shown that the circulating concentrations of several of these molecular forms vary during physiologic or pharmacologic stimulation of gastrin release. The present studies were done to look at the metabolism of gastrins of different chemical compositions and to relate changes in gastric acid secretion to exogenous dose and to changes in circulating gastrin during administration of these hormones in pure form.

Pure gastrin preparations were made available to us by Professor Gregory.[2] These included: nonsulfated and sulfated "little gastrins" which contain 17 amino acids and will be abbreviated G-17-I and G-17-II; "big gastrins", containing 34 amino acids and called G-34-I and G-34-II; and "minigastrins" containing 13 amino acids and called G-13-I and G-13-II. Human gastrinoma tissue was the source of the pure human peptides. Much of this material was purified from a large tumor metastatic to the liver obtained in the immediate postmortem period from a single patient by Dr. Edward Passaro, Jr. Porcine gastrins were purified from extracts of hog antral mucosa.

The steps leading to final purification were discussed in detail by Professor Gregory.[3] A portion of each peptide was reserved for biologic testing and the remainder was taken for amino acid analysis and sequence determinations.

Biologic testing was performed in dogs with chronic gastric fistulas and Heidenhain pouches. The results of these tests have been published.[1,5] Additional studies were carried out in four human subjects, three with duodenal ulcer, and one free of gastrointestinal disease (Walsh and Isenberg, unpublished observations).

Gastrin solutions were prepared in 0.05 M ammonium bicarbonate. Molar concentrations of these pure peptide solutions were measured by determining absorbance at 280 nm and application of calculated molar extinction coefficients.[5] All calculations were based on molar concentrations. When necessary, radioimmunoassay results were adjusted for differences in inhibitory potency of the various peptides with the antibodies employed. This was done by making separate standard curves for each peptide and using the appropriate curve for measurement of changes in serum gastrin during infusion of the same peptide. The two antibodies used, 2604 of Rehfeld[5] and our 1296,[2] showed equal immunopotency for non-sulfated and sulfated gastrins, but G-34 was approximately 60% and G-13 approximately 40% as potent as G-17 on a molar basis with these antibodies.

For comparisons of G-17 and G-34, single doses of each were administered on separate days for 90 minutes by intravenous infusion. Comparisons of G-17 and G-13 were done by administration of stepwise-increasing doses (each dose double the preceding) for 40-minute periods on the same day. Gastric juice was obtained continuously and divided into 10- or 15-minute periods for measurement of acid secretion. Blood was obtained at appropriate time periods, allowed to clot, and centrifuged; serum was stored frozen until all specimens from a single study were available to be tested by radioimmunoassay in the same assay.

Preliminary tests revealed that G-17-I and II from porcine or human sources had equal biologic and immunochemical activity. The following studies were done in dogs to compare porcine G-17-I and G-17-II with human G-34-I and G-34-II. We established that there was a linear relationship between the dose of gastrin infused and plateau increment achieved in immunoreactive serum gastrin (Fig. 1). This argues against any variation in metabolism due to different rates of infusion of gastrin.

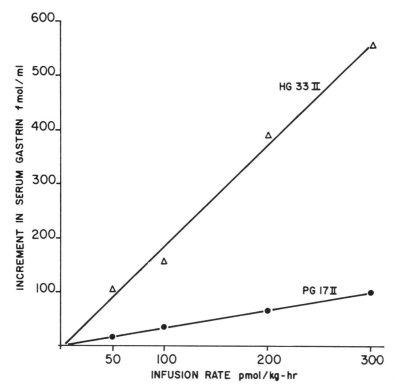

Figure 1. Linear relationships between infusion rates of PG-17-II or HG-34-II and measured increments in immunoreactive serum gastrin. (Reproduced, with permission of the *Journal of Clinical Investigation.*[5])

Disappearance half-time, or half-life, was measured by plotting the change in serum immunoreactive gastrin on a logarithmic scale against time on a linear scale after stopping gastrin infusion at the highest dose given. A typical set of results is illustrated in Figure 2. Over the range which permitted accurate measurement (roughly from 100% to 10% of plateau increment), the points lay on a straight line which could be analyzed by simple linear regression. The half-lives of porcine and human G-17 in the dog ranged between two and four minutes. The half-life of G-13 in a different set of dogs was slightly less than two minutes (Fig. 3). Human G-34-I and II had significantly longer half-lives, approximately 15 to 16 minutes. Thus, the half-life of G-34 in the dog is approximately five times longer than for G-17 or

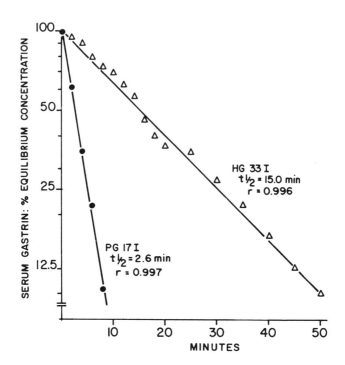

Figure 2. Disappearance of PG-17-I and HG-34-I (immunoreactivity) after cessation of intravenous infusion (basal subtracted). Similar results were obtained with sulfated forms. (Reproduced, with permission of the *Journal of Clinical Investigation*.[5])

G-13, and these differences in half-lives are reflected in the much higher plateau concentrations achieved during infusion of G-34.

Preliminary studies of the half-lives of human G-17 and G-34 in man suggest that the differences are at least as great as in the dog. Values were approximately four minutes for G-17 and approximately 30 minutes for G-34.

The relationships between exogenous dose and acid responses in the dog are shown in the next two figures. Based on exogenous dose administered, G-34 was about 20% more potent than G-17 (Fig. 4). G-13 was only about 40% as potent as G-17 (Fig. 5).

In man, studies have not been completed. It is apparent, however, that equimolar exogenous doses of G-34 and G-13 produce lower acid responses than G-17.

Expression of potency in terms of exogenous dose may be misleading. Although PG-17-II and HG-34-II

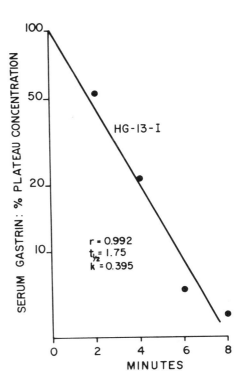

Figure 3. Disappearance of HG-13-I immunoreactivity after cessation of intravenous infusion (basal subtracted). (Reproduced, with permission of *Gut.*[1]).

infused at a rate of 100 pmol/kg/hr produced similar gastric secretory responses, the G-34 produced a substantially higher increase in circulating gastrin. It is apparent that a small increase in circulating G-17 produced acid secretion nearly equal to that produced by a much larger increase in G-34.

This can be expressed formally by plotting acid secretion as a function of increments in circulating gastrin, produced during infusions of different doses of gastrin (Fig. 6). If the plateau circulating concentration is closely related to the concentration available to receptors in the gastric mucosa, this also would be an expression of "endogenous dose" or dose available at the receptor site. Unfortunately, we have no direct information about the partition of gastrin at the receptors relative to circulating concentrations. Since the apparent spaces of distribution of G-17 and G-34 are similar, we can merely infer that these substances are distributed similarly. Based on changes in circulating gastrin, G-17 was

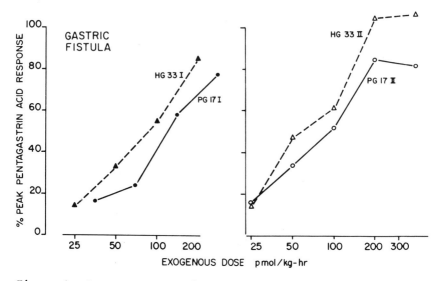

Figure 4. Dose-response relationships for gastric fistula acid secretion as functions of exogenous doses of pure G-17 and G-34 preparations. (Reproduced, with permission of the *Journal of Clinical Investigation*.[5])

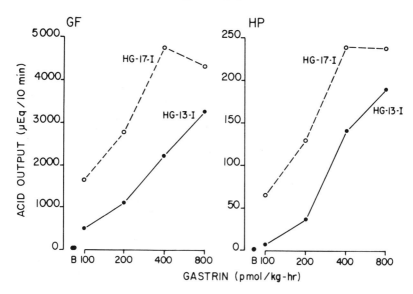

Figure 5. Dose-response relationships for gastric fistula (GF) and Heidenhain pouch (HP) acid secretion as a function of exogenous dose of HG-17-I and HG-13-I. (Reproduced, with permission of *Gut*.[1])

80

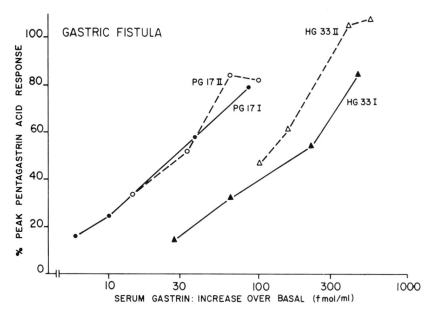

Figure 6. Dose-response relationships for gastric fistula acid secretion as functions of increments in serum immunoreactive gastrin achieved during intravenous infusions of pure G-17 and G-34 preparations (endogenous dose) corrected for differences in immunoreactivity. (Reproduced, with permission of the *Journal of Clinical Investigation.*[5])

approximately five times more potent than G-34 as a stimulant of acid secretion in the dog. Since the plateau increments achieved during infusion of equimolar doses of G-17 and G-13 did not differ significantly, relative "exogenous" and "endogenous" potency was the same, that is, G-17 was 2.5 times as potent as G-13 based on either criterion.

Data are not complete in man. However, the same general relationships appear to hold true for G-17 and G-34, except that G-34 is less potent than G-17 even based on exogenous dose. If G-17 is 1.5 to 2 times as potent by exogenous dose calculations, it is 5 to 10 times as potent based on changes in immunoreactive serum gastrin achieved during infusion.

Our interpretation of physiologic changes in immunoreactive gastrin must take these differences into account. A predominance of G-17 would indicate much greater stimulating capacity than an equivalent change in G-34. Ordinary RIA for gastrin, however, cannot distinguish between these two forms.

Since G-17 is more potent than G-34, it is reasonable to ask if G-34 has any biologic activity or whether it must first be converted to G-17. We have not studied this question directly; however, we performed column chromatography on serum specimens obtained during and after infusion of G-34 in man. As shown in one typical example (Fig. 7), a single peak of G-34 was obtained by chromatography in the same region as G-34 standard. The system was sensitive enough to detect as little as 2% activity in the G-17 region, but no activity was found. Similar results were obtained in other human subjects and suggest at least that no major conversion of G-34 to G-17 occurs in the whole body.

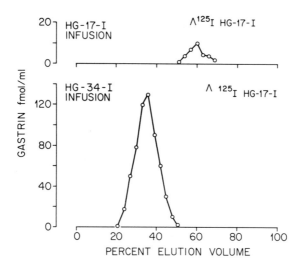

Figure 7. Elution patterns obtained by gel filtration of 0.5 ml serum specimens obtained during infusion of pure HG-17-I and HG-34-I in a human subject. The column was 1 x 100 cm G50 superfine eluted with 0.02 M veronal buffer. Serum protein and conductivity were used to determine void volume and salt peaks (taken as 0 and 100% of elution volume) and a tracer amount of ^{125}I-labeled HG-17-I was added to each serum sample.

SUMMARY

Biologic activity of pure natural human "little gastrin" (G-17), "big gastrin" (G-34) and "minigastrin"
(G-13) was assessed in dog and man by administration
of peptide solutions intravenously and measurement of
gastric acid secretion. Changes in immunoreactive
serum gastrin were determined during and after gastrin
infusions and were used to estimate clearance rate,
half-life and space of distribution for each peptide.
G-34 was cleared more slowly than either G-17 or G-13
and significantly higher serum concentrations of G-34
were achieved at each dose rate. The apparent potency
(rate of gastric acid secretion versus exogenous dose)
of G-34 was similar to G-17 while G-13 was half as
potent. If potency was determined as rate of gastric
acid secretion versus change in serum gastrin, however,
G-17 was several times more potent than G-34. This
discrepancy was due to the much higher gastrin concentrations achieved during G-34 infusion. There was
no evidence of interconversion between G-17 and G-34
in the circulation.

References

1. Debas HT, Walsh JH, Grossman MI: Pure human minigastrin:
       secretory potency and disappearance rate. *Gut* 15:686-
       689, 1974.
2. Dockray GJ: Pattern of serum gastrins at rest and after
       stimulation in man and in dogs, in Thompson JC (ed),
       Gastrointestinal Hormones, Austin: University of Texas
       Press, 1975, pp 59-73.
3. Gregory RA, Tracy HJ: Chemistry of gastrin, in Thompson JC
       (ed), *Gastrointestinal Hormones*, Austin: University of
       Texas Press, 1975, pp 13-24.
4. Rehfeld JF, Stadil F, Malmstrøm J, Miyata M: Gastrin heter-
       ogeneity in serum and tissue, in Thompson JC (ed),
       Gastrointestinal Hormones, Austin: University of Texas
       Press, 1975, pp 43-58.
5. Walsh JH, Debas HT, Grossman MI: Pure human big gastrin:
       immunochemical properties, disappearance half-time, and
       acid-stimulating action in dogs. *J Clin Invest* 54:477-
       485, 1974.
6. Yalow RS: Heterogeneity of peptide hormones with relation to
       gastrin, in Thompson JC (ed), *Gastrointestinal Hormones*,
       Austin: University of Texas Press, 1975, pp 25-41.

BINDING AND MEASUREMENT OF DIFFERENT GASTRIN FORMS BY REGION-SPECIFIC ANTIBODIES TO GASTRIN

James E. McGuigan and Charles A. Herbst

Division of Gastroenterology, University of Florida
College of Medicine, Gainesville, Florida and
Department of Surgery, University of North Carolina
School of Medicine, Chapel Hill, North Carolina

In 1964 Gregory and Tracy[7,8] reported the identification, purification, and structural characterization of two gastrins which they isolated from porcine gastric mucosa. These gastrins were heptadecapeptides (each containing 17 amino acid residues in a single polypeptide chain) and differed only by the presence of sulfation of the tyrosyl residue in position 12. The molecular species in which the tyrosyl was esterified with sulfate was designated as gastrin II and the nonsulfated form as gastrin I. Subsequently, with their colleagues, they identified and characterized the structure of antral gastrins from a variety of other mammalian species including man. In each instance, heptadecapeptides were identified. Human heptadecapeptide gastrins I and II were identical to those of porcine gastrins except for substitution of leucyl in position 5 in human gastrins, in contrast to methionyl in that position in porcine gastrins. Following the elucidation of the primary structure of porcine gastrin heptadecapeptides, Mutt and Jorpes[14] demonstrated that the carboxyl-terminal pentapeptide amide of porcine cholecystokinin-pancreozymin was identical to that of porcine gastrin. This carboxyl-terminal pentapeptide amide contained the terminal tetrapeptide amide which is, or contains, the physiologically active site of the gastrin molecule.
Subsequently, Yalow and Berson,[27,28] by use of Sephadex gel chromatography and starch gel electrophoresis,

85

showed that the major circulating form of gastrin was
larger in molecular weight than heptadecapeptide gastrins and less acidic than the strongly negatively
charged heptadecapeptide gastrin molecules; they
named this larger and less acidic gastrin, big or
basic gastrin. Big gastrin has been shown to have a
molecular weight of approximately 3800, to be composed of 34 amino acid residues, of which the carboxyl-terminal 17 constitutes the heptadecapeptide
amide gastrin form. Subsequently, they demonstrated
that big gastrin was present in the mucosa of the
upper small intestine, constituting an increasing
proportion of the progressively decreasing total
gastrin content with caudad progression through the
duodenum.[2] More recently, Berson and Yalow[29] demonstrated an even larger form of gastrin both in plasma
and in extracts of jejunal mucosa which they designated "big-big" gastrin. This molecular species of
gastrin has a molecular weight of approximately
20,000.[30] Incubation of big gastrin or big-big gastrin with trypsin yields heptadecapeptide gastrin.
An additional gastrin species which has been identified in the antral mucosa, in gastrinoma extracts,
and in sera from patients with gastrinomas appears
to comprise the carboxyl-terminal 13 amino acid residues of heptadecapeptide gastrin and has been designated as "minigastrin".[22] Most recently, immunologic
studies support the presence of a gastrin fragment
in the circulation and in gastrinoma extracts which
is an amino terminal fragment of the gastrin heptadecapeptide and probably represents the amino terminal tridecapeptide of heptadecapeptide gastrins.[6,20]
Thus it appears that there are at least five major
peptide forms of gastrin that can be detected in
tissue extracts and in the circulation; thus far, in
each instance, when examined, these forms appear to
be demonstrable as gastrins I and II. Thus, at least 10
molecular species of gastrin have been identified in
tissue extracts and in serum or plasma (Fig. 1).
A variety of techniques have been evolved for the
production of antibodies to gastrin for use in radioimmunoassay measurement of gastrin. The two principal methods have been immunization of rabbits with
synthetic human gastrin I hexadecapeptide (SHG:2-17)
conjugated to bovine serum albumin by carbodiimide,[16]
and alternatively, immunization of guinea pigs with

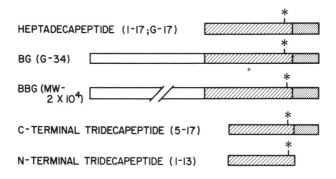

HEPTADECAPEPTIDE (I-17;G-17)

BG (G-34)

BBG (MW~ 2 X 10⁴)

C-TERMINAL TRIDECAPEPTIDE (5-17)

N-TERMINAL TRIDECAPEPTIDE (1-13)

* TYROSYL SULFATED (GASTRIN II) OR NON-SULFATED
(GASTRIN I)

Figure 1. Five major molecular species of gastrin,
each probably existing in either sulfated (gastrin II)
or nonsulfated (gastrin I) forms. All except the
N-terminal tridecapeptide contain the active site
gastrin peptide fragment, the carboxyl-terminal
tetrapeptide amide (   ).

partially purified porcine gastrin.[26] Both techniques
yield antibodies of high titer with specificity for
gastrin and are suitable for radioimmunoassay of gastrin. Additional methods of production of antibodies
to gastrin have included immunization of experimental
animals with peptide fragments of gastrin, including
the carboxyl-terminal tetrapeptide amide,[15,17] pentagastrin,[31] and the amino tridecapeptide of gastrin,[1,19]
in each instance covalently conjugated to carrier
protein molecules by a variety of coupling agents.

Temperley and Stagg[24] examined the immunologic reactivity and acid-stimulating activity of serum gastrin
in a patient with a gastrinoma and demonstrated consistent divergence between biologic activity and
immunologic measurement of gastrin with the antibody
preparation used in their radioimmunoassay. It is
probable that differences between immunoassayability
and biologic activity reflected differences in the
reactivity of the antibody population with various
molecular species of circulating gastrins in that
gastrinoma subject. Using antibodies produced to
pentagastrin, Young and his colleagues[3,5] obtained
serum immunoreactive gastrin levels that were much
higher than those obtained by investigators using

antibodies produced to hexadecapeptide human gastrin I
or partially purified porcine gastrin. In addition,
they reported increased basal serum gastrin levels
in duodenal ulcer patients, whereas most other investigators have found that basal serum gastrin concentrations in duodenal ulcer and normal subjects do
not differ. They also found that immunoreactive
serum gastrin levels in duodenal ulcer patients decreased strikingly after vagotomy,[3] whereas other
investigators have found increased serum gastrin
levels after vagotomy. They suggested that differences in results might be explained by immunoreactive
detection of additional species of gastrin by antibodies to pentagastrin, which were not detected in
other antibody systems.

Hansky and his colleagues[10,13] have reported serum
gastrin levels which, in general, have been somewhat
lower than those observed by most investigators.
Recently, Hansky[11] reported that the antibody preparation that he had used for radioimmunoassay reacted
with gastrin I but not with gastrin II. When he
used a different antibody preparation that exhibited
immunoreactivity with both gastrin II and gastrin I,
he obtained somewhat higher gastrin concentrations.

The multiplicity of tissue and circulating gastrin
forms and fragments and the variety of antibodies
produced to gastrin, oblige careful assessment of
the immunologic reactivity of antibodies utilized
with the various peptide gastrin species. The
studies to be described examined the characteristics
of binding of various forms of gastrin with antibodies that are directed to various portions of a
variety of gastrin peptides.

It should be emphasized that there does not exist
an antibody to the complete gastrin molecule; that
is, no single γG antibody molecule possesses complete specificity for intact gastrin heptadecapeptides
nor for any of the larger gastrin species. In response to immunization with human gastrin I, hexadecapeptide or partially purified gastrin antibodies
to gastrin are elicited which, although heterogeneous
do exhibit maximum specificity for defined regions of
the gastrin molecule. In studies of antibodies produced to amino acid polymers and peptides, and to
repeating saccharide units, it has been shown that
the size of antigenic determinant recognized by a
single antibody molecule, does not exceed six to

eight amino acid residues. Therefore, antibodies
produced to molecules as large as heptadecapeptide
gastrin or larger, would be anticipated to differ
in their recognition properties and in the associated
correlation between immunologic reactivity and biologic activity.

Because of the identity of the carboxyl-terminal
pentapeptide amide of cholecystokinin-pancreozymin
(CCK-PZ) and gastrin, CCK-PZ cross-reactivity could
present problems with immune measurement of gastrin.
Indeed, cross-reactivity of antibodies to gastrin
with cholecystokinin-pancreozymin can be demonstrated
both when antibodies are produced in response to
immunization with hexadecapeptide conjugated gastrin
and with porcine gastrin which has been partially
purified; fortunately, cross-reactivity with antibodies to gastrin, although detectable, is not pro-
hibitive. Results of our studies in assessing immunoreactivity of 18 different preparations of antibodies
to human gastrin (2-17), revealed that the immunologic
potency of CCK-PZ (that is, the inhibition of binding
of radiolabeled gastrin by 75% with human gastrin I
as reference) ranged from 0.020 to 0.001 (median
0.0032). Cross-reactivity with cholecystokinin-
pancreozymin with antibodies produced to partially
purified porcine gastrin has been reported to be
0.00027.[26] The somewhat higher degree of cross-reactivity of antibodies to human gastrin I (2-17) with
CCK-PZ probably reflects somewhat more specificity
for the active site carboxyl-terminal region of gastrin with these antibodies when compared with those
produced to impure porcine gastrin. Antibodies produced to the carboxyl-terminal tetrapeptide amide of
gastrin[15,17] exhibit approximately equivalent immunologic reactivity with cholecystokinin-pancreozymin and
gastrin; therefore, in the presence of significant concentrations of CCK-PZ, these antibodies are not sufficiently specific to be of value in measuring gastrin.

We have extensively examined the immunologic reactivity of a variety of antibody preparations, produced
in response to immunization of rabbits with conjugated-
hexadecapeptide gastrin, in respect to their binding
of human gastrins I and II. In Figure 2 is shown a
calibration curve demonstrating binding of human
gastrin I and human gastrin II by an antibody preparation produced in response to immunization with human
gastrin I (2-17), demonstrating equivalent immunologic

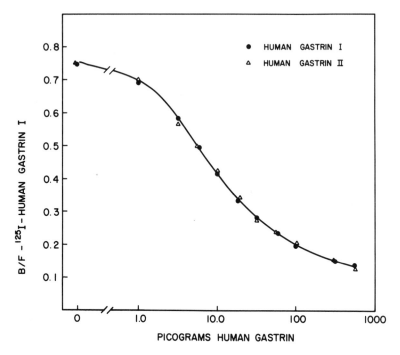

Figure 2. Calibration curve demonstrating equivalent binding
of ^{125}I-human gastrin I by antibodies to human gastrin I (2-17)
in the presence of variable amounts of human gastrin I and
human gastrin II.

reactivity with human gastrins I and II. In the examination of 18 antibody preparations produced to human
gastrin I (2-17) we have found 50% (9/18) of the antibody preparations exhibited equivalent immunologic
reactivity (>90%) with human gastrin I and human
gastrin II. Twenty-eight percent exhibited near equivalent immunologic reactivity (50%-90%) with human
gastrins I and II and 22% showed measurable but reduced (<50%) immunologic reactivity with human gastrin
II. We have not identified, among these antibody populations, any antibodies directed exclusively to human
gastrin I without detectable immunologic reactivity
with human gastrin II.
 We have also examined the immunologic reactivity of
these antibodies to gastrin (2-17) with the human
gastrin I aminotridecapeptide. Results indicated that
most antibodies to human gastrin I (2-17) exhibit

negligible immunoreactivity (immunologic potency
<0.005) with the isolated aminotridecapeptide portion
of gastrin.[18]

It is most important that a high degree of correlation be achieved between immunoreactivity using antibodies to gastrin, and biologic activity of tissue or
circulating gastrin peptides. Removal of the carboxyl-
terminal amide group of pentagastrin or heptadecapeptide amide gastrin, abolishes physiologic activity.
We have examined the immunologic reactivity of antibodies to human gastrin I (2-17) with heptadecapeptide
gastrin, in which the amide group has been removed
(desamidogastrin).[21] Results indicate that desamidogastrin is less than 1% as immunoreactive as intact
heptadecapeptide amide gastrin in inhibiting antibody
binding of radiolabeled gastrin. These observations
are particularly important inasmuch as deamidation of
the gastrin molecule or removal of its carboxyl-
terminal amino acid (phenylalanine-amide) may be
mechanisms by which gastrin molecules are progressively degraded *in vivo*. Therefore, with as subtle a
degradation step as removal of the amide group,>99%
of the immunoreactivity of the gastrin peptide is
abolished, and therefore, within the framework of
this molecular modification of the gastrin molecule,
antibodies to gastrin (2-17) exhibit a high degree
of correlation between immunologic reactivity and
biologic reactivity. This property of antibodies to
gastrin (2-17) reflects a favorable characteristic
of substantial specificity of the antibody for the
active site region of gastrin heptadecapeptide amide.

It has been possible to produce antibodies to gastrin which exhibit no immunologic cross-reactivity
with CCK-PZ.[1,19] This objective has been achieved
by repeated immunization of rabbits with the aminotridecapeptide of gastrin (residues 1-13) covalently
conjugated to bovine serum albumin by triazine linkage.
As would be predicted, antibodies produced in this
manner exhibit no immunologic cross-reactivity with
CCK-PZ, with pentagastrin, nor with tetrapeptide amide
of heptadecapeptide amide gastrins (Fig. 3). They
exhibit approximately equivalent immunoreactivity
with human gastrins I and II. Antibodies produced
exhibit no immunologic cross-reactivity with CCK-PZ
because of direction of their recognition toward the
amino terminal region of the gastrin heptadecapeptide.

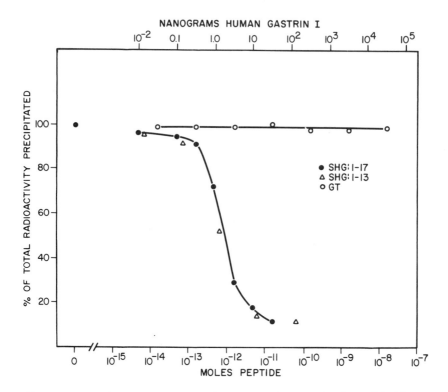

Figure 3. Calibration curve demonstrating equivalent binding of ^{125}I-human gastrin I by antibodies to the amino tridecapeptide of human gastrin I (1-13) in the presence of variable amounts of human gastrin I (1-17) and the amino tridecapeptide. No evidence of immunoreactivity with the C-terminal gastrin tetrapeptide amide (GT).

In addition, we have also produced and examined antibodies to the gastrin tetrapeptide amide which were produced by immunization with the gastrin tetra- peptide (conjugated to bovine serum albumin using carbodiimide). These antibodies exhibit approximately equivalent immunologic reactivity with CCK-PZ and the gastrin tetrapeptide, as well as with human gastrins I and II. Furthermore, antibodies to the tetrapeptide amide of gastrin exhibit exquisite recognition charac- teristics for subtle structural modification of the tetrapeptide amide of gastrin, particularly when these modifications, for example, removal of the amide group, amino acid interposition, deletion, or substitution

occur near the carboxyl-terminus (Ross and McGuigan,
unpublished observations). We have used antibodies
to the tetrapeptide amide of gastrin to measure fasting and postcibal levels of serum gastrin in normal
persons and in patients with duodenal ulcer disease.
Our results indicate that serum gastrin concentrations
measured with antibodies to tetrapeptide amide gastrin, are not significantly higher than those obtained
with antibodies to human gastrin I (residues 2-17).
These results do not support the suggestion that antibodies to the tetrapeptide amide detect gastrin species additional to those measured by antibodies to
human gastrin I (2-17).

We also examined human big or basic gastrin with
three antibody preparations, each with specificity
for different peptide regions of human gastrin; these
included antibodies to human gastrin I (2-17), antibodies to the aminotridecapeptide amide portion of
gastrin (1-13) and antibodies to the gastrin tetrapeptide amide (14-17). Results indicated equivalent
immunologic reactivity of antibodies to human gastrin
I (2-17) and antibodies to the tetrapeptide amide of
gastrin (14-17) with big gastrin and human gastrin
heptadecapeptide. In contrast, antibodies produced
with immunization with the human gastrin I amino
tridecapeptide (1-13) showed no immunologic reactivity
with intact big gastrin, or only a minimal amount
(immunologic potency <0.0005). Incubation of big
gastrin with trypsin (trypsin 1.0 mg/ml, in phosphate
buffer 0.1M, pH 7.4, for 30 min at 37C) restored
complete immunologic reactivity of big gastrin with
antibodies to the aminotridecapeptide.

We have demonstrated that gastrin is present in or
on abundant granules which pack the cytoplasm of
delta cells in the normal human pancreas.[9] Equivalent
specific immunofluorescence is achieved when pancreatic islets are overlain with either fluoroscein-
labeled antibodies to human gastrin I (2-17) or
fluorescein-labeled antibodies to the aminotridecapeptide amide portion of human gastrin I (1-13).
These results are consistent with the conclusion that
the species of gastrin present in pancreatic islet
delta cells is heptadecapeptide amide gastrin and do
not suggest that this is big gastrin.

We have examined the proportion of big gastrin and
heptadecapeptide amide gastrin in Zollinger-Ellison
tumor extracts by subjecting these extracts to separation by starch gel electrophoresis.[12] Results of

these studies indicate that in most instances the
major gastrin component of gastrinoma tissue is heptadecapeptide gastrin and not big gastrin. This is in
agreement with prior chemical and physiologic observations of Gregory and Tracy. In contrast, however,
in these same patients starch gel electrophoretic
separation of circulating gastrin reveals big gastrin,
and not heptadecapeptide amide gastrin as the major
circulating serum component. The explanation for the
divergence between tumor and circulating gastrin
species in Zollinger-Ellison patients is probably
explained by the longer half-life of big gastrin
(9 to 15 min) compared with heptadecapeptide (2.5 to
3.0 min).[23,25] If one assumes equivalent rates of
release of big gastrin and heptadecapeptide gastrin
(per mole gastrin present) from gastrinoma tissues,
the difference in concentration of the two circulating
gastrin species would be dictated by differences in
their rates of biologic removal and would be consistent with the observed excess of the more slowly
removed larger gastrin species.

We have examined serum samples from patients with
gastrinoma that have been subjected to starch gel
electrophoresis by comparative immunoassay with both
antibodies to human gastrin I (2-17) and antibodies
to the amino tridecapeptide of gastrin (1-13).
Results of these studies indicate that the more
slowly migrating big gastrin is not measured by antibodies to the aminotridecapeptide amide (1-13), which
is in accord with our earlier observations upon examining purified human big gastrin. Big gastrin is
readily identified by antibodies to human gastrin I
(2-17). The more rapidly anodally migrating heptadecapeptide amide gastrin is measured both by antibodies to human gastrin I (2-17) and antibodies to
the aminotridecapeptide amide of gastrin (1-13). In
addition, a more rapidly migrating immunoreactive
gastrin species is identified by antibodies to the
amino tridecapeptide amide of gastrin (1-13) but is
not detected by antibodies to the intact human gastrin
I (2-17). The behavior of this most rapidly anodally
migrating species is consistent with an amino peptide
portion of the gastrin molecule, and may well represent the aminotridecapeptide amide portion of human
gastrin.

It is abundantly clear from the discussion and
results described above that a multiplicity of gastrin

species exists both in serum and tissues. Furthermore, a variety of antibodies have been introduced and applied to the immunoassay detection and measurement of gastrin peptides. The molecular species of gastrin differ enormously in their immunoreactivity with the various antibody preparations to gastrin, and these differences are dictated in great part by the region of maximum specificity on the peptide for which the antibody is directed. The highly desired sorting out and clarification of relationships between immunologic and biologic activity will only be achieved through the careful separation, definition, and characterization of biologic activities of various gastrin peptide species and their immunologic activity with precisely defined species of antibodies to gastrin.

SUMMARY

A variety of molecular species of gastrin have been demonstrated in tissue extracts and in the circulation which include heptadecapeptide gastrin, big gastrin, big-big gastrin, and smaller molecular fragments of heptadecapeptide gastrin. Two principal methods for production of antibodies for radioimmunoassay of gastrin have been immunization of rabbits with human gastrin I (residues 2-17) and partially purified porcine gastrin, both of which techniques have produced antibodies sufficiently specific and sensitive for gastrin radioimmunoassay. Divergence between biologic activity of gastrin and radioimmunoassay of gastrin probably reflects differences in specificity of antibody preparation used in these radioimmunoassays. Antibodies to human gastrin I (2-17) exhibit limited, but measurable, cross-reactivity with cholecystokinin-pancreozymin but no immunoreactivity with the amino tridecapeptide of human gastrin I . Antibodies to the tetrapeptide amide of human gastrin I exhibit virtually equivalent immunologic reactivity with intact gastrin, the gastrin tetrapeptide, and cholecystokinin-pancreozymin. Antibodies with major specificity for the amino tridecapeptide of gastrin exhibit a high degree of immunologic reactivity with heptadecapeptide gastrin, but virtually no immunologic reactivity with big gastrin. The highly desired sorting out and clarification of relationships between immunologic and biologic activity of gastrin will be achieved only through careful separation, definition, and characterization of biologic activity of various gastrin peptide species with their immunologic re-activity to precisely defined species of antibodies to gastrin.

References

1. Agarwal KL, Grudzinski S, Kenner GW, Rogers NH, Sheppard RC, McGuigan JE: Immunochemical differentiation between gastrin and related peptide hormones through a novel conjugation of peptides to proteins. *Experientia* 27:514-515, 1971.
2. Berson SA, Yalow RS: Nature of immunoreactive gastrin extracted from tissues of gastrointestinal tract. *Gastroenterology* 60:215-222, 1971.
3. Byrnes DJ, Lazarus L, Young JD: Effect of vagotomy on serum gastrin in patients with duodenal ulceration. *Australas Ann Med* 19:240-243, 1970.
4. Byrnes DJ, Lazarus L, Young JD: The many faces of gastrin. *Australas Ann Med* 19:380-381, 1970.
5. Byrnes DJ, Young JD, Chisholm DJ, Lazarus L: Serum gastrin in patients with peptic ulceration. *Brit Med J* 2:626-629, 1970.
6. Dockray GH, Walsh JH: Identification of a N-terminal fragment of heptadecapeptide gastrin in the serum of patients with Zollinger-Ellison syndrome (ZES), abstracted. *Gastroenterology* 66:874, 1974.
7. Gregory H, Hardy PM, Jones DS, Kenner GW, Sheppard RE: The antral hormone gastrin: Structure of gastrin. *Nature* 204:931-933, 1964.
8. Gregory RA, Tracy HJ: The constitution and properties of two gastrins extracted from hog antral mucosa. *Gut* 5:103-117, 1964.
9. Greider MH, McGuigan JE: Cellular localization of gastrin in the human pancreas. *Diabetes* 20:389-396, 1971.
10. Hansky J, Cain MD: Radioimmunoassay of gastrin in human serum. *Lancet* 2:1388-1390, 1969.
11. Hansky J, Soveny C, Korman MG: What is immunoreactive gastrin? Studies with two antisera, abstracted. *Gastroenterology* 64:740, 1973.
12. Herbst CA, McGuigan JE: Examination of gastrins in Zollinger-Ellison tumor extracts and sera, abstracted. *Gastroenterology* 64:743, 1973.

13. Korman MG, Hansky J, Scott PR: Serum gastrin in duodenal
        ulcer: III. Influence of vagotomy and pylorectomy.
        Gut 13:39-42, 1972.
14. Mutt V, Jorpes JE: Isolation of aspartyl-phenylalanine
        amide from cholecystokinin-pancreozymin. *Biochem
        Biophys Res Commun* 26:392-397, 1967.
15. McGuigan JE: Antibodies to the carboxyl-terminal tetra-
        peptide of gastrin. *Gastroenterology* 53:697-705, 1967.
16. McGuigan JE: Immunochemical studies with synthetic human
        gastrin. *Gastroenterology* 54:1005-1011, 1968.
17. McGuigan JE: Antibodies to the C-terminal tetrapeptide
        amide of gastrin: Assessment of antibody binding to
        cholecystokinin-pancreozymin. *Gastroenterology*
        54:1012-1017, 1968.
18. McGuigan JE: Studies of the immunochemical specificity of
        some antibodies to human gastrin I. *Gastroenterology*
        56:429-438, 1969.
19. McGuigan JE: Production and characterization of specific
        antibodies to gastrin with no cross-reactivity with
        cholecystokinin-pancreozymin. *Am J Med Sci* 260:139-
        149, 1970.
20. McGuigan JE, Herbst CA: Separate immunochemical measure-
        ments of heptadecapeptide and big gastrins by use of
        region-specific antibodies to gastrin, abstracted.
        Gastroenterology 66:854, 1974.
21. McGuigan JE, Thomas HF: Physiological and immunological
        studies with desamidogastrin. *Gastroenterology*
        62:553-558, 1972.
22. Rehfeld JF, Stadil F: Gel filtration studies on immuno-
        reactive gastrin in serum from Zollinger-Ellison
        patients. *Gut* 14:369-373, 1973.
23. Straus E, Yalow RS: Studies on the distribution and
        degradation of heptadecapeptide, big, and big big
        gastrin. *Gastroenterology* 66:936-943, 1974.
24. Temperley JM, Stagg BH: Bioassay and radioimmunoassay of
        plasma gastrin in a case of Zollinger-Ellison syndrome.
        Scand J Gastroent 6:735-738, 1971.
25. Walsh JH, Debas HT, Grossman MI: Pure natural human big
        gastrin: Biological activity and half life in dog,
        abstracted. *Gastroenterology* 64:873, 1973.
26. Yalow RS, Berson SA: Radioimmunoassay of gastrin.
        Gastroenterology 58:1-14, 1970.
27. Yalow RS, Berson SA: Size and charge distinctions between
        endogenous human plasma gastrin in peripheral blood
        and heptadecapeptide gastrins. *Gastroenterology*
        58:609-615, 1970.

28. Yalow RS, Berson SA: Further studies on the nature of
    immunoreactive gastrin in human plasma. *Gastroenter-
    ology* 60:203-214, 1971.
29. Yalow RS, Berson SA: And now, "big, big" gastrin. *Biochem
    Biophys Res Commun* 48:391-395, 1972.
30. Yalow RS, Wu N: Additional studies on the nature of big
    big gastrin. *Gastroenterology* 65:19-27, 1973.
31. Young JD, Byrnes DJ, Chisholm DJ, Griffiths FB, Lazarus L:
    Radioimmunoassay of gastrin in human serum using
    antiserum against pentagastrin. *J Nucl Med* 10:745-
    748, 1969.

DIFFERENTIAL DIAGNOSIS OF HYPERGASTRINEMIA

Eugene Straus and Rosalyn S. Yalow

Solomon A. Berson Research Laboratory,
Bronx Veterans Administration Hospital,
and Mt. Sinai School of Medicine, The
City University of New York, New York

Clinical application of gastrin radioimmunoassay
is principally directed to diagnosis of a gastrin-
secreting tumor. Basal gastrin levels have been reported to be greatly elevated in patients with the
Zollinger-Ellison syndrome (ZE),[10] whereas patients
with ordinary acid-peptic disease have generally been
reported to have basal gastrin concentrations that
are low[8] or within the normal range.[11,17,18] On the
basis of such an analysis, many investigators have
considered basal hypergastrinemia in the presence of
hyperchlorhydria to be diagnostic of ZE.[4,8,13,14,16,18]
The coexistence of hypergastrinemia and hyperchlorhydria, however, has been observed earlier in four
subjects who had no evidence of tumor.[3]

In the present study we describe a larger group of
patients with hypergastrinemic hyperchlorhydria whose
gastrin responses to a number of provocative stimuli
are different from those of patients with proven ZE.
We evaluate the usefulness of provocative stimuli in
differentiating this group we have considered to have
nontumorous hypergastrinemic hyperchlorhydria (NT-HH),
from the group with ZE when basal gastrin concentrations of both groups are within the same range.

In a series of 213 highly selected cases of clinical
acid-peptic disease studied in our laboratory, 48 were
proven to have ZE. More than a quarter of these ZE
patients had fasting gastrin concentrations less than
1.0 ng/ml and overlapped with those of a group of 30
patients who appear to have what we have termed nontumorous hypergastrinemic hyperchlorhydria (NT-HH),
presumably due to overactivity of the gastrin-secreting

Table 1. Gastrin concentrations and acid outputs in duodenal ulcer patients

Patient		Age	Sex	Gastrin (pg/ml) Basal	Acid Output (mEq/hr) BAO	MAO
Patients with basal gastrin <0.1 ng/ml						
1.	Mo	40	M	60	15.0	30.0
2.	De	56	M	39	10.2	38.4
3.	Mi	50	M	86	14.2	45.2
4.	El	33	M	51	5.5	28.0
5.	Ja	28	M	92	5.7	15.9
6.	Gr	35	M	50	16.2	44.0
7.	Di	39	M	62	3.1	17.4
8.	St	32	M	38	7.3	34.0
9.	Av	47	M	29	2.2	26.0
10.	Se	54	M	90	2.2	30.2
11.	La	36	M	71	13.8	59.6
12.	Ro	64	M	22	7.2	
13.	He	20	M	87	4.2	26.0
14.	Le	48	M	11	24.0	55.0
15.	Pi	50	M	82	2.1	14.8
16.	Go	21	M	42	8.6	40.0
17.	Du	46	M	31	22.0	40.0
18.	Ma	46	M	60	22.4	25.8
19.	Bu	49	M	40	3.8	39.9
20.	Gi	45	M	55	15.0	33.0
21.	Mr	11	M	28	6.2	25.3
22.	Th	39	M	10	6.8	28.0
23.	Me	45	M	60	24.0	48.0
24.	Hu	59	M	40	3.0	27.0
25.	Ca	30	M	33	7.9	72.2
26.	Sm	63	M	57	5.0	48.9
27.	Ki	39	M	10	13.2	31.0
28.	Mz	42	M	90	35.0	56.0
29.	Ni	41	M	89	13.7	47.7
30.	Fi	41	M	53	2.4	40.0
31.	Ro	27	M	48	21.2	22.5
32.	Db	23	M	70	22.0	23.8
33.	Os	47	M	33	18.9	15.7
34.	Ve	45	M	90	8.1	9.9
35.	Ca	51	M	30	6.7	34.7
Nontumorous hypergastrinemic hyperchlorhydria. Group A						
1.	Ro	38	M	204	8.5	33.5
2.	Ma	39	M	100	6.0	45.0
3.	Cy	62	M	105	8.0	26.0
4.	St	54	M	205	3.0	30.2
5.	Ri	50	M	115	8.0	35.0

Table 1, continued

Patient		Age	Sex	Gastrin (pg/ml) Basal	Acid Output (mEq/hr) BAO	MAO
6.	By	46	M	133	5.0	24.0
7.	Ed	50	M	185	5.0	25.0
8.	Wo	23	M	150	8.4	44.0
9.	Vi	23	M	138	7.5	20.0
10.	Ta	59	M	400	3.3	36.0
11.	Fl	54	M	143	8.0	29.7
12.	Go	64	M	150	10.0	79.8
13.	Ve	45	M	100	8.0	20.0
14.	Mu	27	M	163	8.0	32.0
15.	Co	56	F	1033	7.5	66.9
16.	Di	24	M	120	9.8	40.0
17.	Cl	36	M	370	5.5	65.0
Nontumorous hypergastrinemic hyperchlorhydria. Group B						
1.	Iv	51	M	105	20.0	20.0
2.	Ha	25	M	100	12.6	25.7
3.	Ma	42	M	100	18.0	20.4
4.	Ka	50	M	105	26.0	29.0

cells of the gastrointestinal mucosa (Fig. 1).
Patients with acid-peptic disease and basal gastrin
levels between 0.1 mg/ml and 1 ng/ml were defined
as having NT-HH on the basis of characteristic response to one or more provocative stimuli. The group
was further classified into two subgroups, A and B,
on the basis of acid studies (Table 1). Subgroup A
includes patients with BAO <10 mEq/hr. Subgroup B
includes those with BAO in excess of 12 mEq/hr. The
pattern of response to provocative stimulation in the
NT-HH patients is similar to that seen in normals and
in duodenal ulcer patients with basal gastrin levels
<0.1 ng/ml. This pattern of response is clearly dis-
tinguishable from that seen in ZE patients including,
most importantly, a group of eight ZE patients whose
basal gastrin levels were all below 0.6 ng/ml. In
this unusual group of ZE patients, selected because
they represent the diagnostic problem for which provocative testing is required, confirmation of the
diagnosis was obtained by surgical proof of tumor or
by the demonstration of persistence of elevated plasma
gastrin levels subsequent to total gastrectomy (Table
2). The failure to find tumor at the time of surgery

in seven of the eight patients reported here is probably due to their lower gastrin levels being associated with small and not easily detectable tumors.

The mean plasma gastrin concentrations in the fasting state (45±9 pg/ml) and after the three provocative
stimuli in normal subjects are shown in Figure 2. Standard test meal (STM) was performed as previously described.[15] Calcium challenge was performed according
to the method of Passaro and associates,[13] and secretin
response was measured in response to an intravenous
injection of a bolus of 4 units Boots secretin/kg body
weight. The maximal increase in plasma gastrin after
the STM was 120% and there was no significant response
to calcium or secretin injection.

Patients with duodenal ulcer, whose basal plasma
gastrin concentrations were below 0.1 ng/ml, demonstrated a pattern of response to the three stimuli
(Fig. 3) which was similar to that seen in normals
except that the mean maximal increase in plasma gastrin concentration after the STM was 190%, even
greater than in normals.

Gastrin concentrations in the basal state and after
the STM and calcium challenge for both subgroups of
the NT-HH patients are shown in Figure 4. In both

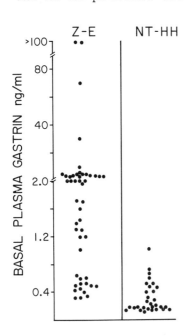

Figure 1. Basal plasma
gastrin concentrations in
patients with proven ZE
(left) and in nontumorous
NT-HH (right). Note the
breaks in scale.

Table 2. Gastrin concentrations and acid outputs in patients with Zollinger-Ellison syndrome in the basal state and following provocative stimuli

Patient		Age	Sex	Gastrin (pg/ml)					Acid Output (mEq/hr)		Tumor found at surgery
				Basal		Peak Concentrations					
				Preop	Post-total gastrectomy	STM*	Ca++	Secretin	BAO	BAO/MAO	
1.	Ha	39	M	550	--	1500	7000	30,000	74	1.0	yes
2.	McC	30	M	580	600	804	1573		30	0.9	no
3.	Wa	45	M	430	270	490			25	0.8	no
							†565				
4.	Wi	32	M	450	175	600		800	20	0.8	no
							†335				
5.	Ra	48	M	325	300	494	1400		35	0.9	no
6.	La	54	M	500	450	850	1129		35	0.6	no
7.	Co	65	M	550	550	610			§5	1.0	no
8.	Ht	55	M	525	400	550			56	0.8	no

* Standard test meal
† Post-total gastrectomy
§ Postsubtotal gastrectomy

Figure 2. Plasma gastrin concentrations in the fasting state and in response to three provocative stimuli in normal subjects.

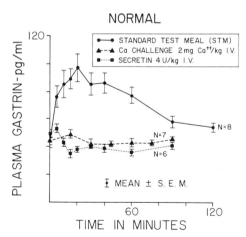

NORMAL

PLASMA GASTRIN-pg/ml

STANDARD TEST MEAL (STM)
Ca CHALLENGE 2mg Ca++/kg I.V.
SECRETIN 4 U/kg I.V.

N=8
N=7
N=6

⟂ MEAN ± S. E. M.

60   120
TIME IN MINUTES

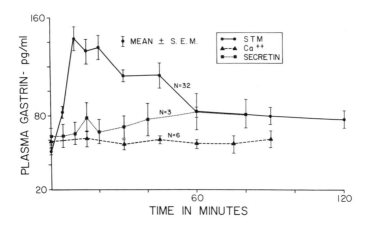

Figure 3. Plasma gastrin concentrations in the fasting state and in response to three provocative stimuli in patients with duodenal ulcer who had basal gastrin concentrations less than 0.1 mg/ml.

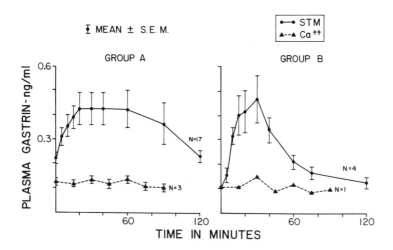

Figure 4. Plasma gastrin concentrations in the fasting state and in response to a test meal and a calcium challenge in non-tumorous (NT-HH) hypersecretors.

subgroups, as in normal subjects and ulcer patients with basal gastrin <0.1 ng/ml, there was no response of plasma gastrin to the calcium injection. The response to the STM was pronounced. In group B the mean increase was greater than 300%.

In contrast to the normal and NT-HH groups, ZE patients responded dramatically to the calcium challenge with a mean maximal increase in gastrin concentration of 350% (Fig. 5). However, the mean maximal increase in gastrin over the basal level following the STM was only 40%. This slight increase might be attributable to release of gastrointestinal gastrin, demonstrable because of the relatively low basal gastrin concentrations in this group.

In Figure 6 are shown the responses to the three provocative stimuli in two representative gastrin hypersecretors; one with ZE syndrome (Ha) and the other (Iv) from the NT-HH group. The ZE patient is hyper-responsive to calcium challenge and even more so to the secretin challenge. Calcium injection

Figure 5. Plasma gastrin concentrations in the fasting state and in response to a test meal and a calcium challenge in patients with proven ZE.

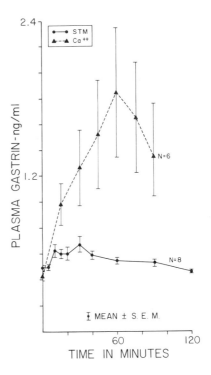

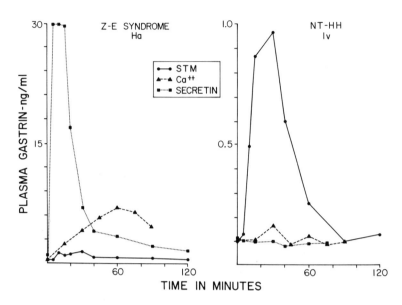

Figure 6. Plasma gastrin concentrations in the fasting state and in response to three provocative stimuli in gastrin hypersecretors; patient Ha (left) has ZE; subject IV (right) is in the nontumorous (NT–HH) group.

provoked a sustained increase from basal gastrin concentrations of 0.4 ng/ml to a peak of 7 ng/ml, 60 minutes after injection. Within five minutes after the secretin injection, gastrin levels increased dramatically to 30 ng/ml. The response to STM in this patient, although minor in comparison to the response to calcium and secretin, was the greatest we have seen in a ZE patient. In contrast, the plasma gastrin of NT-HH patient increased more than 850% following the STM, although he was not responsive to secretin or to calcium.

The effectiveness of secretin in stimulating the release of gastrin in ZE patients appears to be dose-dependent. In a single patient (Wi) the peak increase in gastrin after 1 unit Boots secretin/kg body weight was 65% and was more than twofold greater after the 4 unit/kg dose (Fig. 7). This patient's maximal increase in gastrin concentration (∿100%) after challenge with calcium was the smallest percentage response in our ZE group.

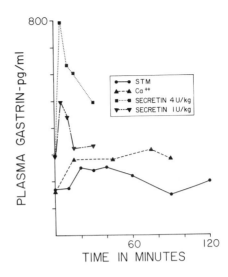

Figure 7. Plasma gastrin concentrations in the fasting state and in response to four provocative stimuli in patient Wi who has ZE.

In order to determine the effects of the various provocative agents on the release of gastrointestinal gastrin in the absence of acid feedback inhibition of gastrin, several patients with pernicious anemia were studied. The gastrin response to the STM in five patients was a prompt increase to a mean maximal value of 140% above basal levels, and to secretin in two patients was a slight though not significant decrease (Fig. 8). The single patient with pernicious anemia challenged with calcium responded with a 150% increase in gastrin.

As yet we have not seen a patient with proven ZE whose basal gastrin levels were below 0.1 ng/ml or an NT-HH patient with basal levels significantly in excess of 1 ng/ml. Basal gastrin concentrations in the range of 0.1 to 1 ng/ml are found in patients with either ZE or NT-HH and provocative tests of gastrin release are required for diagnostic discrimination between these groups. The hormonal form of the circulating gastrin must also be considered. Big gastrin (BG) has been shown to be the predominant circulating form in most gastrin hypersecretors[21] and plasma BG is about fivefold less biologically potent in terms of its stimulatory effect on acid secretion than heptadecapeptide gastrin (HG).[19] Therefore, since a plasma concentration of 40 pg HG/ml would be as potent as 200 pg BG/ml, it is possible that a ZE patient with a small tumor secreting primarily HG, might present immunoreactive

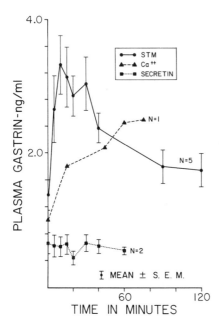

Figure 8. Plasma gastrin concentrations in the fasting state and in response to three provocative stimuli in patients with pernicious anemia.

plasma gastrin levels well within the normal range and pronounced hyperacidity. The provocative tests take advantage of the fact that the stimuli for gastrin release from tumor differ from those for release of gastrin from the gastrointestinal mucosa. Our data indicate that to more than double the plasma gastrin after a STM is evidence against the diagnosis of ZE. In agreement with other workers our data indicate that significant increase in plasma gastrin after calcium or secretin challenge, supports the diagnosis of ZE. The probability of making a valid preoperative diagnosis on the basis of laboratory testing can be expected to increase with the number of diagnostic procedures whose results are consistent with behavior appropriate to the diagnosis.

Preoperative diagnosis of gastrin-secreting tumor is certainly desirable and must frequently be established on physiologic grounds rather than on the basis of structural evidence. If the tumor is not found at surgery, the diagnosis may be confirmed physiologically by the persistence of hypergastrinemia after total gastrectomy. The lack of certainty in the diagnostic power of acid secretory studies[1,5,12,13,20] emphasizes the need for independent criteria based on gastrin radioimmunoassay. Many

patients whose plasma gastrin studies have been referred to our laboratory and who have been shown to
have hypergastrinemia and hyperchlorhydria have been
classified as NT-HH and have not come to surgery.
Generally conservative medical management has sufficed.
Nonetheless, only more prolonged follow-up can attest
to the accuracy of the diagnosis based on laboratory
testing.

Patients who have undergone Billroth II partial
gastrectomy and in whom postoperative basal hypergastrinemia requires a differentiation between ZE
and retained gastric antrum, also represent a diagnostic problem. We have studied two patients with
proven retained gastric antrum in whom elevated
basal gastrin levels fell to below normal levels
after removal of antral tissue. One patient responded to the STM and not to calcium, whereas the
other had the opposite response (Fig. 9). We
suggest that this difference in response might be
explained by hypothesizing that reflux of gastric
contents into the afferent loop took place in one
(Ba) but not in the other (Ma). If reflux were to
occur, there could be mucosal gastrin released by
feeding and feedback inhibition of gastrin secretion

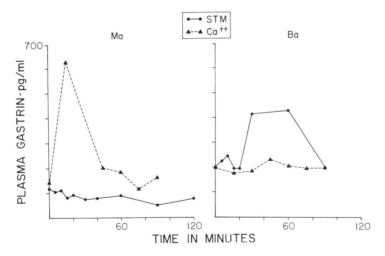

Figure 9. Plasma gastrin concentration in the fasting
state and in response to stimuli in two patients with
retained gastric antrum.

by acid after calcium injection. It was not possible
for us to study their responses to secretin but it
may well be that secretin would provide a better
provocative test for differentiating between retained
antrum and ZE,[7] since secretin does not release
gastrointestinal gastrin.

We have recently demonstrated hypersecretion of
gastrin in association with the short bowel syndrome.[15]
In four consecutive patients with this syndrome, which
is frequently complicated by acid peptic disease, both
fasting gastrin concentrations and integrated gastrin
responses to a test meal were greatly elevated (Fig.10).

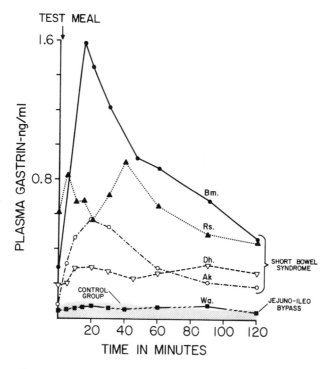

Figure 10. Plasma gastrin concentrations in the fasting state
and in response to a test meal in four patients with short
bowel syndrome, and in one patient with a jejunoileal bypass.
The mean value for the eight control subjects is shown in
the stippled area.   (Reproduced, with permission of
Gastroenterology.[15])

In an additional five patients with short bowel syndrome, basal gastrin concentrations were elevated and ranged from 100 to 400 pg/ml. Some workers have suggested that the small intestine is a major site of gastrin catabolism[2] and that the hypergastrinemia in short bowel syndrome may be due to diminished catabolism. Hypergastrinemia due to diminished catabolism can occur in renal failure[6] and in anephric patients.[9] But consideration of the absolute concentrations of gastrin reached in the fasting and peak-stimulated state, and the time course of appearance and disappearance of plasma gastrin (Fig. 10) unequivocally militate against the hypothesis of a significant role for decreased catabolism in short bowel syndrome. Assuming that the gastrin secretory rates remained unchanged, then the degradation rates would have had to decrease by a factor of three to almost 20 to account for the observed hypergastrinemia. A decreased degradation rate would result in a delay both in achieving the peak gastrin concentration and in the rate of return towards basal levels. Yet the peak gastrin concentrations were achieved at the same time as in the control group and the subsequent fall-off appeared even more rapid. We have speculated that the hypergastrinemia demonstrated in these short bowel patients may be due to the absence of some factor in the small intestine that may play a role in inhibiting gastrin release.

Hypergastrinemia in patients with acid peptic disease can be due to hypersecretion of gastrin from tumor (ZE) or gastrointestinal sources (NT-HH or short bowel syndrome) or to diminished gastrin catabolism (renal disease). Provocative testing is of value in discriminating among these groups.

SUMMARY

The presence of hypergastrinemia and hyperchlorhydria was documented in a group of 21 duodenal ulcer patients whose responses to one or more provocative stimuli clearly distinguish them from patients with proven Zollinger-Ellison syndrome (ZE). Patients in the former group, with basal gastrin levels as high as 1 ng/ml, are defined as having nontumorous hypergastrinemic hyperchlorhydria (NT-HH). Patients with NT-HH had a greater than normal increase of plasma

gastrin levels in response to a meal and no significant response to injections of calcium or secretin.
ZE patients with basal gastrin levels within the same
range were hyper-responsive to injections of secretin
and calcium but had little response to the test meal.
Because the clinical management of patients with ZE
differs from that of patients with NT-HH, diagnostic
differentiation between these two groups is necessary.
When basal gastrin concentrations are less than 1
ng/ml, responses to provocative stimuli provide the
basis for differentiation.

Acknowledgments

This work is supported in part by Mt. Sinai Genetics Center
Grant GM 19-443.

References

1. Aoyagi T, Summerskill WHJ: Gastric secretion with ulcero-
       genic islet cell tumor. Importance of basal acid
       output. *Arch Intern Med* 117:667-672, 1966.
2. Becker HD, Reeder DD, Thompson JC: Extraction of circula-
       ting endogenous gastrin by the small bowel. *Gastro-
       enterology* 65:903-906, 1973.
3. Berson SA, Yalow RS: Radioimmunoassay in gastroenterology.
       Gastroenterology 62:1061-1084, 1972.
4. Isenberg JI, Walsh JH, Passaro E Jr, Moore EW, Grossman MI:
       Unusual effect of secretin on serum gastrin, serum
       calcium, and gastric acid secretion in a patient with
       suspected Zollinger-Ellison syndrome. *Gastroenterology*
       62:626-631, 1972.
5. Kaye MD, Rhodes J, Beck P: Gastric secretion in duodenal
       ulcer, with particular reference to the diagnosis of
       Zollinger-Ellison syndrome. *Gastroenterology* 58:476-
       481, 1970.
6. Korman MG, Laver MC, Hansky J: Hypergastrinemia in chronic
       renal failure. *Br Med J* 1:209-210, 1972.
7. Korman MG, Scott DF, Hansky J, Wilson H: Hypergastrinemia
       due to an excluded gastric antrum: A proposed method
       for differentiation from the Zollinger-Ellison syndrome.
       Aust NZ J Med 2:266-271, 1972.
8. Korman MG, Soveny C, Hansky J: Serum gastrin in duodenal
       ulcer. *Gut* 12:899-902, 1971.

9. Maxwell JG, Moore JG, Dixon J, Stevens LE: Gastrin levels in anephric patients. *Surg Forum* 22:305-306, 1971.

10. McGuigan JE, Trudeau WL: Immunochemical measurement of elevated levels of gastrin in the serum of patients with pancreatic tumors of the Zollinger-Ellison variety. *N Engl J Med* 278:1308-1313, 1968.

11. McGuigan JE, Trudeau WL: Differences in rates of gastrin release in normal persons and patients with duodenal-ulcer disease. *N Engl J Med* 288:64-66, 1973.

12. Passaro E Jr, Basso N, Sanchez RE, Gordon HE: Newer studies in the Zollinger-Ellison syndrome. *Am J Surg* 120:138-143, 1970.

13. Passaro E Jr, Basso N, Walsh JH: Calcium challenge in the Zollinger-Ellison syndrome. *Surgery* 72:60-67, 1972.

14. Polak JM, Stagg B, Pearse AGE: Two types of Zollinger-Ellison syndrome: Immunofluorescent, cytochemical and ultrastructural studies of the antral and pancreatic gastrin cells in different clinical states. *Gut* 13:501-512, 1972.

15. Straus E, Gerson CD, Yalow RS: Hypersecretion of gastrin associated with the short bowel syndrome. *Gastroenterology* 66:175-180, 1974.

16. Thompson JC, Reeder DD, Bunchman HH: Clinical role of serum gastrin measurements in the Zollinger-Ellison syndrome. *Am J Surg* 124:250-261, 1972.

17. Trudeau WL, McGuigan JE: Serum gastrin levels in patients with peptic ulcer disease. *Gastroenterology* 59:6-12, 1970.

18. Trudeau WL, McGuigan JE: Relations between serum gastrin levels and rates of gastric hydrochloric acid secretion. *N Engl J Med* 284:408-412, 1971.

19. Walsh JH, Debas HT, Grossman MI: Pure human big gastrin: Immunochemical properties, disappearance half-time and acid-stimulating action in dogs. *J Clin Invest* 54:477-485, 1974.

20. Winship DH, Ellison EH: Variability of gastric secretion in patients with and without the Zollinger-Ellison syndrome. *Lancet* 1:1128-1130, 1967.

21. Yalow RS, Berson SA: Further studies on the nature of immunoreactive gastrin in human plasma. *Gastroenterology* 60:203-214, 1971.

SERUM GASTRIN IN CHRONIC RENAL FAILURE

J. Hansky, R.W. King, S. Holdsworth

Monash University, Department of Medicine
and Renal Unit, Prince Henry's Hospital,
Melbourne, Australia

Although other sites have been implicated in the metabolic breakdown or excretion of gastrin,[5,9,10] the kidney is thought to have a major role in this process.[1,2,7] Indeed, Newton and Jaffe[7] first suggested that metabolic degradation of radioiodinated gastrin I occurred in the renal cortex and Clendinnen and associates[1] showed that renal uptake of injected gastrin was 40% and that bilateral nephrectomy in dogs resulted in an elevation of serum gastrin levels. These studies were soon followed by reports which suggested that serum gastrin levels were increased in patients with chronic renal failure[4] and in anephric patients.[6] The latter group also measured postcibal gastrin values in anephric patients and reported no increment in gastrin following a meal.

In view of the above studies it was considered that the kidney is a major site of gastrin breakdown and that the hypergastrinemia of chronic renal failure was due to defective breakdown of gastrin with prolongation of its half-life.

We have studied immunoreactive gastrin in chronic renal failure from the following aspects:

1. Fasting levels in relationship to other parameters of renal function.
2. Measurement of postcibal responses to ascertain whether there is increased production of gastrin.
3. Response of serum gastrin to secretin injection.
4. Determination of the molecular species of gastrin in chronic renal failure (CRF).

5. The effect of hemodialysis on gastrin
    levels in CRF.
6. The effect of renal transplantation
    on serum gastrin and whether serum
    gastrin levels can predict transplant
    rejection.
7. Whether the hypergastrinemia is re-
    lated to the reported increased inci-
    dence of duodenal ulcer in chronic
    renal failure.

These studies were performed in patients from the
renal unit at Prince Henry's Hospital and informed
consent was obtained from all patients studied.
Immunoreactive gastrin was measured by radioimmunoassay with use of antibodies to synthetic human
gastrin I (1-17) designated AS4 at a final dilution
of 1:25,000.

The relationship between fasting serum gastrin and
plasma creatinine in 89 patients with renal failure
is shown in Figure 1. The differences in serum
gastrin of patients with severe renal failure
(creatinine >3 mg/100 ml) and mild renal failure
(creatinine <3 mg/100 ml), are significant at $p < 0.025$.
These results indicate that serum gastrin levels are
significantly raised in patients with severe chronic
renal failure and that there is a relationship between the gastrin level and the degree of renal
failure.

To determine whether there is an increased gastrin-
secreting cell (G-cell) mass in patients with chronic
renal failure, the serum gastrin response to a standard protein-bicarbonate meal was assessed. Figure 2

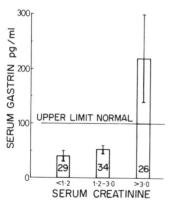

Figure 1. Serum gastrin in
relation to serum creatinine
in patients with chronic renal
failure. Numbers in the
columns refer to number of
patients and all values shown
as mean ± SEM.

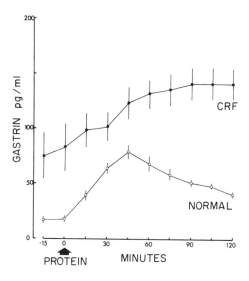

Figure 2. Serum gastrin response to protein meal in six patients with chronic renal failure and 10 normal subjects. All values mean ± SEM.

compares the response in six patients with CRF to that in normal subjects. The amount of gastrin released is not significantly different in the two groups, which suggests that the G-cell mass in CRF is not increased, or alternatively that its release is depressed. Not only is the G-cell mass "normal" but the peak occurs later (75 minutes in CRF compared with 45 minutes in normals) and the response is prolonged. This indicates slower release and defective excretion of the released gastrin.

It has been shown that the intravenous injection of secretin will cause a decrease in serum gastrin in normal subjects or in the hypergastrinemia due to pernicious anemia, antral hyperplasia, or retained excluded antrum. By contrast, such an injection will result in no alteration in serum gastrin or a significant rise in patients with gastrinoma. The mechanism of the decrease in gastrin in normals is unknown, but may be due to either an inhibition of gastrin release or promotion of its excretion.

We have studied the effect of secretin on basal serum gastrin in a small number of patients with chronic renal failure. The fasting patient was given 2 U/kg body weight of secretin intravenously as a bolus injection and blood collected at -15, 0, 5, 10, 15, 30, 45 and 60 minutes after injection. Five patients had elevated basal gastrin and four patients had a normal basal gastrin at the time of study, and the results are shown in Figure 3. In

117

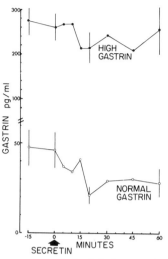

Figure 3. Serum gastrin response to secretin injection (2 U/kg body weight) in patients with chronic renal failure with high and normal fasting gastrin. All values mean ± SEM. Note change in scale on vertical axis.

the group with high gastrin, there is a fall in serum gastrin towards the end of the study period, but this is not significant. In the group with normal fasting gastrin levels, the fall occurs earlier and is significant. These results suggest that the presence of renal failure modifies the response to secretin and may indicate that the fall in gastrin observed in normals is partially due to a promotion of its renal excretion, but defective inhibition of its release cannot be excluded as a mechanism.

Yalow[11] has shown that multiple molecular forms of immunoreactive gastrin are found in plasma and that the relative proportions of the different molecular forms differ widely under different physiologic conditions. Fractionation of the serum of one patient with uremia on Sephadex G50 showed that the gastrin was big (G-34) gastrin. We have fractionated serum from patients with chronic renal failure on Sephadex G50 superfine columns 100x1.6 cm, eluted with 0.02 M veronal buffer pH 8.6 and collected in 2-ml aliquots. Sera studied were fasting, postcibal, and after incubation with trypsin. Figure 4 shows basal serum gastrin thus fractionated. The bulk of gastrin immunoreactivity is in the big or G-34 fraction with less than 10% as the heptadecapeptide. Prior trypsinization shows that this is all converted to heptadecapeptide gastrin but there is a peak in the region of minigastrin (Fig. 5). Postcibal gastrin is also predominantly big (or G-34) gastrin (Fig. 6). Thus, unlike normal subjects or patients with duodenal ulcer

118

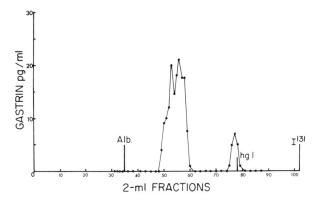

Figure 4. Elution pattern of 1 ml fasting serum
from patient with CRF, showing immunoreactive gastrin
on the ordinate and 2-ml fractions on the abscissa.
Albumin (Alb) and iodide (I^{131}) show void value and
salt peak and position of human gastrin I (HgI) is
also shown. Column is 100 × 1.6 cm Sephadex G50
superfine.

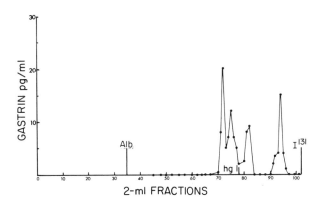

Figure 5. Elution pattern of 1 ml fasting serum
from patient with CRF after incubation with trypsin.
Same column as in Figure 4.

119

whose fasting serum immunoreactive gastrin is the big-
big variety which elutes in the void volume, patients
with CRF have predominantly big (G-34) gastrin. They
therefore have an elution pattern similar to patients
with gastrinoma or pernicious anemia. The significance
of this is not apparent but one possible explanation
is that the kidney degrades only big gastrin.

*THE EFFECT OF HEMODIALYSIS AND RENAL TRANSPLANTATION
ON SERUM GASTRIN*

Although we originally suggested that hemodialysis
does not significantly alter fasting serum gastrin
levels in patients with CRF, a study in a larger
group of patients shows that serum gastrin falls with
hemodialysis. Successful renal transplantation is
associated with a more pronounced decrease in serum
gastrin to levels found in normal subjects (Fig. 7).
We have followed daily fasting serum gastrin levels
in patients after renal transplantation and consider
that the gastrin level is a sensitive index of return
of renal function.
Figures 8 and 9 show the daily serum gastrin and
creatinine in two subjects before and after transplantation. In Figure 8, transplantation was successful and the creatinine and gastrin levels decreased

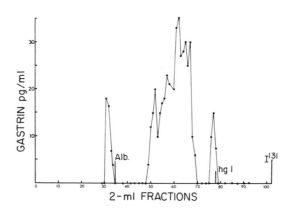

Figure 6. Elution pattern of 1-ml postcibal
serum after protein meal in patient with CRF
taken 90 minutes after ingestion. Same
column as in Figure 4.

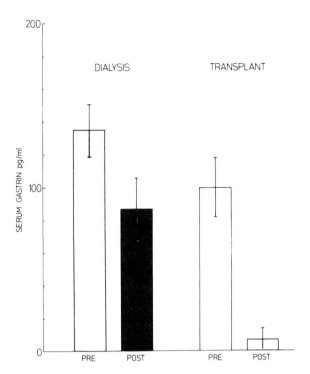

Figure 7. Serum gastrin (mean ± SEM) before
and after hemodialysis and renal transplantation.

Figure 8. Serum crea-
tinine (C) and serum
gastrin (G) in a pa-
tient with chronic
renal failure after
successful renal
transplantation. Hori-
zontal lines mark
normal values for
gastrin (—) and
creatinine (---).

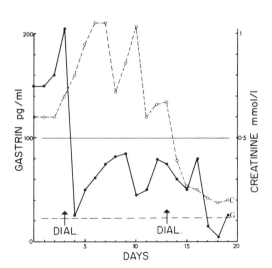

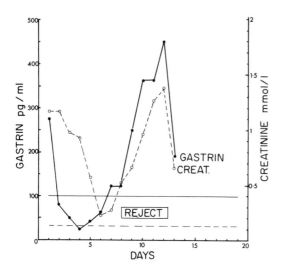

Figure 9. Serum creatinine (C) and serum gastrin (G) in a patient with chronic renal failure after renal transplantation showing effect of episode of transplant rejection. Horizontal lines indicate normal values as in Figure 8.

to normal. By contrast, in Figure 9, although the serum gastrin decreased initially, an increase was associated with a rejection episode, which was finally overcome by immunosuppressive therapy with a decrease in gastrin to normal.

Finally we have to consider the role of this hypergastrinemia in relationship to the reported increased incidence of duodenal ulcer in chronic renal failure. Controversy exists as to the frequency of duodenal ulcer and the levels of basal and stimulated gastric acid secretion in chronic renal failure. Gingell and associates[3] reported that in 45 patients with chronic uremia, both basal acid output and maximal acid output were normal and that after renal transplantation, two of seven patients developed duodenal ulceration and showed a considerable increase in acid output. By contrast, Shepherd and associates[8] reported high overnight acid secretion and a 53% incidence of duodenal ulcer in 15 patients with chronic renal failure on maintenance hemodialysis. We have found no clear correlation between acid secretion and serum gastrin levels in our patients with chronic renal failure and the incidence of duodenal ulcer is not higher than in control populations. Shepherd and associates[8] also showed that secretin injection caused a profound decrease in basal acid output in their group of patients. These results taken in conjunction with our demonstration of no significant change in basal serum

122

gastrin after secretin injection, would indicate that the hypergastrinemia of CRF is not responsible for any duodenal ulcer or increase in acid secretion seen in this disease. Indeed the demonstration that gastrin decreases significantly after renal transplantation would suggest that duodenal ulcer seen after transplantation may be due to steroids, immunosuppressive therapy, or the stress of surgery.

SUMMARY

These studies have indicated that renal inactivation of gastrin is an important mechanism for its degradation, that elevated levels in chronic renal failure are due to defective degradation rather than increased production and that the response of serum gastrin to secretin injection is abnormal. Like patients with gastrinoma and pernicious anemia, the molecular species of gastrin is BG (G-34) and this is convertible to G-17 or smaller fragments with trypsinization of the serum. Elevated levels of serum gastrin can be decreased by hemodialysis and renal transplantation and the serum gastrin is a sensitive index of successful (or failed) renal transplantation.

References

1. Clendinnen BG, Davidson WD, Reeder DD, Jackson BM, Thompson JC: Renal uptake and excretion of gastrin in the dog. *Surg Gynecol Obstet* 132:1039-1043, 1971.
2. Davidson WD, Springberg PD: Renal extraction of endogenous gastrin in the dog, abstracted. *Clin Res* 20:181, 1972.
3. Gingell JC, Burns GP, Chisholm GD: Gastric acid secretion in chronic uremia and after renal transplantation. *Br Med J* 4:424-426, 1968.
4. Korman MG, Laver MC, Hansky J: Hypergastrinaemia in chronic renal failure. *Br Med J* 1:209-210, 1972.
5. Korman MG, Hansky J, Ritchie B, Watts J McK Maloney JE: Disappearance of gastrin across the lung. *Aust J Exp Biol Med Sci* 51:679-687, 1973.
6. Maxwell JG, Moore JG, Dixon J, Stevens LE: Gastrin levels in anephric patients. *Surg Forum* 22:305-306, 1971.
7. Newton WT, Jaffe BM: The fate of intravenously administered radiolabeled gastrin. *Surgery* 69:34-40, 1971.

8. Shepherd AMM, Stewart WK, Wormsley KG: Peptic ulceration
    in chronic renal failure. *Lancet* 1:1357–1359, 1973.
9. Temperley JM, Stagg BH, Wyllie JH: Disappearance of gastrin
    and pentagastrin in the portal circulation. *Gut*
    12:372–376, 1971.
10. Thompson JC, Reeder DD, Davidson WD, Charters AC, Brückner
    WL, Lemmi CAE, Miller JH: Effect of hepatic transit of
    gastrin, pentagastrin and histamine measured by gastric
    secretion and by assay of hepatic vein blood. *Ann Surg*
    170:493–503, 1969.
11. Yalow RS: Gastrins: Small, big and big-big, in Chey WY,
    Brooks FP (eds), *Endocrinology of the Gut*, Thorofare,
    NJ: Charles B. Slack Inc., 1974, pp 261–276.

PATTERNS OF RELEASE AND UPTAKE OF HETEROGENEOUS FORMS OF GASTRIN

James C. Thompson, Phillip L. Rayford,
N. Ian Ramus, H. Roberts Fender,
Hugo V. Villar

Department of Surgery, The University of Texas
Medical Branch, Galveston, Texas

The duration of the physiologic effects of gastrin are brief, which suggests that there are efficient mechanisms for catabolism of gastrin. We have shown that the half-life of exogenously infused heptadeca-peptide gastrin is 2.1 minutes,[25] and Yalow and Berson[35] demonstrated a disappearance half-time for endogenous plasma gastrin in pernicious anemia patients (after antral acidification) of seven minutes. We have previously shown that the kidney is a major site for the deactivation or uptake of exogenous[4,5] and endogenous[3] gastrin. Endogenous gastrin is apparently not extracted by the liver,[24] but there is evidence that it is extracted or inactivated by the small bowel[1] and the secreting gastric fundus.[13]

The early concept of a single circulating form of gastrin, which now seems almost naively idyllic, was changed when Yalow and Berson demonstrated a larger form of gastrin in circulation[36,37] and in gastro-intestinal mucosa.[2] The larger form, called big gastrin, was found to be much more basic than hepta-decapeptide gastrin (G-17); Gregory and Tracy[17] showed that the big form contained G-17 as a C-terminal sequence and they later demonstrated that big gastrin has 34 amino acids and a molecular weight of about 3870.[18] Big gastrin (BG) has been shown to have a disappearance half-time of 15 minutes.[32] BG produces a higher plateau of serum gastrin concentration than does G-17 for each molecular weight infused, but the molar potency of G-17 was much greater than that of BG.[32]

The concept has been made more complex by the report of Yalow and colleagues[38],[39] of a big-big gastrin with a molecular weight at least five times that of big gastrin and a disappearance half-time of about 90 minutes.[30]

The end is not in sight. Rehfeld and associates[26-28] have reported at least two more immunoreactive gastrin components in human serum. One, which Rehfeld has designated Component I, is larger than big gastrin (presumably not as large as big-big gastrin); another, minigastrin, has been shown subsequently to be gastrin 5-17.[16] The disappearance half-time of minigastrin has been shown to be 1.8 minutes.[9]

The great heterogeneity of circulating forms of gastrin and the suggestion that each has a separate rate of catabolism and separate molecular potency (which suggestions have been partially demonstrated), is evidence that in any study on the metabolism of endogenous gastrin, the relative concentrations of the various molecular components must be determined and we must be alert to the possibility that the various forms are treated in a differential fashion. Specifically, in studies on the catabolism or uptake of gastrin by individual organs, it is necessary to determine the uptake of each of the various molecular forms of gastrin.[30]

In the present study, we have determined the disappearance half-time of endogenous, that is, mixed molecular gastrin, we have measured uptake of gastrin by individual organs, and we have attempted to study the patterns of the various molecular forms of gastrin exhibited during gastrin release and during uptake by the kidney.

MATERIALS AND METHODS

Eleven adult healthy mongrel dogs weighing between 17 and 28 kg were used in the studies. Operative procedures and acute experimental procedures were performed with the dogs anesthetized with intravenous pentobarbital. After the experiments, the dogs were killed.

Disappearance Half-time of Endogenous Gastrin

In five dogs, isolated antral pouches were constructed by creating a double mucosal barrier at the antrofundic junction and by ligating the pylorus about a catheter that had been introduced into the antrum via a stab wound in the duodenum. The catheter was brought through the abdominal wall and a gastric fistula was made. The vessels providing blood supply on the greater and lesser curvature of the antrum were carefully mobilized and polyethylene chokers were placed loosely about the entire vascular pedicle on both the greater and lesser curvatures. Experiments were conducted 72 hours later with the dogs awake and alert. Release of gastrin was stimulated by irrigating the pouch with 0.5% acetylcholine solution. Blood samples were obtained from the peripheral vein before and at regular intervals after initiation of antral irrigation with acetylcholine. After 60 minutes of antral stimulation, the chokers were tightened simultaneously to occlude the arterial and venous supply of the antrum. Peripheral blood samples were obtained at frequent intervals after occlusion.

Organ Catabolism of Gastrin and Molecular Patterns of Gastrin During Release, Renal Transit, and Acid Suppression

Six dogs were prepared as diagrammed in Figure 1. The gastric antrum was isolated by placing a clamp across the antrofundic junction and by ligating the pylorus about a catheter introduced via the duodenum. Catheters were placed into the common bile duct and the right ureter, which were ligated distal to the point of catheterization. Catheters for blood sampling were placed into the aorta, mesenteric vein, portal vein, hepatic vein,[29] right renal vein, and jugular vein (which was used to sample peripheral blood). Noncannulating electromagnetic flow probes of appropriate size were placed about the hepatic artery, portal vein, and right renal artery. Blood flow in these vessels was measured with a simultaneous two-channel square-wave electromagnetic flowmeter (Carolina Medical Electronics Inc., Winston-Salem, N.C.). The masses of gastrin entering and

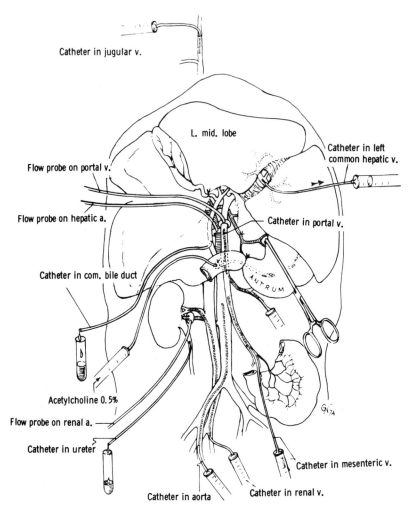

Catheter in jugular v.

L. mid. lobe

Catheter in left
common hepatic v.

Flow probe on portal v.

Flow probe on hepatic a.

Catheter in portal v.

Catheter in com. bile duct

ANTRUM

Acetylcholine 0.5%

Flow probe on renal a.

Catheter in ureter

GN₇₄

Catheter in mesenteric v.

Catheter in aorta

Catheter in renal v.

Figure 1. Experimental preparation for: 1) determining the effect of transit of liver, kidney, small bowel and head on total immunoreactive concentrations of gastrin, and 2) determining the patterns of the different molecular forms of gastrin during basal period, periods of antral stimulation and antral suppression. Catheters were placed into aorta, renal vein, mesenteric vein, portal vein, common hepatic vein, jugular vein, common bile duct, ureter and excluded gastric antrum. Noncannulating flow probes of appropriate sizes were placed around the hepatic artery, portal vein, and renal artery.

leaving the liver were calculated by use of a standard formula.[24] Blood flow determinations were made five minutes before blood samples were obtained, which was near the end of each 40-minute period. Blood flow was reduced to zero by occluding the vessel with a vascular clamp.

The study was divided into three 40-minute periods. Bile and urine were collected during each period. At the end of each of the three periods, 25-ml blood samples were obtained simultaneously from each vascular catheter. After the initial basal period, the antrum was continuously irrigated for 40 minutes with 0.5% acetylcholine solution to stimulate the release of endogenous gastrin. After that, the antrum was irrigated continuously for 40 minutes with 0.1 N HCl. Blood specimens were centrifuged immediately and the serum was frozen. Aliquots were taken later for radioimmunoassay and 5-ml samples of serum from each specimen were applied later to G50 Sephadex superfine columns for gel filtration.

Chromatographic Fractionation Procedure

Serum samples were applied to a Sephadex G50 superfine column measuring 1.5 x 102 cm. Fractionation was carried out at 15C and the columns were eluted with 0.2 M sodium phosphate solution at pH 7.5 containing 0.15 M NaCl and 1% sodium azide. The columns were equilibrated with blue dextran, radioiodinated growth hormone (^{125}I HGH), radioiodinated cholecystokinin (^{125}I CCK), and radioiodinated synthetic human heptadecapeptide gastrin I (^{125}I SHG-17). Fractions of 2 ml were collected and counted in a gamma spectrometer (Picker). The chromatographic pattern of the various marker substances is illustrated in Figure 2. Five separate columns were used in random sequence.

In test studies of serum, 5 ml of serum were applied to the column and eluted. Two-milliliter fractions were collected and the immunoreactive gastrin in 500 μl of each eluate was determined by radioimmunoassay. Gastrin immunoreactivity was arbitrarily assigned to different gastrin molecular components according to the fraction in which it was eluted from the column. That is, fractions appearing in the void volume, marked by blue dextran and by ^{125}I HGH, were designated as big-big gastrin (BBG); fractions

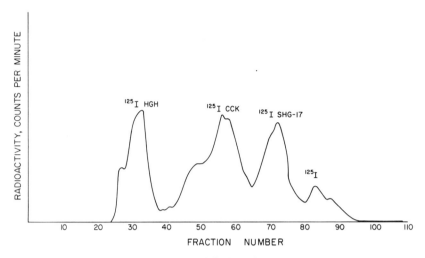

Figure 2. Elution patterns of ^{125}I, ^{125}I synthetic human gastrin 17, ^{125}I porcine cholecystokinin and ^{125}I human growth hormone from a 1.5 x 102 cm column of superfine Sephadex G50.

appearing in the area between the void volume and the ^{125}I CCK peak were designated as Rehfeld's Component I (Comp I); fractions appearing in the ^{125}I CCK peak were designated as big gastrin (BG); fractions appearing in the area of the ^{125}I SHG-17 peak were designated as heptadecapeptide gastrin (G-17); and fractions appearing between the ^{125}I SHG-17 peak and the iodide (^{125}I) peak were designated as mini-gastrin (MG). The five components thus appear in a sequence similar to that used in a schematic elution diagram composed by Walsh.[33]

Radioimmunoassay of Gastrin

Gastrin was measured in either 300 µl of serum obtained before chromatography or 500 µl of each column fraction obtained by chromatography, by our radioimmunoassay technique (described elsewhere in detail[20,23]). Antibodies against gastrin were obtained in rabbits by using human synthetic gastrin 2-17, conjugated to bovine serum albumin. The assay uses the double antibody system described by Odell and associates.[22] G-17-1 is radioiodinated in the assay by means of the technique of Greenwood and associates.[15] The antiserum used (UT-55) has been characterized; it recognizes all known molecular forms of gastrin (Walsh, personal communication). Gastrin concentrations were calculated as picograms per milliliter (pg/ml) of serum or total picograms of gastrin immunoreactivity in each column fraction.

Student's "t" test for paired samples was used to determine the significance of differences between means. Differences with *p* values of less than 0.05 were considered significant.

RESULTS

Disappearance Half-time of Endogenous Gastrin

Basal gastrin values were 100 pg/ml. Gastrin concentration rose to a plateau of 300 pg/ml during antral irrigation with acetylcholine. After the chokers were tightened, levels fell precipitously, and near baseline concentrations were obtained about one hour later (Fig. 3).

Disappearance half-time was calculated by the method of Walsh and associates.[32] After subtraction of basal gastrin values, all individual values were converted to the natural logarithm. The regression of the natural logarithm of the serum gastrin value versus time, was computed to yield a slope in which the half-life was determined by dividing into 0.693 (the natural logarithm of 2). The calculated half-life for endogenous gastrin by this method was 8.6 minutes (Fig. 4).

Catabolism of Total Immunoreactive Serum Gastrin by Various Organs

Average serum concentrations of total immunoreactive gastrin in specimens taken from six different vessels in six dogs during the basal period, during the period of antral stimulation with local acetylcholine solution, and during the period of antral suppression with irrigation of 0.1 N hydrochloric acid are shown in Figure 5. The basal concentration of gastrin in the aorta was 87±12 pg/ml. Gastrin concentration increased to 195±26 pg/ml during antral stimulation and decreased to 78±10 pg/ml during suppression of gastrin release by acidification of the antrum. There was no significant

difference in the concentration of gastrin among samples from the six vessels during either the basal or
the suppressed periods. During antral stimulation,
however, there was a significant increase in gastrin
concentration in the portal vein (304±27 pg/ml) and
the hepatic vein (269±39 pg/ml), as compared to the
aorta (Table 1). The concentration in the renal vein
(RV) was 130±13 pg/ml, which was significantly less
than the concentration in the aorta and represented
an extraction of 30% of the gastrin presented to the
kidney. Gastrin appearing in the urine accounted
for less than 0.4% of that entering the kidney.

Gastrin concentration in the mesenteric vein (MV)
during the period of antral stimulation was 185±40
pg/ml, which provides no evidence of uptake of
gastrin by the small bowel. If the data from dog I

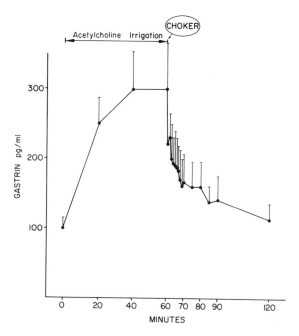

Figure 3. Serum gastrin concentrations during a
basal period, during a period of antral irrigation
with 0.5% acetylcholine solution, and after instan-
taneous occlusion of the antral blood supply by
chokers. Mean values from five dogs.

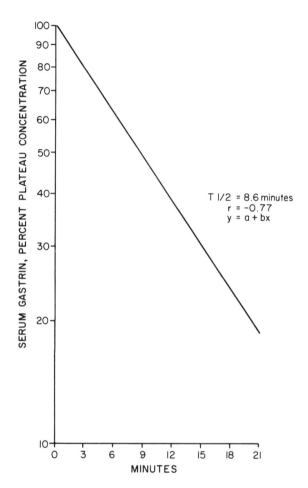

Figure 4. Linear regression analysis of disappearance half-time utilizing data from Figure 3, with basal levels subtracted, converted to natural logarithm.

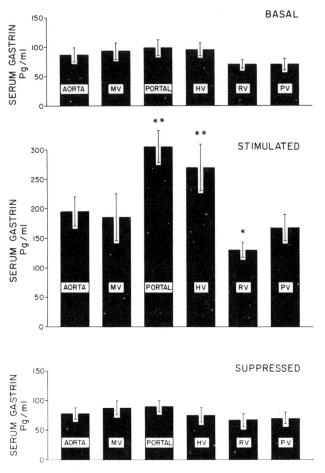

Figure 5. Total immunoreactive concentrations of serum
gastrin in samples obtained from six vascular catheters
during the basal period, during period of antral stimulation with 0.5% acetylcholine stimulation, and during
antral suppression with 0.1 HCl; mean values from six
dogs. There were no significant differences in the
concentrations of gastrin in samples obtained from any
site during either the basal period or the period of
antral suppression. During periods of stimulation,
concentrations of gastrin in the portal vein and in the
hepatic vein were significantly higher than in the
aorta (**). During the stimulated period, concentrations
of gastrin in the renal vein were significantly less
than in the aorta (*).

134

Table 1. Serum gastrin concentration, pg/ml, in samples from
six vessels during stimulated (antral irrigation
with 0.5% acetylcholine) state. All six specimens
were withdrawn exactly simultaneously.

Dog	Aorta	Mesenteric vein	Portal vein	Hepatic vein	Renal vein	Peripheral vein
I	269	378	336	364	107	192
II	204	169	314	247	166	151
III	250	165	388	400	164	266
IV	151	128	309	198	113	154
V	201	175	187	251	143	139
A	97	98	290	157	89	103
Mean	195	185	304*	269*	130*	167
S.E.	26	40	27	39	13	23

* denotes values which are significantly different ($p < 0.05$)
from the simultaneous concentration of serum gastrin in
the aorta

(Table 1) were removed from this group, however, a
dog in which the concentration of gastrin in the
mesenteric vein was much higher than in the aorta,
small bowel extraction of gastrin would equal about
20% of the gastrin presented to the small bowel.
The difference would be of borderline significance.

The hepatic clearance of gastrin was calculated by
determining the mass of gastrin entering the liver
and leaving the liver. Plasma flows in the hepatic
artery and portal vein were first calculated by mul-
tiplying the measured blood flow in each vessel ×
(1-hematocrit). The following quantities were
calculated by the formulas given below:[24]

1. Afferent hepatic plasma flow (AH_F),
    considered to be equal to efferent
    hepatic venous (HV_F) plasma flow:
    $AH_F = PV_F + HA_F = HV_F$.

2. Afferent hepatic plasma concentration
    of gastrin (AH_C):

$$AH_C = \frac{PV_C \cdot PV_F + HA_C \cdot HA_F}{HA_F + PV_F}$$

3. Afferent hepatic mass (AH_M) of gastrin
    per minute (picograms per minute):
    $AH_M = AH_C \cdot AH_F$.

135

    4.   Hepatic venous mass (HV_M), representing the mass of gastrin (picograms per minute) leaving the liver per minute:

$$HV_M = HV_F \cdot HV_C.$$

Blood flow measurements were not obtained in one dog because of equipment malfunction.

The mean of the plasma flows in the five remaining dogs (ml/min) in the hepatic artery (HA) and the portal vein (PV) are as follows: basal period, HA-98±11, PV-245±34; stimulated period, HA-96±22, PV-191±31; suppressed, HA-124±42, PV-188±37.

The mass of endogenous gastrin entering and leaving the liver was not significantly different during any of the three periods (Fig. 6). The mass of gastrin entering the liver increased from a basal level of

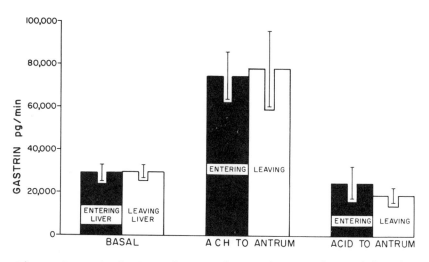

Figure 6. Calculation of mass of gastrin entering and leaving the liver in five dogs during basal period, during period of acetylcholine stimulation in the antrum, and during period of antral acidification. The amount of gastrin entering and leaving the liver rose significantly from basal during antral stimulation. There was no significant difference between the amount of gastrin entering and leaving the liver during any of the three periods.

29,000 pg/min to 75,000 pg/min during antral stimulation and decreased to 25,000 pg/min during antral acidification. Gastrin appearing in the bile amounted to less than 0.2% of the afferent hepatic mass of gastrin in each of the three periods.

Patterns of Molecular Forms of Gastrin During Antral Stimulation and After Transit of the Kidney

Gel filtration elution patterns were determined on all specimens from all dogs but we will present only a few individual samples of molecular patterns in the aorta and renal vein. Other data will be the basis for future communications.

A typical elution pattern taken from a portal vein sample during the period of acetylcholine stimulation of the antrum in dog I is shown in Figure 7. In this and subsequent figures, the fine-line graph depicts, from right to left on the ordinate, the measured radioactivity of first the ^{125}I peak and then the larger labeled G-17 peak. At about fraction 30 there is a small peak in the void volume found whenever labeled synthetic human gastrin was placed on the column; the significance of the peak is unknown. At the bottom of the figure are designated those fractions labeled big-big gastrin (BBG), Rehfeld's Component I (Comp I), big gastrin (BG), heptadecapeptide gastrin (G-17) and minigastrin (MG), corresponding to the areas of the labeled marker substances shown in Figure 2. The largest amount of immunoreactivity in Figure 7 is in the G-17 fraction.

Gel filtration elution patterns from aortic samples, taken from dog 1 during basal, stimulated and acid-suppressed periods, are shown in Figure 8. In the basal sample (Fig. 8A) the major component is big-big gastrin and there are only small peaks (which may be artifactual) in other areas. During antral stimulation, there was a great increase in big gastrin and especially in G-17 (Fig. 8B). The notched peak of G-17 presumably represents separation into sulfated and nonsulfated forms of G-17. After antral acidification (Fig. 8C) the relative amounts of big gastrin and G-17 have diminished and BBG is relatively larger. Several of the problems encountered during this aspect of the study, especially in samples obtained after antral acidification, are illustrated in Figure 8C.

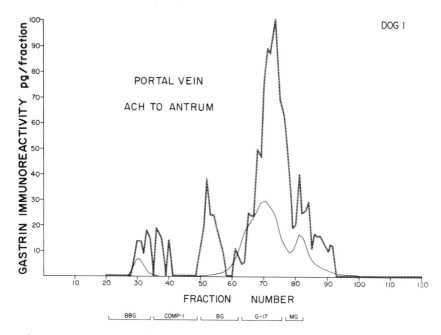

Figure 7. Typical elution pattern from the portal vein sample
of Dog I during period of acetylcholine stimulation of the antrum.
The fine-line graph on the ordinate depicts, from right to left,
the measured radioactivity of first the ^{125}I peak and then the
larger labeled G-17 peak. Gastrin immunoreactivity of eluate
fractions determined by gastrin radioimmunoassay. The fraction
labeled BBG (big-big gastrin), Comp-1 (Rehfeld's Component 1),
BG (big gastrin), G-17 (heptadecapeptide gastrin), and MG (minigastrin) are derived from markers in Figure 2. This figure
demonstrates that the major gastrin-like immunoreactivity in
the portal vein is in the G-17 fragment.

Figure 8. Elution pattern of gastrin immunoreactivity
in samples obtained from the aorta of Dog 1 during
basal period (8A), during stimulation of the antrum (8B),
and during suppression of the antrum (8C). Big-big
gastrin is an important component during basal periods
and periods of antral suppression. G-17 is again seen
to be the major component during periods of antral
stimulation.

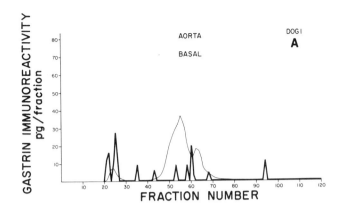

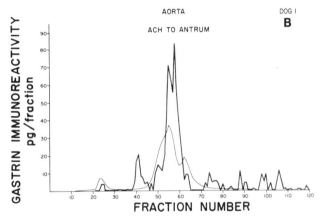

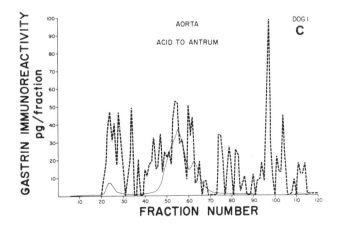

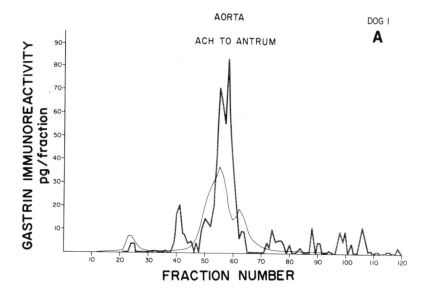

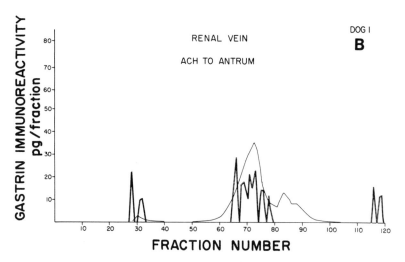

Figure 9. Elution patterns of gastrin immunoreactivity in samples obtained from Dog 1 during periods of antral stimulation from the aorta (9A) and from the renal vein (9B). Vascular transit of the kidney apparently resulted in nearly complete uptake of big gastrin and in uptake of the majority of G-17. Big-big gastrin appeared relatively more prominent in the renal vein samples.

First is the number of narrow peaks: since iodide is
the most pure substance applied to the column, many
investigators believe that any peak that is less wide
than the iodide fraction is artifactual. Second, although after antral acidification the total amount of
gastrin diminished in measurements of the total amount
of immunoreactive gastrin (Fig. 5), this diminution is
not always reflected in the amount of gastrin immunoreactivity detected in column samples (Figs. 8B & 8C).
We are aware of assay errors that may be introduced by
buffer systems and have taken care to perform all
assays of column eluates and of reference preparations
in identical buffer systems. Another interesting finding in many specimens obtained after antral acidification is the large amount of spiking immunoreactivity
to the right of the iodide peak, that is, to the right
of fraction 70 in Figure 8C. The identity of this
material is unknown.

The effect of passage through the kidney on various
molecular forms of gastrin during periods of antral
stimulation of release of gastrin is shown in Figure 9.
The aortic sample shows clean peaks in the areas of
big gastrin and G-17 (Fig. 9A), but after passage
through the kidney the big gastrin peak has disappeared, the G-17 peak is much smaller, and the big-
big gastrin peak is more prominent.

The qualitative changes occurring after antral stimulation and after antral acidification and after passage of stimulated levels of gastrin through the kidney, are easily appreciated from Figures 8 and 9. This
presentation of the data, however, does not allow relation of one elution pattern to another in a quantitative fashion, nor does it allow for accumulation of
quantitative data by performance of multiple studies.
In order to relate the amount of gastrin in each peak
to the total amount of immunoreactive gastrin originally applied to the column, we have calculated a new
value for each peak (P_2) which would be a function of
the total immunoreactivity of the original sample and
would, therefore, allow accumulation of data among several individuals. The following formula was used:

$$P_2 = \frac{P_1 \times G_s}{G_f}$$

where: P_1 = amount of gastrin measured under
              each peak after chromatography and

G_s = amount of gastrin in 5 ml of serum
applied to columns and

G_f = total immunoreactive gastrin in
all fractions after chromatography
including material under five
discrete peaks plus all other
immunoreactivity in column eluates.

This value for each peak (BBG, Comp I, BG, G-17, MG) is plotted as picograms of gastrin immunoreactivity per 5 ml of serum.

Data from eluate fractions from the aorta and renal vein from each of five dogs (an accident in handling led to loss of material from one dog) during the basal period, during the period of acetylcholine irrigation of the antrum, and during the period of antral acidification. The mean and standard errors for these calculated fractions during each period are illustrated in Figure 10.

Comparison of the amount of immunoreactivity in each molecular peak in each period illustrates several points. The largest molecular component during the basal period and during the period of antral acidification is big-big gastrin. Stimulation of gastrin release did not cause an increase of this fraction, but there was a statistically significant increase of big gastrin, G-17, and minigastrin on antral stimulation. G-17 is the largest peak during antral stimulation; it comprises 47% of the immunoreactivity in aortic samples during antral stimulation. The apparent increase in Component I during antral stimulation is not significant. There was no significant renal uptake of any of the five molecular forms of gastrin during either the basal or suppressed periods. During the period of acetylcholine stimulation of the antrum, however, the kidney extracted 60% of big gastrin, 42% of G-17, and 65% of minigastrin. Renal extractions of big gastrin and of G-17 are statistically significant. Aortic and renal concentrations of big gastrin and Component I were unchanged. The renal extraction of total immunoreactive gastrin measured from serum samples before gel filtration for these five dogs was 36%. The mean of the sum of the percent uptake of the five molecular peaks during antral stimulation in these five dogs is 36.9%.

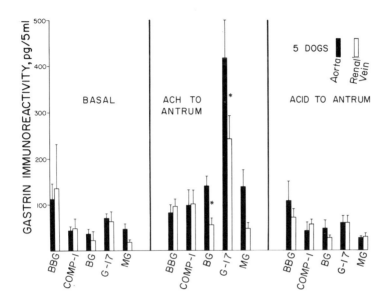

Figure 10. Schema for presentation of patterns of gastrin
molecular heterogeneity in sample obtained from the aorta
and renal vein in five dogs. There were no significant
differences in the concentrations of any of the five molecular components between the aorta and renal vein during
the basal period or during the period of antral acidification. There was uptake of 60% of big gastrin, 42% of G-17,
and 65% of minigastrin on transit of the kidney during
antral stimulation. The differences in the big gastrin
and G-17 fractions were significant (*). Big-big gastrin
is relatively prominent during basal period and period of
antral acidification, whereas big gastrin, G-17, and minigastrin are relatively prominent during antral stimulation.
The increases of big gastrin, G-17, and minigastrin during
antral stimulation were statistically significant.

DISCUSSION

Circulating gastrin is a heterogeneous mixture of various molecular forms of the hormone. The half-life of 8.6 minutes for endogenous gastrin determined in this study is intermediate between that of big-big gastrin and big gastrin on one hand and G-17 and mini-gastrin on the other (Table 2). Since basal gastrin values (which in our measurements have a relatively high percentage of BBG and Comp I) are subtracted from the total stimulated levels of gastrin in computing disappearance half-time, the majority of gastrin involved in the computations is comprised of BG, G-17, and MG, and the half-life of 8.6 minutes represents the disappearance half-time of this mixture.

The results of this study confirm our previous findings[24] as well as those of Dencker and colleagues[11] on the lack of hepatic uptake of endogenous gastrin.[22] Debas and Grossman[8] have bioassay evidence of slight hepatic inactivation of G-17. There is no evidence to support this on measurement of total immunoreactivity (Fig. 6). Specific evidence must await future analysis of the effect of hepatic transport on the various molecular forms of gastrin.

The failure to demonstrate uptake of circulating endogenous gastrin by the small bowel is at variance with our previous experience.[1] The variation may be due to differences in experimental preparations. In the earlier study, the superior mesenteric vein was cannulated retrogradely via the splenic vein and all

Table 2.   Disappearance half-time of various molecular forms of gastrin

Molecular forms of gastrin	Half-time
Big-big gastrin[30]	90 minutes
Big gastrin[32]	15 minutes
Endogenous gastrin (this study)	8.6 minutes
G-17[25]	2.1 minutes
Minigastrin[10]	1.8 minutes

venous tributaries to the superior mesenteric vein
from the duodenum and large bowel were ligated. In
the present study, the mesenteric vein was catheter-
ized in an antegrade fashion and the catheter tip
may have been in a sufficiently cephalad position
so as to receive blood from the stimulated gastric
antrum. This may account for the high gastrin value
in the mesenteric vein sample in dog 1 (Table 1),
for example.

The present study confirms previous suggestions
that renal uptake of gastrin may be an important
catabolic mechanism.[3,5,6] The fate of gastrin picked
up by the kidneys is unknown; it may be simply altered (by renal parenchymal cells) and returned in
an immunochemically unrecognizable form. Urinary
excretion is not important; we have shown repeatedly
that only small amounts of gastrin appear in the
urine. Davidson and associates[7] have shown that gastrin levels rise in nephrectomized rats but not in
rats with bilateral ureteral ligation; they have
provided evidence that gastrin is removed by a process
other than glomerular filtration and they suggest that
gastrin is removed at least partially by direct uptake
from peritubular blood.[14]

It seems unlikely that the kidneys, which receive
only 25% of the cardiac output and clear only 30%-
35% of the stimulated levels of gastrin, can account
entirely for the rapid turnover of endogenous gastrin.
Even if basal values are subtracted from stimulated
values (as they are in calculation of disappearance
half-time), the renal uptake of the *stimulated* fraction
of gastrin is only 45%. Other sites for degradation
or uptake must be considered. We have previously
shown small but significant uptake of gastrin by the
secreting gastric fundus.[13] These studies are difficult to perform because sufficient volumes of blood
are hard to come by and stimulation of gastrin secretion is difficult to achieve in anesthetized animals.

Data from the present study and from previous
studies on catabolism of gastrin suggest that loss
of gastrin is not a nonspecific result of tissue
transit. Although Korman and associates[21] have
suggested that the lung may be an important site for
removal of gastrin from circulation, we and others
have provided direct measurements which indicate that
there is no uptake of gastrin on transit of the

lung.[12,31] We have also demonstrated that gastrin is
not taken up on passage through the liver,[24] the hind
limb[31] or the head (present study).

Most previous reports of fractionation of serum
gastrin into molecular components have used serum
from patients with the Zollinger-Ellison syndrome
in which the high concentrations of gastrin have
facilitated clear separation of peaks because of the
large amounts of immunoreactivity present. In order
to achieve separation of different molecular forms
of gastrin from normal dog serum, it was necessary
to load each column with 5 ml of serum and to determine immunoreactivity in 500-µl aliquots of 2 ml
fractions from the column. Even so, only small
amounts of immunoreactivity were detectable in some
basal samples.

Division of gastrin immunoreactivity into five
"peaks" was an arbitrary choice for this study, but
we have found immunoreactive fractions, especially
in samples obtained during antral stimulation, in
the area of each of the five designated peaks.
There is controversy about the two larger molecular
sizes of gastrin. Yalow[34] was unable to find significant immunoreactivity in the region of Rehfeld's
Component I on fractionation of several plasmas on
1 x 200 cm G50 superfine Sephadex columns. She was
able to detect Component I-like immunoreactivity in
eluates from a Zollinger-Ellison tumor. Rehfeld and
associates[28] note that Yalow and colleagues have
failed to describe Components I and IV (minigastrin);
they ascribe their success in separating these fractions to their use of extralong Sephadex G50 superfine columns. In further disagreement, they were
unable to detect big-big gastrin in a variety of
sera.[28] We were able to detect immunoreactivity in
the void volume as well as in the Component I area
between the void volume and ^{125}I-labeled cholecystokinin (the marker for big gastrin).

Analysis of different molecular components on
antral stimulation, antral acidification, and on
transit of the kidney (Fig. 10), provides an insight
into the changing patterns of gastrin heterogeneity
during different physiologic states. The observations that big-big gastrin is the major fraction of
total immunoreactive gastrin during fasting and
that it is not altered by antral stimulation[30,39]
are confirmed. There is a significant increase in

big gastrin, G-17, and minigastrin on antral stimulation and a significant decrease in each of those
components on application of acid to the antrum.
Renal uptake was greatest in BG, G-17, and MG. This
would suggest that these three forms are physiologically kinetic, whereas BBG and Comp I are perhaps
static. In the only previous study of the effect of
feeding on molecular patterns in dog plasma,[39] the
largest postprandial component found in the single dog
studied was G-17. We found that G-17 comprised almost
half of all immunoreactivity from aortic specimens
during the period of stimulation. The method of
analysis of different molecular forms of gastrin
used in this study may be useful in investigating
patterns of gastrin response to different physiologic
states (for example, a minute-by-minute analysis of
antral vein samples after antral stimulation or, the
comparison of patterns in the portal vein and hepatic
artery with those in the hepatic vein).

When we first studied the uptake of endogenous
gastrin by the kidney,[3,19] the failure to show renal
inactivation of gastrin during the basal state and
during antral acidification was perplexing. When
the small bowel was found to take up stimulated but
not basal levels of gastrin,[1] we suggested that the
trigger for the processes of degradation might be
activated simply by achievement of a threshold concentration or by changes in the relative concentrations of the various molecular forms of gastrin.
Our present study validates the latter suggestion.

SUMMARY

Studies on the release of gastrin into the circulation and disappearance of gastrin from the circulation
were performed acutely in 11 anesthetized dogs. Under
the conditions of the experiment, the disappearance
half-time of endogenous (mixed molecular forms) gastrin is 8.6 minutes. There was no change in the
total measurable gastrin immunoreactivity after transit of the liver. Intestinal extraction of total
gastrin immunoreactivity is probable. Renal uptake
of serum gastrin did not occur during basal periods
and during periods of antral suppression with acid,
but renal uptake of stimulated total immunoreactive
endogenous gastrin was significant (30%).

Fractionation of serum samples obtained during basal periods, during periods of antral stimulation, and during periods of antral suppression, yielded immunoreactivity that was divided into five peaks (big-big gastrin, Rehfeld's Component I, big gastrin, heptadecapeptide, and minigastrin). Big-big gastrin was the largest peak in basal and suppressed samples. Big gastrin, heptadecapeptide gastrin, and minigastrin rose significantly in stimulated samples. Heptadeca-peptide gastrin was the largest peak in stimulated samples. There was no significant uptake of any of the five molecular forms of gastrin on transit of the kidney during basal periods or during periods of antral suppression. During periods of antral stimu-lation, however, the kidney extracted 60% of big gastrin, 42% of heptadecapeptide gastrin, and 65% of minigastrin. Concentrations of big-big gastrin and of Component I were unchanged. The findings would suggest that the larger forms of gastrin are relative-ly inactive physiologically, whereas big gastrin, heptadecapeptide gastrin, and minigastrin are physio-logically kinetic.

Acknowledgments

This work was supported by a grant from the National Insti-tutes of Health (AM 15241) and by a grant from the John A. Hartford Foundation, Inc. Dr. Ramus is the recipient of a Wellcome Research Travel Grant.

References

1. Becker HD, Reeder DD, Thompson JC: Extraction of circula-ting endogenous gastrin by the small bowel. *Gastroent-erology* 65:903-906, 1973.
2. Berson SA, Yalow RS: Nature of immunoreactive gastrin ex-tracted from tissues of gastrointestinal tract. *Gastroenterology* 60:215-222, 1971.
3. Booth RAD, Reeder DD, Hjelmquist UB, Brandt EN Jr, Thompson JC: Renal inactivation of endogenous gastrin in dogs. *Arch Surg* 106:851-854, 1973.
4. Clendinnen BG, Davidson WD, Reeder DD, Jackson BM, Thompson JC: Renal uptake and excretion of gastrin in the dog. *Surg Gynecol Obstet* 132:1039-1043, 1971.

5. Clendinnen BG, Reeder DD, Brandt EN Jr, Thompson JC: Effect of nephrectomy on the rate and pattern of the disappearance of exogenous gastrin in dogs. *Gut* 14:462-467, 1973.

6. Davidson WD, Springberg PD, Falkinburg NR: Renal extraction and excretion of endogenous gastrin in the dog. *Gastroenterology* 64:955-961, 1973.

7. Davidson WD, Moore TC, Shippey W, Conovaloff AJ: Effect of bilateral nephrectomy and bilateral ureteral ligation on serum gastrin levels in the rat. *Gastroenterology* 66:522-525, 1974.

8. Debas HT, Grossman MI: Hepatic inactivation of gastrointestinal hormones. Presented, V World Congress of Gastroenterology, Mexico City, October, 1974.

9. Debas HT, Walsh JH, Grossman MI: Pure human minigastrin: Secretory potency and disappearance rate. *Gut* 15: 686-689, 1974.

10. Debas HT, Walsh JH, Grossman MI: Pure natural human "minigastrin": Biological activity and half life, abstracted. *Gastroenterology* 66:837, 1974.

11. Dencker H, Håkanson R, Liedberg G, Norryd C, Oscarson J, Rehfeld JF, Stadil F: Gastrin in portal and peripheral venous blood after feeding in man. *Gut* 14:856-860, 1973.

12. Dent RI, Levine B, James JH, Hirsch H, Fischer JE: Effects of isolated perfused canine lung and kidney on gastrin heptadecapeptide. *Am J Physiol* 225:1038-1044, 1973.

13. Evans JCW, Reeder DD, Becker HD, Thompson JC: Extraction of circulating endogenous gastrin by the gastric fundus. *Gut* 15:112-115, 1974.

14. Grace, SG, Davidson WD, State D: Renal mechanisms for removal of gastrin from the circulation. *Surg Forum* 25:323-325, 1974.

15. Greenwood FC, Hunter WM, Glover JS: The preparation of of ^{131}I-labeled human growth hormone of high specific radioactivity. *Biochem J* 89:114-123, 1963.

16. Gregory RA: The gastrointestinal hormones. A review of recent advances. (The Bayliss-Starling Lecture 1973). *J Physiol* 241:1-32, 1974.

17. Gregory RA, Tracy HJ: Isolation of two "big gastrins" from Zollinger-Ellison tumour tissue. *Lancet* 2:797-799, 1972.

18. Gregory RA, Tracy HJ: Big gastrin. *Mt Sinai J Med* 40: 359-364, 1973.

19. Hjelmquist UBE, Reeder DD, Brandt EN Jr, Thompson JC: Effect of the kidney on endogenous gastrin. *Surg Forum* 23:318-320, 1972.

20. Jackson BM, Reeder DD, Thompson JC: Dynamic characteristics of gastrin release. *Am J Surg* 123:137-142, 1972.

21. Korman MG, Hansky J, Ritchie BC, Watts J McK Maloney JE:
    Disappearance of gastrin across the lung. *Aust J
    Exper Biol Med Sci* 51:679-687, 1973.
22. Odell WD, Rayford PL, Ross GT: Simplified, partially auto-
    mated method for radioimmunoassay of human thyroid-
    stimulating, growth, luteinizing and follicle stimulating
    hormones. *J Lab Clin Med* 70:973-980, 1967.
23. Rayford PL, Reeder DD, Thompson JC: Interlaboratory
    reproducibility of gastrin measurements by radioimmuno-
    assay. *J Lab Clin Med*, in press.
24. Reeder DD, Brandt EN Jr, Watson LC, Hjelmquist UBE, Thompson
    JC: Pre- and posthepatic measurements of mass of endog-
    enous gastrin. *Surgery* 72:34-41, 1972.
25. Reeder DD, Jackson BM, Brandt EN Jr, Thompson JC: Rate
    and pattern of disappearance of exogenous gastrin in
    dogs. *Am J Physiol* 222:1571-1574, 1972.
26. Rehfeld JF: Three components of gastrin in human serum.
    Gel filtration studies on the molecular size of
    immunoreactive serum gastrin. *Biochim Biophys Acta*
    285:364-372, 1972.
27. Rehfeld JF, Stadil F: Gel filtration studies on immuno-
    reactive gastrin in serum from Zollinger-Ellison
    patients. *Gut* 14:369-373, 1973.
28. Rehfeld JF, Stadil F, Vikelsøe J: Immunoreactive gastrin
    components in human serum. *Gut* 15:102-111, 1974.
29. Shoemaker WC, Walker WF, Van Itallie TB, Moore FD: A
    method for simultaneous catheterization of major
    hepatic vessels in a chronic canine preparation.
    Am J Physiol 196:311-314, 1959.
30. Straus E, Yalow RS: Studies on the distribution and
    degradation of heptadecapeptide, big, and big big
    gastrin. *Gastroenterology* 66:936-943, 1974.
31. Thompson JC, Becker HD, Evans JCW, Hjelmquist UBE, Brandt
    EN, Reeder DD: Studies on the catabolism of gastrin,
    in Chey WY and Brooks FP (eds), *Endocrinology of the
    Gut*, Thorofare, NJ: Charles B. Slack Inc., 1974,
    pp 295-303.
32. Walsh JH, Debas HT, Grossman MI: Pure human big gastrin.
    Immunochemical properties, disappearance half-time
    and acid-stimulating action in dogs. *J Clin Invest*
    54:477-485, 1974.
33. Walsh JH, Trout HH III, Debas HT, Grossman MI: Immuno-
    chemical and biological properties of gastrins obtained
    from different species and of different molecular
    species of gastrins, in Chey WY and Brooks FP (eds),
    Endocrinology of the Gut, Thorofare, NJ: Charles B.
    Slack, Inc., 1974, pp 277-289.

34. Yalow RS: Gastrins: Small, big and big-big, in Chey WY
    and Brooks FP (eds), *Endocrinology of the Gut,*
    Thorofare, NJ: Charles B. Slack, Inc., 1974, pp 261-276.
35. Yalow RS, Berson SA: Radioimmunoassay of gastrin.
    Gastroenterology 58:1-14, 1970.
36. Yalow RS, Berson SA: Size and charge distinctions be-
    tween endogenous human plasma gastrin in peripheral
    blood and heptadecapeptide gastrins. *Gastroenterology*
    58:609-615, 1970.
37. Yalow RS, Berson SA: Further studies on the nature of
    immunoreactive gastrin in human plasma. *Gastroenterology*
    60:203-214, 1971.
38. Yalow RS, Berson SA: And now, "big, big" gastrin. *Biochem
    Biophys Res Commun* 48:391-395, 1972.
39. Yalow RS, Wu N: Additional studies on the nature of big
    big gastrin. *Gastroenterology* 65:19-27, 1973.

ENDOCRINE CELLS

ENDOCRINE CELLS OF THE INTESTINAL MUCOSA

Enrico Solcia, Julia M. Polak, Roberto Buffa,
Carlo Capella, A.G.E. Pearse

Institute of Pathological Anatomy, University of Pavia,
Pavia, Italy; Histopathology, Histochemistry and Ultrastructure Center, University of Pavia-Varese, Varese,
Italy; and Royal Postgraduate Medical School, Hammersmith Hospital, London, England

The endocrine cells of the gastrointestinal mucosa
have been the subject of many studies in the last
few years.[6,7,9,12,15,17,19,28,29,37,39] Ultrastructurally and histochemically, several types of endocrine cells have been identified in the stomach,
including 5-hydroxytryptamine (5HT) producing cells
(EC-cells), gastrin (G) cells, A-like cells, reputed
to store gastric glucagon-like immunoreactive material (GLI), and other types of cells whose function
is poorly understood (ECL,D,D_1 and X-cells).[31]
Despite the fact that several established or candidate hormones have been purified from the intestinal
mucosa, morphologic studies on the intestinal endocrine cells have been less conclusive.[3,5,8,13,18,31,34]
The availability of specific antisera against several
intestinal hormones, which led to the detection of
specialized immunoreactive cells,[3,23-26,32] prompted
us to consider the possibility of comparing these
immunoreactive cells with the various cell types
identified in ultrastructural investigations.

MATERIAL AND METHODS

Light Microscopy

An indirect immunofluorescence technique with appropriate control tests[23-25,32] was applied to sections
of human, pig, and dog gastrointestinal mucosa fixed

155

in a series of cross-linking agents recently introduced in histochemical practice.[20,23,24,26] Both
vapor fixation of freeze-dried specimens and immer-
sion in liquid fixative solutions were tested. The
usual aldehyde fixatives were also used.

Antibodies against pure natural porcine secretin,
glucagon, GIP, VIP and motilin, or synthetic human
gastrin I, were used.[21,23-27]

The sections were photographed under fluorescence
microscopy, refixed in Bouin's fluid and restained
with Grimelius' silver[11] or Sevier-Munger's silver;[30]
other sections were refixed in aldehyde solutions
and restained with Masson's argentaffin reaction or
diazonium reaction for 5HT.[33]

Electron Microscopy

Small samples of the above tissues were fixed in a
mixture of 2% paraformaldehyde and 2.5% glutaraldehyde in 0.1 M phosphate buffer pH 7.3. Some of these
specimens were postfixed in 1% osmium tetroxide, dehydrated in ethanol and embedded in Epon 812; ultramicrotome sections were stained with uranyl acetate
and lead citrate. Other specimens were cut with a
Smith-Farquhar tissue sectioner (Sorvall); 100-150 µ
thick sections were stained with Masson's argentaffin
reaction, Sevier-Munger's silver or Grimelius' silver,
as already reported,[3,5,36-38] and then dehydrated
and embedded in Epon. Ultramicrotome sections of
silver-treated material were observed in the electron
microscope with and without uranyl counterstaining.

RESULTS

Light Microscopy

The findings of light microscopic studies are summarized in Table 1. The application of immunofluorescence
tests with motilin antibodies to sections of human,
dog, and pig intestine, allowed endocrine-like cells
scattered in the epithelium lining the crypts and
villi of the duodenum and jejunum to be stained
selectively. On restaining the sections with Sevier-
Munger's and Grimelius' silver, all motilin cells were
heavily blackened (Fig. 1). Motilin immunofluorescent
cells of aldehyde-fixed sections also reacted with

Table 1. Intestinal immunofluorescent cells, their staining patterns and ultrastructural equivalents

Immuno-fluorescence	Sevier-Munger	Grimelius	5HT methods	Electron microscopy
Intestine				
Motilin	+++	+++	+++	EC-cell
GIP	+++	+++	–	K-cell
Secretin	±	+	–	S-cell ?
Glucagon	–	+	–	L-cell ?
VIP	–	±	–	H-cell ?
Gastrin	–/+	–	–	I-cell ?
Antrum				
Gastrin	–	+	–	G-cell

the argentaffin and diazonium reactions.

Use of GIP antibodies allowed detection of numerous medium-sized immunofluorescent cells in the jejunum and duodenum of man, pig, and dog; they were less numerous in the ileum. On restaining with silver techniques, GIP-cells were heavily blackened (Fig. 2).

Small immunofluorescent cells reacting with anti-secretin antibodies have been detected in the duodenal and (although less numerous) in the jejunal mucosa of man, pig, and dog. On restaining with Sevier-Munger's silver, secretin cells showed poor reactivity or none at all (Fig. 3); slight yellow-brown reactivity was obtained with Grimelius' silver.

Small cells, which react with VIP antibodies, have been found along the whole small intestine (especially in the ileum) as well as in the colon. When the sections were restained with silver techniques VIP-cells gave poor reactivity or none at all.

Numerous medium-sized cells of the jejunum, ileum, and colon showed selective immunofluorescence using glucagon antibodies. The same cells, which were interpreted as enteroglucagon (EG) cells, failed to react with Sevier-Munger's silver and were stained only slightly with Grimelius' silver.

Fairly numerous cells reacting with gastrin antibodies have been detected in the duodenum and jejunum; very few of them have been observed in the ileum. In freeze-dried, vapor-fixed sections, a minority of such cells showed some reactivity with Sevier-Munger's silver (brown staining); usually no reactivity was

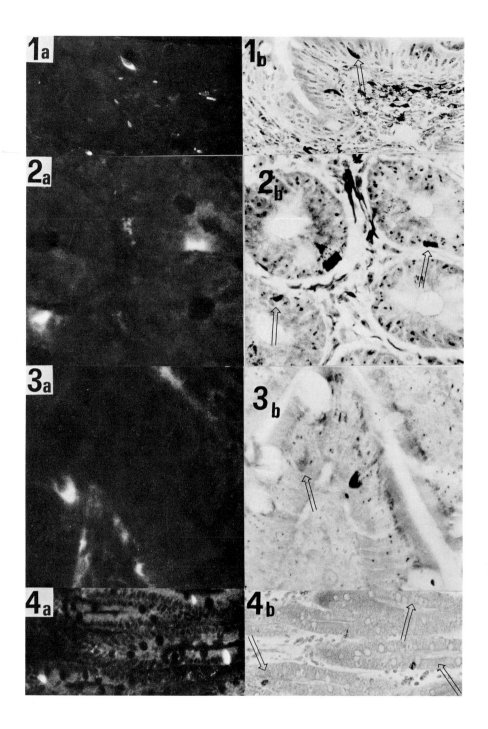

found in sections fixed with conventional aldehyde solutions. Unlike gastrin cells of the pyloric mucosa, most gastrin cells of the intestinal mucosa failed to react with Grimelius' silver, despite appropriate fixation in Bouin's fluid (Fig. 4).

Electron Microscopy

The results of electron microscopic studies are summarized in Table 1. Direct application of Sevier-Munger's and Grimelius' silver to electron microscopy allowed detection in the intestinal mucosa of two types of endocrine cells with heavily reactive granules (Figs. 5 & 6). These cells reproduced the ultrastructural features of previously identified EC- and K-cells.[6,9,31,34,39] As in previous studies, EC-cells reacted also with Masson's argentaffin reaction, whereas K-cells failed to react.

←————————

Figure 1. Motilin cell (arrow) of pig jejunum stained with immunofluorescence (a) and restained with Sevier-Munger's silver (b). Note that, besides the motilin cell, a nonmotilin (GIP?) cell is also blackened by silver (×340).

Figure 2. Two GIP-cells (arrows) of human jejunum stained with immunofluorescence (a) and restained with Sevier-Munger's silver (b). Note blackening of the two GIP-cells, as well as of a non-GIP (motilin?) cell (×380).

Figure 3. Secretin cell of human jejunum stained with immunofluorescence (a) and restained with Sevier-Munger's (b). Note very poor reactivity of the secretin cell to the silver technique (arrow) whereas another endocrine cell (motilin cell? GIP-cell?) is blackened (×380).

Figure 4. Gastrin cells of the dog jejunum: a) immunofluorescence, b) Grimelius' silver. Note failure of the gastrin cells to react with the silver method (×250).

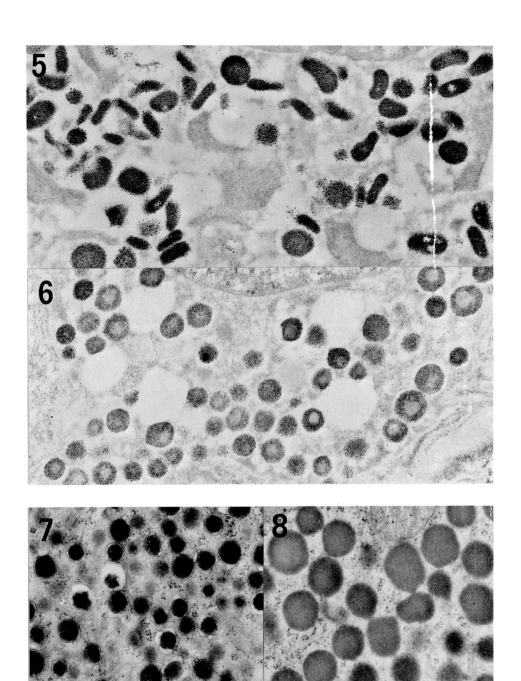

EC-cells showed peculiar pleomorphic granules: round, oblonged, pyriform, rod-like, kidney-shaped, and biconcave. They were found in all portions of the gut, from the stomach to the rectum. As noted before, however,[5,6,31,39] gastric EC-cells showed evident ultrastructural differences in respect to duodenojejunal EC-cells, including smaller granules of more complex internal structure. Some ultrastructural difference was also noted between EC-cells of the proximal and distal intestine.

K-cells showed moderately large, round-to-ovoid granules, with an osmiophilic, argyrophobe body surrounded by a less osmiophilic, heavily argyrophil matrix (Fig. 6). They were mainly found in the duodenum and jejunum; a few were also observed in the ileum. This distribution, coupled with the intense reactivity with Sevier-Munger's silver, reproduced closely the behavior of immunofluorescent GIP cells in light microscopy sections.

The remaining endocrine cells showed poor reactivity or none with the Sevier-Munger technique at the ultrastructural level; some of them showed slight reactivity with Grimelius' silver. Among these cells,

Figure 5. EC granules stained with Sevier-Munger's silver at ultrastructural level. Note the pleomorphism of the granules, which are covered with very thin silver grains. Uranyl counterstaining (×20,200).

Figure 6. Granules of a K-cell stained with Sevier-Munger's silver and counterstained with uranyl. Note deposition of silver grains in the peripheral matrix of the granules, whereas the argyrophobe core reacts with uranyl (×20,200).

Figure 7. Granules of an S-cell under conventional electron microscopy. Dog duodenum (×20,200).

Figure 8. Granules of an L-cell of the dog colon (×20,200).

conventional electron microscopy allowed L-cells
(Fig. 7) which are distributed in the jejunum, ileum
and colon and reproduce the morphology of immunofluorescent EC-cells to be distinguished from S-cells
(Fig. 8), (which are mostly restricted to the duodenum
and jejunum and apparently reproduce the morphology
of secretin cells). Besides EC and L-cells, a third
type of endocrine cell has been regularly found in
the human colon and rectum by electron microscopy.
This cell, tentatively labeled H-cell,[31] showed
small to medium-sized, fairly regular or angular
granules of moderate osmiophilia. A similar cell
seemed also to be represented in the small intestine.
A relationship of this cell with VIP immunofluorescent
cells, although possible, was neither supported nor
disproved by available morphologic data.

Cells reproducing the ultrastructural features of
G-cells, known to correspond to gastrin immunofluorescent cells of the pyloric mucosa,[2,4,6,7,9,11,14,29,31,34,]
[37,39] were found only in the human duodenum, and
in very limited numbers. In contrast with gastrin
immunofluorescent cells, no G-cells have been observed
in the jejunum or ileum. Some cells reproducing the
features of previously described I-cells,[3,5,31] have
been regularly found in the duodenum and jejunum;
their morphology and distribution, as well as their
unreactivity with Grimelius' silver, seemed to parallel those of most intestinal gastrin immunoreactive
cells.

Besides the above cells, D-cells, mostly duodenal,
and a few D_1-cells have been observed in ultrastructural studies. Both D- and D_1-cells have been found
also in the gastric mucosa and pancreas.[5,13,19,29,31,]
[37,38]

DISCUSSION

The hormonal status of the active peptides recently
purified from the intestine is strongly supported by
their storage in specialized cells showing staining
and ultrastructural features that unequivocally reproduce those of well-known endocrine cells.

The different size, shape, number, distribution,
and staining patterns of the cells storing the various
peptides, suggest that each peptide hormone is stored
in a distinct cell type. The attribution of motilin

to the argentaffin EC-cells of the upper small intestine has already been proved by the argentaffinity and ultrastructural pattern of motilin-immunofluorescent cells.[21] The intense reactivity of motilin cells with argyrophil techniques is in keeping with this conclusion. The failure of gastric EC-cells to react with motilin antibodies fits well with the ultrastructural differences between these cells and duodenojejunal motilin-storing EC-cells.

Despite the well-known abundance of EC-cells in the ileum and colon,[3,5,8,9,15,31,34,39] very few or no motilin cells have been found in these intestinal tracts. In the rabbit, some ultrastructural difference was observed between EC-cells of the proximal and distal intestine.[6] Preliminary studies suggest that a similar pattern might occur even in man and other species. If so, the nonreactivity of several argentaffin carcinoids from the lower intestine in respect to motilin antisera[22] could be explained. The rare argentaffin carcinoids of the upper small intestine remain to be investigated with respect to their possible motilin production.

The close relationship of GIP-cells with ultrastructurally-identified K-cells seems likely also, given their similar morphology, distribution, and reactivity with argyrophil techniques. Their failure to react with 5HT-related techniques distinguishes them from motilin and nonmotilin EC-cells.

The poor reactivity or the unreactivity of secretin, enteroglucagon, and VIP-cells with Sevier-Munger's silver, clearly separates such cells from 5HT, motilin, and GIP-cells, as well as from ultrastructurally-identified EC- and K-cells. The different reactivity of the two groups of cells in respect to Grimelius' silver is also evident, although somewhat less sharply than with Sevier-Munger's technique.

The attribution of enteroglucagon to ultrastructurally-identified L-cells is supported by the close parallelism of their distribution in various intestinal tracts with respect to the distribution of glucagon immunofluorescent (EG) cells. Both cells were numerous in the colon, ileum and lower jejunum, but very scarce in the duodenum. This distribution was distinctive in respect to all other types of immunofluorescent cells or ultrastructurally-identified cells, apart from VIP-cells and H-cells. VIP-cells were less numerous and smaller than EG-cells, however, and showed different zonal distribution in the mucosa.[27]

The occurrence of VIP-cells in the lower intestinal tracts, including the colon, is at variance with that of several types of immunofluorescent or ultrastructurally-identified endocrine cells, including secretin immunofluorescent cells and ultrastructurally-defined S-cells. As noted before,[3,5,24,31,32,39] available data on distributive and staining patterns may support the storage of secretin in S-cells. The possible origin of VIP from H-cells deserves investigation.

The lack of ultrastructurally-defined G-cells in most samples of intestinal mucosa that show consistent amounts of gastrin immunoreactive cells, as well as the failure of the latter cells to react with Grimelius' silver, suggests that a large proportion of intestinal cells reacting with antigastrin antisera are morphologically different from pyloric-type gastrin (G) cells. In fact, intestinal gastrin showed some chemical difference with respect to pyloric gastrin, with prevalence of large-molecule gastrins over heptadecapeptide gastrin.[1] Moreover, HCl seems unable to block the release of intestinal gastrin, although it effectively blocks the release of gastrin from the pyloric mucosa.[35]

The possibility that ultrastructurally-defined I-cells correspond to intestinal non-G gastrin cells seems to be considered. Moreover, the possibility that some gastrin-like cross-reacting peptide is involved (CCK or a CCK-related peptide?) should be investigated.

Pancreatic D-cells, which in some tests have been shown to react with gastrin antibodies,[10,16,38] certainly differ ultrastructurally and histochemically (in being heavily reactive with Davenport's silver, as well as in other ways) from pyloric-type G-cells and also from the non-G gastrin cell of the intestinal mucosa. So far, convincing evidence is lacking for the existence of G-cells in the normal pancreas.

SUMMARY

It is concluded that the use of the same argentaffin and argyrophil techniques for restaining immunofluorescent cells in histologic sections and

for staining endocrine cell granules at the ultrastructural level, allows identification of at least
two types of intestinal hormone-producing cells, the
motilin cell and the GIP-cell. For a reliable identification of the remaining immunoreactive cells
(including secretin, enteroglucagon, VIP and gastrin
cells), some other approach seems needed.

Acknowledgments

The authors wish to thank Dr. JC Brown for generous gifts of
motilin and GIP antiserum, Drs. V Mutt and S Said for generous
gifts of secretin and VIP, and Dr. S Bloom for his help in
producing specific antisera.

References

1. Berson SA, Yalow RS: Nature of immunoreactive gastrin
      extracted from tissues of gastrointestinal tract.
      Gastroenterology 60:215-222, 1971.
2. Bussolati G, Canese MG: Electron microscopical identifi-
      cation of the immunofluorescent gastrin cells in the
      cat pyloric mucosa. *Histochemie* 29:198-206, 1972.
3. Bussolati G, Capella C, Solcia E, Vassallo G, Vezzadini P:
      Ultrastructural and immunofluorescent investigations
      on the secretin cell in the dog intestinal mucosa.
      Histochemie 26:218-227, 1971.
4. Bussolati G, Pearse AGE: Immunofluorescent localization
      of the gastrin-secreting G cells in the pyloric antrum
      of the pig. *Histochemie* 21:1-4, 1970.
5. Capella C, Solcia E: The endocrine cells of the pig
      gastrointestinal mucosa and pancreas. *Arch Histol Jap*
      35:1-29, 1972.
6. Capella C, Solcia E, Vassallo G: Identification of six
      types of endocrine cells in the gastrointestinal
      mucosa of the rabbit. *Arch Histol Jap* 30:479-495, 1969.
7. Creutzfeldt W, Arnold R, Creutzfeldt C, Feurle G, Ketterer
      H: Gastrin and G-cells in the antral mucosa of patients
      with pernicious anaemia, acromegaly and hyperparathyroid-
      ism and in a Zollinger-Ellison tumour of the pancreas.
      Eur J Clin Invest 1:461-479, 1971.

8. Ferreira MN: Argentaffin and other "endocrine" cells of the small intestine in the adult mouse: I. Ultrastructure and classification. *Am J Anat* 131:315-330, 1971.

9. Forssmann WG, Orci L, Pictet R, Renold AE, Rouiller C: The endocrine cells in the epithelium of the gastrointestinal mucosa of the rat: An electron microscope study. *J Cell Biol* 40:692-715, 1969.

10. Greider MH, McGuigan JE: Cellular localization of gastrin in the human pancreas. *Diabetes* 20:389-396, 1971.

11. Grimelius L: A silver nitrate stain for α_2 cells in human pancreatic islets. *Acta Soc Med Uppsala* 73:243-270, 1968.

12. Håkanson R, Owman C, Sjöberg NO, Sporrong B: Amine mechanisms in enterochromaffin and enterochromaffin-like cells of the gastric mucosa in various mammals. *Histochemie* 21:189-220, 1970.

13. Kobayashi S, Fujita T, Sasagawa T: The endocrine cells of human duodenal mucosa. An electron microscope study. *Arch Histol Jap* 31:477-494, 1970.

14. Larsson LI, Sundler F, Håkanson R, Grimelius L, Rehfeld JF, Stadil F: Histochemical properties of the antral gastrin cell. *J Histochem Cytochem* 22:419-427, 1974.

15. Lechago J, Bencosme SA: The endocrine elements of the digestive system. *Int Rev Exp Pathol* 12:119-201, 1973.

16. Lomsky RF, Langr F, Vortel V: Immunohistochemical demonstration of gastrin in mammalian islets of Langerhans. *Nature* 223:618-619, 1969.

17. McGuigan JE: Gastric mucosal intracellular localization of gastrin by immunofluorescence. *Gastroenterology* 55:315-327, 1968.

18. Osaka M, Sasagawa T, Fujita T: Endocrine cells in human jejunum and ileum: An electron microscope study of biopsy materials. *Arch Histol Jap* 35:235-248, 1973.

19. Pearse AGE, Coulling I, Weavers B, Friesen S: The endocrine polypeptide cells of the human stomach, duodenum and jejunum. *Gut* 11:649-658, 1970.

20. Pearse AGE, Polak JM: Cross linking agents for use in immunohistochemistry. *Proc R Micro Soc* , in press.

21. Pearse AGE, Polak JM, Bloom SR, Adams C, Dryburgh JR, Brown JC: Enterochromaffin cells of the mammalian small intestine as the source of motilin. *Virchows Arch [Zellpathol]* 16:111-120, 1974.

22. Pearse AGE, Polak JM, Heath CM: Polypeptide hormone production by "carcinoid" apudomas and their relevant cytochemistry. *Virchows Arch [Zellpathol]* 16:95-109, 1974.

23. Polak JM, Bloom S, Coulling I, Pearse AGE: Immunofluorescent localization of enteroglucagon cells in the gastrointestinal tract of the dog. *Gut* 12:311-318, 1971.

24. Polak JM, Bloom S, Coulling I, Pearse AGE: Immunofluorescent localization of secretin in the canine duodenum. *Gut* 12:605-610, 1971.

25. Polak JM, Bloom S, Kuzio M, Brown JC, Pearse AGE: Cellular localization of gastric inhibitory polypeptide in the duodenum and jejunum. *Gut* 14:284-288, 1973.

26. Polak JM, Pearse AGE, Adams C, Garaud JC: Immunohistochemical and ultrastructural studies on the endocrine polypeptide (APUD) cells of the avian gastrointestinal tract. *Experientia* 30:564-567, 1974.

27. Polak JM, Pearse AGE, Garaud JC, Bloom SR: Cellular localization of a vasoactive intestinal peptide in the mammalian and avian gastrointestinal tract. *Gut* 15:720-724, 1974.

28. Rubin W: Endocrine cells in the normal human stomach. A fine structural study. *Gastroenterology* 63:784-800, 1972.

29. Sasagawa T, Kobayashi S, Fujita T: The endocrine cells in the human pyloric antrum. An electron microscope study of biopsy materials. *Arch Histol Jap* 32:275-288, 1970.

30. Sevier AC, Munger BL: A silver method for paraffin sections of neural tissue. *J Neuropathol Exp Neurol* 24:130-135, 1965.

31. Solcia E, Capella C, Vassallo G, Buffa R: Endocrine cells of the gastric mucosa. *Int Rev Cytol,* in press.

32. Solcia E, Capella C, Vezzadini P, Barbara L, Bussolati G: Immunohistochemical and ultrastructural detection of the secretin cell in the pig intestinal mucosa. *Experientia* 28:549-550, 1972.

33. Solcia E, Sampietro R, Capella C: Differential staining of catecholamines, 5-hydroxytryptamine and related compounds in aldehyde-fixed tissues. *Histochemie* 17:273-283, 1969.

34. Solcia E, Sampietro R, Capella C: Cytology and cytochemistry of hormone producing cells of the upper gastrointestinal tract, in Creutzfeldt W (ed), *Origin, Chemistry, Physiology and Pathophysiology of the Gastrointestinal Hormones.* Stuttgart: Schattauer, 1970, pp 3-29.

35. Stern DH, Walsh JH: Gastrin release in postoperative ulcer patients: Evidence for release of duodenal gastrin. *Gastroenterology* 64:363-369, 1973.

36. Vassallo G, Capella C, Solcia E: Grimelius' silver stain
       for endocrine cell granules, as shown by electron
       microscopy. *Stain Technol* 46:7-13, 1971.
37. Vassallo G, Capella C, Solcia E: Endocrine cells of the
       human gastric mucosa. *Z Zellforsch Mikrosk Anat*
       118:49-67, 1971.
38. Vassallo G, Solcia E, Bussolati G, Polak J, Pearse AGE:
       Non-G cell gastrin-producing tumours of the pancreas.
       Virchows Arch [Zellpathol] 11:66-79, 1972.
39. Vassallo G, Solcia E, Capella C: Light and electron
       microscopic identification of several types of endo-
       crine cells in the gastrointestinal mucosa of the cat.
       Z Zellforsch Mikrosk Anat 98:333-356, 1969.

FLUORESCENCE HISTOCHEMISTRY OF POLYPEPTIDE HORMONE-SECRETING CELLS IN THE GASTROINTESTINAL MUCOSA

L.-I. Larsson, F. Sundler, R. Håkanson

Departments of Histology and Pharmacology,
University of Lund, Lund, Sweden

Immunohistochemistry has opened up new avenues for the study of polypeptide hormone-secreting cells. Most profound has been its impact in the field of gastrointestinal endocrinology. The immunohistochemical localization of a certain polypeptide hormone provides a basis for the characterization of the hormone-storing cell by histologic, histochemical, and electronmicroscopic techniques. Of particular importance in this respect is the use of histochemical procedures, since they may provide much additional information concerning both hormonal and nonhormonal components of the endocrine cells. This information may, for instance, throw light on the way peptide hormones are produced and stored in the cells. Fluorescence microscopic techniques are noteworthy among histochemical methods for their high sensitivity. In the last decade a number of such techniques have been developed for the demonstration of several biogenic amines and of peptides or proteins with certain distinctive features. In the following, we will review our experience with such methods when applied to the endocrine cells of the gut.

FLUORESCENCE HISTOCHEMISTRY OF AMINES

Formaldehyde-Induced Fluorescence

In 1961-1962 Falck and Hillarp[17],[18] developed a fluorescence histochemical procedure for the demonstration of arylethylamines at the cellular level. The
method is based on the capacity of formaldehyde gas
to convert certain biogenic monoamines, such as catecholamines and 5-hydroxytryptamine (5-HT), into highly
fluorescent compounds. This reaction is favored by
the presence of protein. In the initial step, formaldehyde engages in a Pictet-Spengler cyclization
reaction with the arylethylamine (phenylethylamine or
indolethylamine), whereby tetrahydroisoquinoline or
tetrahydro-β-carboline derivatives, respectively, are
formed via a Schiff's base. In a second step, these
weakly fluorescent compounds are dehydrogenated to
the corresponding, intensely fluorescent dihydro derivatives. This may occur in two different ways:
a) via an autoxidative step to 6,7-dihydroisoquinoline
or 3,4-dihydro-β-carboline or b) via a second, acid-
catalyzed reaction with formaldehyde, yielding the 2-
methylated dihydro derivatives (Fig. 1).[8] The histochemical procedure makes use of freeze-dried tissue
specimens and condensation in the dry state to ensure
that the condensation of the amines with formaldehyde
takes place at their cellular storage sites without
displacement. The sensitivity of the Falck-Hillarp
method can be expressed as the lowest amount of substance that is detectable. It appears from the work
of Jonsson[42] and Fuxe and Jonsson[20] that as little
as 5×10^{-6} pmol of noradrenaline can be detected
within one nerve terminal varicosity. Dopa and the
catecholamines are transformed into fluorophores that
emit light with a maximum at about 480 nm, whereas
indolethylamines, such as 5-hydroxytryptophan and
5-HT emit formaldehyde-induced fluorescence with a
maximum at about 535 nm (Fig. 2). These spectral
differences make it possible to distinguish between
catecholamines and 5-HT by microspectrofluorometry.
Dopamine, moreover, can be distinguished from noradrenaline and adrenaline by a characteristic acid-
induced shift in the excitation spectrum.[6] The histochemical and microspectrofluorometric procedure
has been described in detail by Björklund and associates.[9]

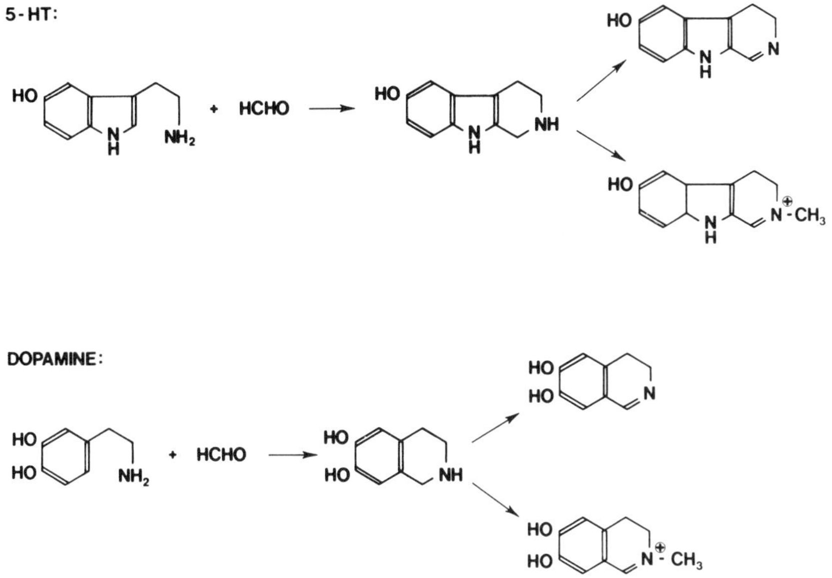

Figure 1. Postulated reaction mechanism for the condensation between formaldehyde and arylethylamines. The end products are intensely fluorescent. For details see text.

OPT-Induced Fluorescence

The fluorometric assay of histamine involves its condensation with o-phthalaldehyde (OPT).[65] This reaction has been adapted for the fluorescence microscopic demonstration of histamine.[16,30,43] The procedure of Ehinger and Thunberg[16] and Håkanson and Owman[30] is sensitive enough to allow the demonstration of histamine also in non-mast-cell stores.[13] The reaction sequence that leads to the formation of the fluorophore and the nature of fluorophore is largely unknown. The spectral characteristics of the OPT-induced histamine fluorophores have been defined in tissues as well as in various model systems (Fig. 3).[26] It should be noted, however, that since the specificity of the OPT method is low, biogenic compounds other than histamine may account for OPT-induced fluorescence (more about this later). The spectral properties of the OPT-induced histamine fluorescence are characteristically concentration-dependent (Fig. 3). Therefore, cytospectrofluorometry will not unequivocally identify the fluorogenic compound. It

171

must be emphasized that although the OPT histofluorescence method can visualize histamine, it is not
capable of identifying the amine, even in conjunction with cytospectrofluorometry. For final identification of the fluorogenic compound, chemical
analysis is necessary.

Amines in Tissues

Catecholamines, histamine and 5-HT occur ubiqui-
tously in the tissues of both vertebrates and inver-
tebrates. To interpret the physiologic roles of
these amines it is essential to know their cellular
storage sites. The fluorescence microscopic technique of Falck and Hillarp[18] has been paramount in
providing such information. As a result amines are
now known to be constituents of many peptide hormone-
secreting cells,[57] as well as of numerous cells which

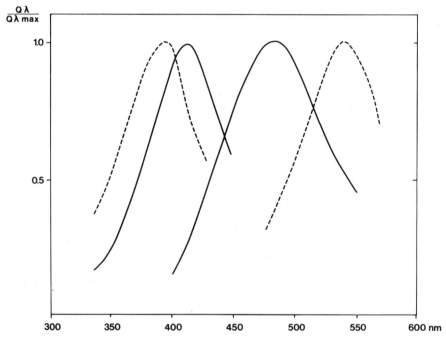

Figure 2. Excitation (left) and emission (right) spectra of
the formaldehyde-induced fluorescence of authentic dopamine
(——) and 5-HT (----) in protein droplet models.

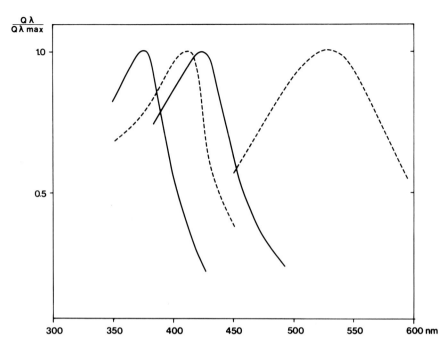

Figure 3. Excitation (left) and emission (right) spectra of
the OPT-induced fluorescence of histamine in two different
concentrations on silica gel models: ——, 0.5 μg/cm^2;
----, 0.5 mg/cm^2.

have an unknown function and are classified as endocrine on morphologic evidence alone. All these cells
are characterized by the presence of narrow cisternae
of endoplasmic reticulum and numerous free ribosomes,
an often-prominent Golgi apparatus, numerous small,
elongated mitochondria, microfilaments, microtubules,
and most important, abundant cytoplasmic membrane-
bound granules (1000-3000 Å). The cells, moreover,
often exhibit a distinct polarity, in that the
cytoplasmic granules predominate in those parts of
the cell facing the capillary bed. 5-HT is present
in the enterochromaffin cells (Fig. 4), which constitute the largest source of 5-HT in the body, in
pancreatic islet cells of several animal species,
and in the calcitonin cells of sheep and goats.[57]
In addition to having been found in adrenomedullary
cells, catecholamines have been found in pancreatic
islet cells, and in few scattered endocrine-like

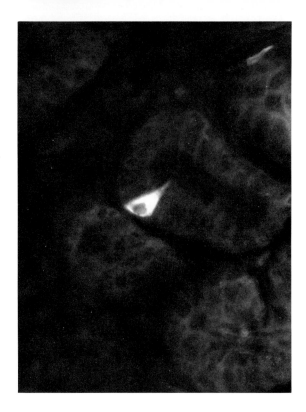

Figure 4a. Yellow-fluorescent endocrine-like cell of the enterochromaffin type in the duodenum of pig. The formaldehyde-induced yellow fluorescence reflects the 5-HT contained in the cell (×500).

Figure 4b. Excitation (left) and emission (right) spectra of the formaldehyde-induced fluorescence.

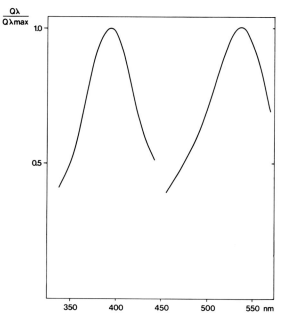

cells of the gastric mucosa of rabbit and cat (Fig. 5), and in the calcitonin cells of the chicken and cow. From cytospectrofluorometry in conjunction with chemical analysis, it appears that the catecholamine in these latter cells is dopamine.[57]

Histamine has been detected by the OPT histofluorescence method (and identified chemically) in a large population of epithelial, argyrophil cells in the oxyntic mucosa of rat and mouse stomach (Fig. 6).[30,31,69] In electron micrographs, they have the characteristics of cells producing peptide hormones.[33] Ultrastructurally, they comprise two different cell types, one with vesicular-type granules and the other with rounded, uniformly electron-dense granules.[33]

In all probability the endocrine and endocrine-like cells produce the amine they contain. Available evidence suggests that the amine is stored in the secretory granules together with the hormone. This conclusion has been reached by electron microscopic histochemistry,[34,40,41] and has been confirmed by subcellular fractionation.[4] The association between the amine and the peptide hormone in the secretory granules suggests a functional role for the amines in the formation, storage, or release of the peptide hormone.[57] So far, however, this is only conjecture.

Most peptide hormone-secreting cells contain no demonstrable amine. It has been known for quite some time, however, that dopa and 5-hydroxy-tryptophan are taken up by the majority of these cells where they are converted into dopamine (Fig. 7) or 5-HT, respectively, which is stored in the secretory granules for at least a few hours.[57] This feature of "amine precursor uptake and decarboxylation" led Pearse[60] to group these cells under the name "APUD-cells." There is no evidence that they differ in any important fashion from those previously discussed endocrine cells which are known to store endogenous dopamine or 5-HT. It is possible that the formation and storage of fluorogenic amines from exogenous precursors in such cells, mimic the elaboration of an endogenous amine which cannot be visualized by available histochemical procedures. The physiologic meaning of the so-called APUD mechanism is unclear, but it has offered convenient means for the fluorescence microscopic detection of polypeptide hormone-producing cells that do not contain histochemically

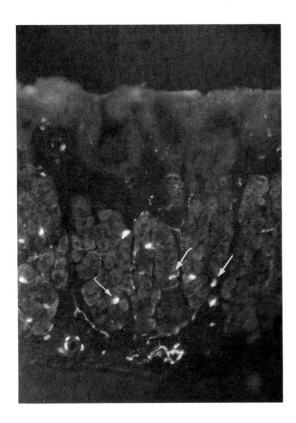

Figure 5a. Green-fluorescent endocrine-like cells (arrows) of the enterochromaffin type (together with yellow-fluorescent enterochromaffin cells) in the oxyntic mucosa of a young cat. The formaldehyde-induced green fluorescence reflects the dopamine contained in the cells (×120).

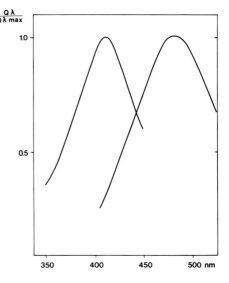

Figure 5b. Excitation (left) and emission (right) spectra of the formaldehyde-induced fluorescence.

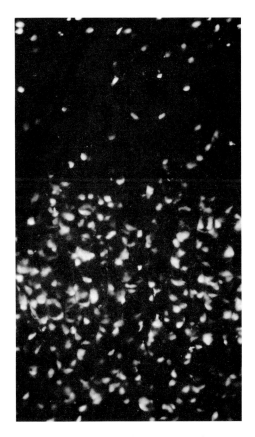

Figure 6. OPT-induced fluorescence in endocrine-like cells of the enterochromaffin-like type[24] in the oxyntic mucosa of the rat. The OPT-induced fluorescence reflects the presence of histamine in these cells (×170).

demonstrable arylethyl amines. It should be noted, however, that the APUD mechanism is shared also by other actively protein-synthesizing cells such as the pancreatic exocrine cells,[2,3] gastric chief cells,[32] and Paneth's cells.[1]

The mucosa of the digestive tract is rich in endocrine-like cells. On the basis of their amine content, they can be divided into two systems, which differ from each other with respect to their chemical and histological properties. The first system - the enterochromaffin cell system - contains 5-HT (Fig. 4) or dopamine (Fig. 5) and stain argentaffin as well as argyrophil. (The dopamine-storing cells in gastric mucosa of rabbit and cat[32] have never actually been shown to be chromaffin or argentaffin; this is merely anticipated, because they are rich in dopamine which - like 5-HT - is a reducing compound.) By immunohistochemistry the motilin cell has recently been shown to be a member of the enterochromaffin cell system.[61] This adds to previous evidence that the enterochromaffin cells in fact comprise several

177

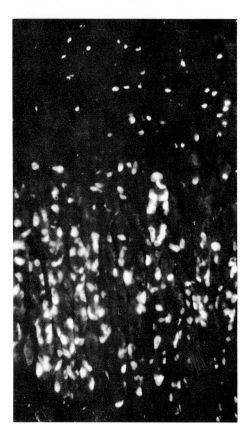

Figure 7. Formaldehyde-
induced green fluorescence
in endocrine-like cells of
rat stomach two hours after
the injection of *L*-dopa.
The fluorescence reflects
the presence of dopamine in
the cytoplasm. Without pretreatment with *L*-dopa,
these cells do not display
formaldehyde-induced fluorescence. Because of their
morphologic resemblance to
the enterochromaffin cells
they are referred to as
enterochromaffin-like
(×170).

distinct cell types.[10,19,32,71] The second system
(enterochromaffin-like according to the terminology
of Håkanson[24]) is made up of epithelial cells which
stain argyrophil but not argentaffin. With argyrophil
staining they are morphologically indistinguishable
from the enterochromaffin cells at the light microscopic level. The enterochromaffin-like cells are
devoid of histochemically detectable arylethylamines.
After treatment of the animal with *L*-dopa, these
cells, which now contain dopamine, can be readily
detected by their typical catecholamine fluorescence
(Fig. 7). In the oxyntic gland area of the rat and
mouse, the enterochromaffin-like cells contain histamine, detectable by its OPT-induced fluorescence
(Fig. 6). Besides these cells, the system of enterochromaffin-like cells (according to the above terminology) have been shown to include the antral gastrin
cells (Larsson, Sundler, Håkanson, unpublished data)
and probably also many other gastrointestinal hormone-
producing cell types.

FLUORESCENCE HISTOCHEMISTRY OF PEPTIDES

On theoretical grounds it appeared likely that formaldehyde would yield fluorophores not only with
certain arylethylamines and their precursor amino
acids, but also with peptides that have these amino
acids in NH_2-terminal position. Of the amino acids
that can be visualized with the Falck-Hillarp technique, dopa and 5-HTP are not common constituents of
peptides or proteins. Tryptophan, however, might be
expected to exist as NH_2-terminus in certain peptides
and proteins. According to an analogous reasoning,
peptides with NH_2-terminal histidine might be expected
to give fluorescence with OPT. These assumptions have
been fully confirmed in model experiments.[25,35-38]

The Formaldehyde-Ozone Method

Tryptamine and tryptophan give weak fluorescence
only upon formaldehyde treatment. The fluorescence
yield of these two compounds, tryptamine in particular,
is much enhanced by the introduction of an oxidant
such as ozone.[7] In model experiments we could show
that this applies also to peptides that contain NH_2-
terminal tryptophan.[37,38] The chemical reaction
sequence is thought to be analogous (Fig. 8) to the
formaldehyde condensation of catecholamines and 5-HT.
With the formaldehyde-ozone method, 5-HT can be
detected with about the same sensitivity as with the
conventional Falck-Hillarp procedure, whereas the
catecholamines give no visible fluorescence. When
this method was applied to specimens from the digestive tract, a number of endocrine and endocrine-
like cells were found to emit strong and characteristic fluorescence (Fig. 9). Such fluorescence was

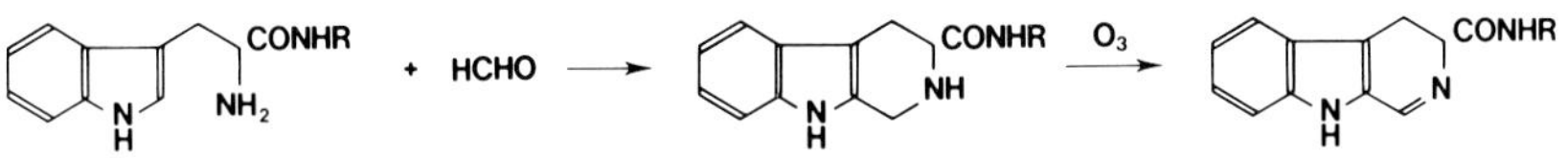

Figure 8. Postulated reaction mechanism for the condensation
between formaldehyde and peptides with NH_2-terminal tryptophan.
The formation of the highly fluorescent end product requires
the presence of an oxidant.

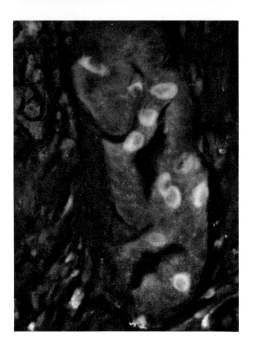

Figure 9a. Formaldehyde-ozone-induced fluorescence in endocrine-like cells in the antropyloric mucosa of rabbit. These cells have been identified as gastrin cells by immunohistochemistry (×340).

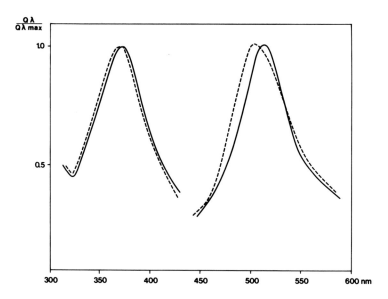

Figure 9b. Excitation (left) and emission (right) of formaldehyde-ozone-induced fluorescence of a gastrin cell in the rabbit antrum (----) and of authentic tryptophyl-glycine in protein droplet models (——).

observed, for instance, in a large population of epithelial cells in antral mucosa of man, pig, rabbit, and cat.[29,51,52] By restaining formaldehyde-ozone-treated sections with antigastrin serum we were able to show that these cells are identical with the gastrin cells.[51,52] As tryptamine cannot be measured chemically in antral mucosa,[29] the cells of the abovementioned species probably contain a peptide (or protein) with NH_2-terminal tryptophan. Studies on fetal rabbits showed that formaldehyde-ozone-induced fluorescence in these cells appears at the same time as does gastrin immunoreactivity.[46] In human fetuses, gastrin cells appear first in duodenal and much later in antral mucosa. In both locations they emit formaldehyde-ozone-induced fluorescence of moderate intensity.[45] Also in pancreatic and duodenal gastrinomas, formaldehyde-ozone treatment induces fluorescence in the gastrin-immunoreactive tumor cells.[47] Subcellular fractionation of such tumors as well as of rabbit antral mucosa, has shown that formaldehyde-ozone-induced fluorescence and peptides with NH_2-terminal tryptophan occur in the fraction containing the gastrin-storing granules.[44] Thus, the secretory granules of the gastrin cells of a number of mammals, including man, appear to contain an unidentified peptide with NH_2-terminal tryptophan. The gastrin components hitherto isolated from antral mucosa (of which heptadecapeptide gastrin is by far the predominant form) do not have tryptophan in the NH_2-terminal position.[22] Thus, some other granular component is probably responsible for the formaldehyde-ozone-induced fluorescence.

The A_1 cells of the human pancreatic islets have been claimed to store compounds with gastrin immunoreactivity.[23,54] No formaldehyde-ozone-induced fluorescence could be detected in these cells.[45] Formaldehyde-ozone treatment induces strong fluorescence in the glucagon-containing A_2-cells of the pancreatic islets of man but not of other species investigated.[45] Conceivably, the human glucagon cells store a peptide with NH_2-terminal tryptophan, although the possibility that these cells store tryptamine cannot as yet be ruled out.

In the small and large intestine of man and cat, scattered epithelial cells showing typical formaldehyde-ozone-induced fluorescence have been observed (unpublished data). Their identity is unknown.

The Formaldehyde-HCl Method

Recently we found that 5 to 10 minutes exposure of formaldehyde gas-treated sections to the fumes of concentrated hydrochloric acid induces strong and characteristic cytoplasmic fluorescence in several different cell systems (Fig. 10).[27,48] From recent model experiments it appears that this method demonstrates tryptophan in peptides and proteins regardless of the position of this amino acid in the molecule.[48,49]

The formaldehyde-HCl method induces strong fluorescence in the gastrin cells of man and cats but not of pigs, rabbits, rats,or chickens.[27,45,48,53] The reason for its failure to demonstrate pig and rabbit gastrin cells which have been shown to contain peptides with NH_2-terminal tryptophan may be that the formaldehyde-HCl method is of lower sensitivity than the formaldehyde-ozone method. Also the duodenal gastrin cells of man display formaldehyde-HCl-induced fluorescence[45] as do gastrin-producing pancreatic tumors (Larsson, unpublished data). The human pancreatic A_1 (or D) cells are nonfluorescent with this method.[45] Formaldehyde-HCl treatment induces instead strong fluorescence in the glucagon cells of the pancreatic islets and in the zymogen granules of pancreatic acinar cells.[45,48] This is not unexpected, since indole stains have long been used to demonstrate these cells.[21,62] It may be noted, however, that the formaldehyde-HCl method is superior to the indole stains in sensitivity and resolution.

In the small and large intestine of man, pigs, and cats, the formaldehyde-HCl method demonstrates a number of disseminated epithelial cells of an endocrine-like appearance (unpublished data). These cells seem to be more numerous than those demonstrated with the formaldehyde-ozone technique. In addition to the endocrine-like cells, Paneth's cells of the small intestine give intense fluorescence upon formaldehyde-HCl treatment.

Tryptophan is found in two positions in the heptadecapeptide gastrin molecule,[22] and the hormone may therefore contribute to the formaldehyde-HCl-induced fluorescence. The gastrin cells of many species, however, do not yield fluorescence upon formaldehyde-HCl treatment, an observation that is difficult to reconcile with the assumption that heptadecapeptide

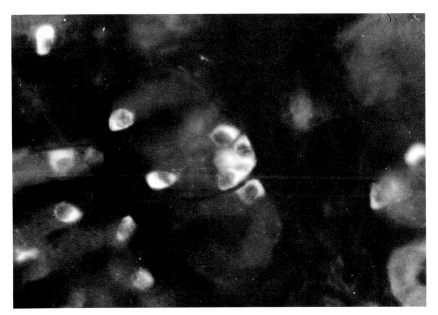

Figure 10a. Formaldehyde-HCl-induced fluorescence in endocrine-like cells in the antropyloric mucosa of cat. These cells have been identified as gastrin cells by immunohistochemistry (×420).

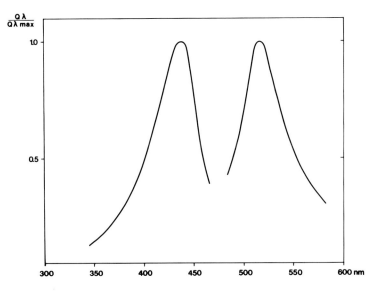

Figure 10b. Excitation (left) and emission (right) of formaldehyde-HCl-induced fluorescence of a gastrin cell in the cat antrum.

gastrin alone is responsible for the formaldehyde-
HCl-induced fluorescence. It is perhaps more likely
that it demonstrates tryptophan also present in additional peptides that are in the secretory granules.
An analogous reasoning may be applied to the glucagon
cells which also give intense fluorescence upon treatment with formaldehyde-HCl; the fact that glucagon
contains only one tryptophan residue speaks against
glucagon being the main contributor to the fluorescence observed. Another glucagon-immunoreactive
peptide, however, has been recognized in glucagon
cells.[39] This molecule, which may represent "pro-
glucagon", has been demonstrated by its ability to
incorporate labeled tryptophan. The contribution
of this peptide to the formaldehyde-HCl-induced
fluorescence is unknown.

The OPT Method

   From model experiments we know that OPT induces
fluorescence not only with histamine, but also with
peptides having histidine in the NH_2-terminal position.[14,25,35] Compared with histamine the peptides
require more vigorous reaction conditions to yield
optimal fluorescence with OPT.[13] OPT-induced fluoresence with spectral properties similar to those
of authentic glucagon has been observed in the glucagon cells of the pancreatic islets (Table 1).[12,15,68]
This fluorescence may be explained by the fact that
the glucagon molecule has NH_2-terminal histidine. The
spectral properties of the OPT-induced fluorescence
of such peptides in histochemical models are similar,
but not identical, to those of the histamine fluorophore (Table 1).[35] OPT readily forms fluorophores
with peptides that have NH_2-terminal histidine also
after formaldehyde treatment,[35] a feature that is not
shared with histamine. This discrepancy between
histamine and peptides with NH_2-terminal histidine is
of importance in the discrimination between these compounds in tissue sections. Another discrepancy of
practical importance is that whereas histamine easily
diffuses in the presence of water and therefore requires strictly controlled conditions for its proper
histochemical visualization, the hitherto demonstrated
peptides do not seem to diffuse. OPT-induced fluorescence occurs in scattered cells in the mucosa within

Table 1. Spectral characteristics of OPT-induced fluoresence of histamine and other cellular constituents

Source	Excitation max. (nm)	Emission max. (nm)**
Gastric endocrine cell (rat)	370	425
Authentic histamine (0.5 µg)*	365	430
Mast cell	370, 410	540
Authentic histamine (0.5 mg)*	375, 410	540
Pancreatic A$_2$-cell (rat)	370, 420	430, 490
Authentic glucagon (1 µg)*	415	490

* Concentration per cm^2 on silica gel model[26]
** The emission spectra were recorded using the mercury lines closest to the values of maximum excitation of the individual fluorophores (i.e., the 365 nm or 405 nm lines).

wide areas of the gastrointestinal tract.[63,64] This fluorescence has been attributed to peptides with NH$_2$-terminal histidine on the basis of criteria specified above.[35] We have observed OPT-reactive cells (probably storing peptides with NH$_2$-terminal histidine) in the fundic mucosa of the canine stomach and in the proventriculus of the chicken.[67] In addition, such cells are frequent in the lower part of the intestine (studied in cats, pigs and humans) (Fig. 11). The OPT-reactive cells in the mucosa of the digestive tract stain argyrophil with the Grimelius silver technique (unpublished data). The identity of the fluorogenic compounds has not yet been established, although hormones known to have NH$_2$-terminal histidine (enteroglucagon, secretin, and vasoactive intestinal peptide, VIP) are the most likely candidates. It should be noted, however, that the OPT-induced fluorescence may reflect the presence of histidyl-peptides other than the recognized hormones.

The Fluorescamine Method

Fluorescamine was introduced a few years ago as a highly sensitive detection reagent for the fluorometric determination of primary amino groups in amines, amino acids, peptides, proteins, phospholipids and

185

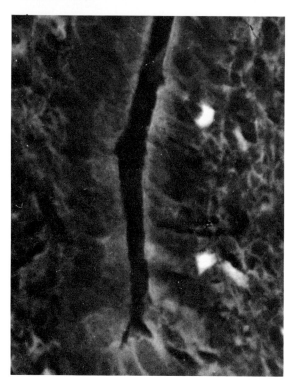

Figure 11. OPT-induced fluorescence in two endocrine-like cells in the ileal mucosa of the cat. The specimen was fixed with gaseous formaldehyde (×420).

amino sugars.[11,56,70] The postulated reaction mechanism is illustrated in Figure 12. Recently we found that fluorescamine was useful also as a histochemical reagent for the demonstration of amino groups.[28] When used in histochemistry, fluorescamine probably does not demonstrate free amines or amino acids since it is to be expected that such compounds are extracted by the handling in aqueous media. Rather, the fluorescamine-induced fluorescence observed in tissue sections derives from larger molecules such as peptides

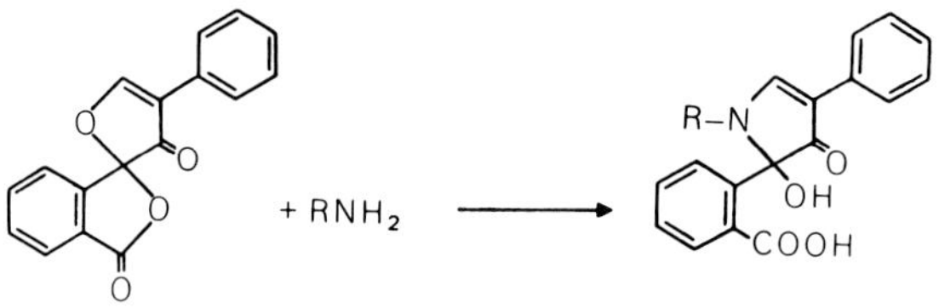

+ RNH₂ ⟶

Figure 12. Postulated reaction sequence for the condensation between primary amines and fluorescamine. The fluorescent end product is water-stable, whereas fluorescamine itself is rapidly broken down by water.

or proteins. From model experiments it appears that
the amidine group of arginine[11] and the ε-amino group
of lysine[55] add only little to the total fluorescence
of peptides and proteins, whereas the NH_2-terminal
amino groups and the amino groups of phospholipids
are the most likely candidates. During the initial
trials with this method, we observed that fixation
with gaseous formaldehyde, known to block amino groups,
did not prevent fluorescamine from inducing intense
fluorescence in certain cell systems, most of which
have an established or anticipated endocrine function.[28,66] Our results indicate that in these cells
certain amino groups are in some way protected from
reacting with formaldehyde, and are thus available
for reaction with fluorescamine. Earlier histochemical results suggest that formaldehyde does not block
all amino groups.[5,58,59] One explanation may be that
the steric configuration "protects" certain amino
groups. The nature of the peptide or protein that
emits fluorescamine-induced fluorescence in the peptide hormone-secreting cells is unknown. A clue to
its function may be offered by observations on thyroid C cells which in some species display strong
fluorescamine-induced fluorescence. In the C cells
of the cat the fluorescence was found to disappear
upon degranulation, which suggests that the fluorescamine-induced fluorescence is given by some granular
component.[50]
    When applied to the gastrointestinal tract, fluores-
camine was found to induce intense fluorescence in a
rich population of cells in the antropyloric mucosa
of a number of species (Fig. 13a), including man, as
well as in scattered cells along the intestinal mucosa (Fig. 13b). In the antrum of chickens and dogs
the fluorescent cells have been identified as the
gastrin cells by restaining fluorescamine-treated
sections with antigastrin serum by using the immunoperoxidase technique for visualization.[50] The distribution of cells emitting fluorescamine-induced fluorescence in the intestinal epithelium has been extensively
studied in cats. Only few fluorescent cells occur in
the upper part of the intestines, whereas they are considerably more numerous in the terminal ileum and
colon. By restaining sections with silver (Grimelius'
technique) the cells were found to be argyrophil.
The fluorescamine-induced fluorescence shows a characteristic distribution to the basal part of the cells,

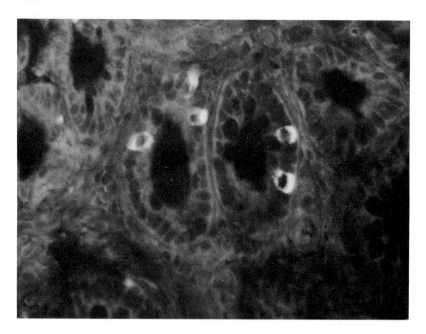

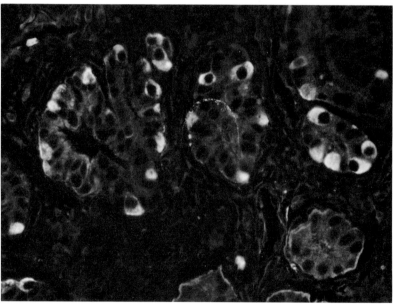

Figure 13a and b. Fluorescamine-induced fluorescence in endocrine-like cells of the gastrointestinal mucosa. a) Section from cat ileum. b) Section from chicken antrum (gizzard-duodenal junction). The specimens were fixed with gaseous formaldehyde and embedded in Araldite (×340).

suggesting that the compound(s) responsible for the fluorescence are stored in the secretory granules.[50] In the gastrin cell, heptadecapeptide gastrin is the main secretory product. This molecule does not possess any free amino groups (pyroglutamic acid is the NH_2-terminus) and therefore cannot be expected to give fluorescamine-induced fluorescence. It is possible that other gastrin components are responsible for the fluorescence. As fluorescamine does not induce fluorescence in the gastrin cells of all species, however, (not in those of the rat, for instance) it is perhaps more likely that the fluorescence derives from some nonhormonal component of the gastrin granules.

SUMMARY

The Nature of the Peptides or Proteins Demonstrated

In the preceding we have described certain properties of polypeptide hormone-secreting cells as conceived by fluorescence histochemical procedures. Many of these properties are shared by several different populations of polypeptide-secreting cells, giving the impression that these cells have many features in common, perhaps reflecting a common ancestry. The intense fluorescence displayed by the different endocrine or endocrine-like cell systems upon treatment with the histochemical methods described, makes it tempting to assume that the compounds demonstrated are present in fairly high concentrations within the cells. The secretory granules are the obvious candidates for storing peptides in such high concentrations. Indeed, subcellular fractionations have shown that the formaldehyde-ozone-[44] and formaldehyde-HCl-induced (unpublished data) fluorescence observed in gastrin cells, is given by some granular component. In studies on the thyroid C-cells we have shown that degranulation abolishes the fluorescamine-induced fluorescence. In all cases, however, the nature of the demonstrated peptide or protein is unknown. It is evident that quite often the fluorescence histochemical findings cannot be explained in terms of the granular content of identified peptide hormones. Therefore the reactions displayed by these cells must reflect the presence of other components in the secretory granules, such as hormone precursors, non-hormonal peptides or proteins engaged in storage of the hormone.

No doubt, histochemistry will prove to be of great value in defining the granular content of the different types of polypeptide hormone-secreting cells. This will help us to understand how these cells function, what they have in common and how they differ from each other.

Acknowledgments

The work described was supported by grants from the Swedish Medical Research Council (04X-1007, 04X-3764) and Riksföreningen mot Cancer (04X-4499).

References

1. Ahonen A: Histochemical and electron microscopic observations on the development, neural control and function of the Paneth cells of the mouse. *Acta Physiol Scand* (suppl 398):5-71, 1973.

2. Alm P: Fluorescence microscopy of the 5-HTP turnover in the exocrine pancreas of mice and rats. *Z Zellforsch Mikrosk Anat* 96:212-221, 1969.

3. Alm P, Ehinger B, Falck B: Histochemical studies on the metabolism of *L*-DOPA and some related substance in the exocrine pancreas. *Acta Physiol Scand* 76:106-120, 1969.

4. Atack CV, Ericson LE, Melander A: Intracellular distribution of amines and calcitonin in the sheep thyroid gland. *J Ultrastruct Res* 41:484-498, 1972.

5. Baker JR: *Principles of Biological Microtechnique: A Study of Fixation and Dyeing*, London: Methuen, 1970.

6. Björklund A, Ehinger B, Falck B: A method for differentiating dopamine from noradrenaline in tissue sections by microspectrofluorometry. *J Histochem Cytochem* 16:263-270, 1968.

7. Björklund A, Falck B, Håkanson R: Histochemical demonstration of tryptamine: Properties of the formaldehyde-induced fluorophores of tryptamine and related indole compounds in models. *Acta Physiol Scand* 74 (suppl 318): 1-31, 1968.

8. Björklund A, Falck B, Lindvall O, Svensson LA: New aspects on reaction mechanisms in the formaldehyde histofluorescence method for monoamines. *J Histochem Cytochem* 21:17-25, 1973.

9. Björklund A, Falck B, Owman C: Fluorescence microscopic and microspectrofluorometric techniques for the cellular localization and characterization of biogenic amines, in Berson SA (ed), *Methods of Investigative and Diagnostic Endocrinology*, vol 1, Amsterdam: North-Holland Publishing Co, 1972, pp 318-368.

10. Black WC 3rd: Enterochromaffin cell types and corresponding carcinoid tumors. *Lab Invest* 19:473-486, 1968.

11. Böhlen P, Stein S, Dairman W, Udenfriend S: Fluorometric assay of proteins in the nanogram range. *Arch Biochem Biophys* 155:213-220, 1973.

12. Brody MJ, Håkanson R, Lundquist I, Owman C, Sundler F: Cellular localization of glucagon by fluorescence microscopy: Reaction of NH2-terminal histidine with o-phthaldialdehyde. *J Histochem Cytochem* 21:13-16, 1973.

13. Brody MJ, Håkanson R, Owman C, Sundler F: An improved method for the histochemical demonstration of histamine and other compounds producing fluorophores with o-phthaldialdehyde. *J Histochem Cytochem* 20:945-948, 1972.

14. Edvinsson L, Håkanson R, Rönnberg AL, Sundler F: Separation of histidyl-peptides by thin-layer chromatography and microspectrofluorometric characterization of their o-phthalaldehyde-induced fluorescence. *J Chromatogr* 67:81-85, 1972.

15. Ehinger B, Håkanson R, Owman C, Sporrong B: Histochemical demonstration of histamine in paraffin sections by a fluorescence method. *Biochem Pharmacol* 17:1997-1998, 1968.

16. Ehinger B, Thunberg R: Induction of fluorescence in histamine-containing cells. *Exp Cell Res* 47:116-122, 1967.

17. Falck B: Observations on the possibilities of the cellular localization of monoamines by a fluorescence method. *Acta Physiol Scand* 56 (suppl 197):1-25, 1962.

18. Falck B, Hillarp NA, Thieme G, Torp A: Fluorescence of catechol amines and related compounds condensed with formaldehyde. *J Histochem Cytochem* 10:348-354, 1962.

19. Ferreira MN: Argentaffin and other "endocrine" cells of the small intestine in the adult mouse: I. Ultrastructure and classification. *Am J Anat* 131:315-330, 1971.

20. Fuxe K, Jonsson G: The histochemical fluorescence method
    for the demonstration of catecholamines: Theory, prac-
    tice, and application. *J Histochem Cytochem* 21:293–
    311, 1973.
21. Glenner GG, Lillie RD: The histochemical demonstration of
    indole derivatives by the post-coupled p–dimethylamino-
    benzylidene reaction. *J Histochem Cytochem* 5:279–296,
    1957.
22. Gregory RA: The gastrointestinal hormones: A review of
    recent advances. (The Bayliss-Starling Lecture, 1973).
    J Physiol 241:1–32, 1974.
23. Greider MH, McGuigan JE: Cellular localization of gastrin
    in the human pancreas. *Diabetes* 20:389–396, 1971.
24. Håkanson R: New aspects of the formation and function of
    histamine, 5-hydroxytryptamine and dopamine in gastric
    mucosa. *Acta Physiol Scand* 79 (suppl 340):1–134, 1970.
25. Håkanson R, Johansson H, Rönnberg AL: OPT-induced fluores-
    cence of glucagon and secretin. *Acta Physiol Scand*
    83:427–429, 1971.
26. Håkanson R, Juhlin L, Owman C, Sporrong B: Histochemistry
    of histamine: Microspectrofluorometric characterization
    of the fluorophores induced by o-phthaldialdehyde.
    J Histochem Cytochem 18:93–99, 1970.
27. Håkanson R, Larsson LI, Nishizaki H, Owman C, Sundler F: A
    new type of formaldehyde-induced fluorescence in a popu-
    lation of endocrine cells in cat antro-pyloric mucosa.
    Histochemie 34:1–9, 1973.
28. Håkanson R, Larsson LI, Sundler F: Fluorescamine: A novel
    reagent for the histochemical detection of amino groups.
    Histochemistry 39:15–23, 1974.
29. Håkanson R, Lindstrand K, Owman C, Sundler F: Tryptamine
    or tryptophyl-peptides in endocrine cells of rabbit
    gastric antrum. *Biochem Pharmacol* 21:1703–1712, 1972.
30. Håkanson R, Owman C: Concomitant histochemical demonstration
    of histamine and catecholamines in enterochromaffin-like
    cells of gastric mucosa. *Life Sci* 6:759–766, 1967.
31. Håkanson R, Owman C: Argyrophilic reaction of histamine-
    containing epithelial cells in murine gastric mucosa.
    Experientia 25:625–626, 1969.
32. Håkanson R, Owman C, Sjöberg NO, Sporrong B: Amine mecha-
    nisms in enterochromaffin and enterochromaffin-like
    cells of gastric mucosa in various mammals. *Histochemie*
    21:189–220, 1970.
33. Håkanson R, Owman C, Sporrong B, Sundler F: Electron micro-
    scopic identification of the histamine-storing argyrophil
    (enterochromaffin-like) cells in the rat stomach.
    Z Zellforsch Mikrosk Anat 122:460–466, 1971.

34. Håkanson R, Owman C, Sporrong B, Sundler F: Electron micro-scopic classification of amine producing endocrine cells by selective staining of ultra-thin sections. *Histo-chemie* 27:226-242, 1971.
35. Håkanson R, Owman C, Sundler F: o-Phthalaldehyde (OPT). A sensitive detection reagent for glucagon, secretin and vasoactive intestinal peptide. *J Histochem Cytochem* 20:138-140, 1972.
36. Håkanson R, Sjöberg AK, Sundler F: Formaldehyde-induced fluorescence of peptides with N-terminal 3,4-dihydroxy-phenylalanine and 5-hydroxytryptophan. *Histochemie* 28:367-371, 1971.
37. Håkanson R, Sundler F: Formaldehyde condensation: A method for the fluorescence microscopic demonstration of pep-tides with NH_2-terminal tryptophan residues. *J Histo-chem Cytochem* 19:477-482, 1971.
38. Håkanson R, Sundler F: Formaldehyde-induced fluorescence of a tryptophyl tetrapeptide. *J Histochem Cytochem* 19:693-695, 1971.
39. Hellerström C, Howell SL, Edwards JC, Andersson A, Östenson CG: Biosynthesis of glucagon in isolated pancreatic islets of guinea pigs. *Biochem J* 140:13-23, 1974.
40. Jaim-Etcheverry G, Zieher LM: Electron microscopic cyto-chemistry of 5-hydroxytryptamine (5-HT) in the beta cells of guinea pig endocrine pancreas. *Endocrinology* 83:917-923, 1968.
41. Jaim-Etcheverry G, Zieher LM: Cytochemical localization of monoamine stores in sheep thyroid gland at the electron microscope level. *Experientia* 24:593-595, 1968.
42. Jonsson G: Microfluorimetric studies on the formaldehyde-induced fluorescence of noradrenaline in adrenergic nerves of rat iris. *J Histochem Cytochem* 17:714-733, 1969.
43. Juhlin L, Shelley WB: Detection of histamine by a new fluorescent o-phthalaldehyde stain. *J Histochem Cyto-chem* 14:525-528, 1966.
44. Larsson LI, Håkanson R, Sundler F: Formaldehyde-ozone-induced fluorescence in isolated gastrin granules, submitted.
45. Larsson LI, Håkanson R, Sjöberg NO, Sundler F: Fluorescence histochemistry of the gastrin cell in foetal and adult man, submitted.
46. Larsson LI, Rehfeld JF, Sundler F, Håkanson R, Stadil F: Concomitant development of gastrin immunoreactivity and formaldehyde-ozone-induced fluorescence in gastrin cells of rabbit antropyloric mucosa. *Cell Tiss Res* 149:329-332, 1974.

47. Larsson LI, Sundler F, Grimelius L, Håkanson R, Buffa R,
    Solcia E: Formaldehyde-ozone-induced fluorescence in
    gastrin-producing tumours. *Virchows Arch [Pathol Anat]*,
    in press.
48. Larsson LI, Sundler F, Håkanson R: Formaldehyde-HCl treat-
    ment: A fluorescence histochemical method for the
    demonstration of tryptophan residues in peptides and
    proteins, submitted.
49. Larsson LI, Sundler F, Håkanson R: Microspectrofluorometric
    characterization of tryptophan-containing peptides on
    paper or silica gel after treatment with formaldehyde,
    formaldehyde-ozone or formaldehyde-HCl, submitted.
50. Larsson LI, Sundler F, Håkanson R: Fluorescamine as a
    histochemical reagent: Observations on the possibili-
    ties of demonstrating polypeptide hormone-secreting
    cells, submitted.
51. Larsson LI, Sundler F, Håkanson R, Grimelius L, Rehfeld JF,
    Stadil F: Histochemical properties of the antral gastrin
    cell. *J Histochem Cytochem* 22:419-427, 1974.
52. Larsson LI, Sundler F, Håkanson R, Rehfeld JF, Stadil F:
    Immunofluorescent localization of gastrin in rabbit
    antropyloric mucosa to argyrophil cells exhibiting
    formaldehyde-ozone-induced fluorescence. *Histochemie*
    37:81-87, 1973.
53. Larsson LI, Sundler F, Håkanson R, Rehfeld JF, Stadil F:
    Distribution and properties of gastrin in the gastro-
    intestinal tract of chicken. *Cell Tiss Res*, in
    press.
54. Lomsky R, Langr F, Vortel V: Immunohistochemical demon-
    stration of gastrin in mammalian islets of Langerhans.
    Nature 223:618-619, 1969.
55. Nakai N, Lai CY, Horecker BL: Use of fluorescamine in the
    chromatographic analysis of peptides from proteins.
    Anal Biochem 58:563-570, 1974.
56. Naoi M, Lee YC, Roseman S: Rapid and sensitive determina-
    tion of sphingosine bases and sphingolipids with fluores-
    camine. *Anal Biochem* 58:571-577, 1974.
57. Owman C, Håkanson R, Sundler F: Occurrence and function
    of amines in endocrine cells producing polypeptide
    hormones. *Fed Proc* 32:1785-1791, 1973.
58. Pearse AGE: *Histochemistry: Theoretical and Applied*, ed 2,
    London: J&A Churchill, 1960, p 122.
59. Pearse AGE: *Histochemistry. Theoretical and Applied*, ed 3,
    vol 1, London: J&A Churchill, 1968.
60. Pearse AGE: The cytochemistry and ultrastructure of poly-
    peptide hormone-producing cells of the APUD series and
    the embryologic, physiologic and pathologic implications
    of the concept. *J Histochem Cytochem* 17:303-313, 1969.

61. Pearse AGE, Polak JM, Bloom SR, Adams C, Dryburgh JR, Brown JC: Enterochromaffin cells of the mammalian small intestine as the source of motilin. *Virchows Arch[Zellpathol]* 16:111–120, 1974.
62. Petersson B, Hellerström C, Hellman B: Some characteristics of two types of A-cells in the islets of Langerhans of guinea pigs. *Z Zellforsch Mikrosk Anat* 57:559–566, 1962.
63. Polak JM, Bloom S, Coulling I, Pearse AGE: Immunofluorescent localization of enteroglucagon cells in the gastrointestinal tract of the dog. *Gut* 12:311–318, 1971.
64. Polak JM, Coulling I, Bloom S, Pearse AGE: Immunofluorescent localization of secretin and enteroglucagon in human intestinal mucosa. *Scand J Gastroent* 6:739–744, 1971.
65. Shore PA, Burkhalter A, Cohn VH: A method for the fluorometric assay of histamine in tissues. *J Pharmacol Exp Ther* 127:182–186, 1959.
66. Sundler F, Larsson LI, Håkanson R, Ljungberg O: Fluorescamine-induced fluorescence in C cell tumours of the thyroid. *Virchows Arch [Pathol Anat]* 363:17–20, 1974.
67. Sundler F, Larsson LI, Håkanson R, Rehfeld JF, Holst J, Stadil F: OPT-reactive cells and gastrin cells in the digestive tract of the chicken. *Agents Actions* 4:208–209, 1974.
68. Takaya K: A new fluorescent stain with o-phthalaldehyde for A cells of the pancreatic islets. *J Histochem Cytochem* 18:178–183, 1970.
69. Thunberg R: Localization of cells containing and forming histamine in the gastric mucosa of the rat. *Exp Cell Res* 47:108–115, 1967.
70. Udenfriend S, Stein S, Böhlen P, Dairman W, Leimgruber W, Weigele M: Fluorescamine: A reagent for assay of amino acids, peptides, proteins and primary amines in the picomole range. *Science* 178:871–872, 1972.
71. Zbinden G, Pletscher A, Studer A: Regionäre Unterschiede der Reserpinwirkung auf enterochromaffine Zellen und 5-Hydroxytryptamin-Gehalt im Magendarmtrakt. *Schweiz Med Wochenschr* 87:629–631, 1957.

THE SECRETORY CYCLE OF THE G-CELL: ULTRASTRUCTURAL AND BIOCHEMICAL INVESTIGATIONS OF THE EFFECT OF FEEDING IN RATS

W. Creutzfeldt, N.S. Track,
C. Creutzfeldt, R. Arnold

Division of Gastroenterology and Metabolism, Department of Medicine, University of Göttingen, Göttingen, Germany

Patients with duodenal ulcer (DU) have a normal number of antral G-cells and at the same time, as a group, an increased immunoreactive gastrin (IRG) concentration of the antral mucosa if compared with healthy controls (Fig. 1).[1] According to the secretory cycle of the G-cell formulated by Forssmann and Orci,[5] the number of electron-dense secretory granules of the G-cells would be expected to be higher in DU patients than in controls. Forssmann and Orci had observed in cats and rats that, in the fasting state, the G-cells contained predominantly electron-dense secretory granules and after feeding, predominantly electron-lucent membranous sacs. This had been interpreted as discharge of the stored hormone from the granules into the cytoplasm and from there into the bloodstream. Despite an increased IRG concentration of the antral mucosa, however, and a normal number of G-cells, DU patients had less electron-dense secretory granules and more electron-lucent membranous sacs in their G-cells (Fig. 2).[1]

The ultrastructural studies of Forssmann and Orci had not been correlated to biochemical findings. Conflicting reports have been presented concerning the effect of feeding upon the antral gastrin content. Fyrö,[6] using a bioassay, described a decrease of the antral gastrin activity 90 and 180 minutes after feeding in cats. Evans, Reeder and Thompson[4] found

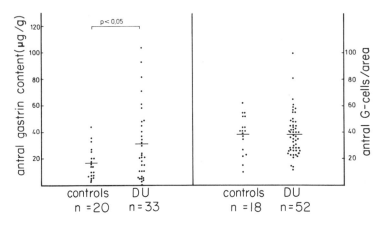

Figure 1. Gastrin (IRG) concentration of extracts from boiled
antral mucosal biopsies (left panel) and number of antral G-
cells (right panel) in controls and in patients with duodenal
ulcer (DU). The G-cells are counted in 5 to 10 different areas
of the mucosal biopsies in each case (mean ± SEM).

no change of the IRG concentration in dogs 90 minutes
after feeding. Lichtenberger and associates[9] detected
a decrease of the antral IRG concentration in rats
during starvation or intravenous alimentation, and an
increase after feeding for longer periods.
    This study was designed to determine how the ultra-
structural changes in G-cell granule appearance in
response to feeding are related to the biosynthesis
and release of IRG from rat antral mucosa.

MATERIAL AND METHODS

    Male Wistar rats (200 to 230 g) were kept on a liq-
uid diet for 72 hours and then fasted for 48 hours.
Fasted rats were fed by intragastric instillation of
2 ml Vivasorb[R] (an amino acid, carbohydrate, fat
solution) and killed by neck dislocation after specific time intervals up to 120 minutes. Serum IRG was
estimated by radioimmunoassay.[10] The antrum was excised and several small pieces were immersed immediately in 3% glutaraldehyde and processed for ultrastructural analysis;[2] the remainder was homogenized
in 10 mM phosphate buffer (pH 7.5). In some experiments, the antrum was homogenized in 0.3 M sucrose
(5 mM phosphate buffer, pH 6.0) at 4C and centrifuged

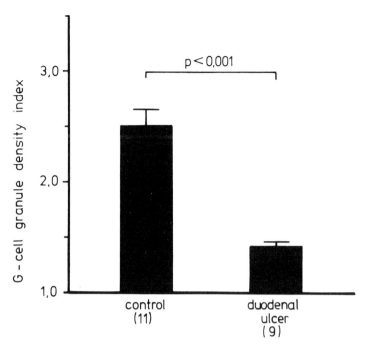

Figure 2. G-cell granule density index (scoring of electron-dense material in G-cell granules) of duodenal ulcer patients and controls. Granules of 10 G-cells per case were counted and scored as follows: empty = 1; intermediate-empty = 2; intermediate-full = 3; full = 4.

at 100,000 g for 60 minutes. All extracts were boiled for 10 minutes and centrifuged, and the IRG and protein content of the supernatant were determined. Antral IRG contents are expressed as ng IRG/mg protein. To calculate the proportion of the total antral IRG in the 100,000-g supernatant (S-100), the S-100 IRG content was divided by the sum of the 100,000-g pellet and supernatant IRG contents.

In an attempt to obtain a quantitative assessment of the overall granule population in the different G-cell activity states, a G-cell granule density index, based upon the electron density of the granule content, was devised. A "full" granule scored 4, an "intermediate full" 3, an "intermediate-empty" 2, and an "empty" granule, 1. Five rats were investigated from each of the following conditions: fasting, 5 minutes, 60 minutes and 120 minutes after feeding.

The secretory granules of 10 antral G-cells were
scored for each rat.

RESULTS

  The fasting serum IRG level was 33.3±1.7 pg/ml
(m ± SEM). A first, minor serum response was detected 10 minutes after feeding (41.1±3.2), and the major

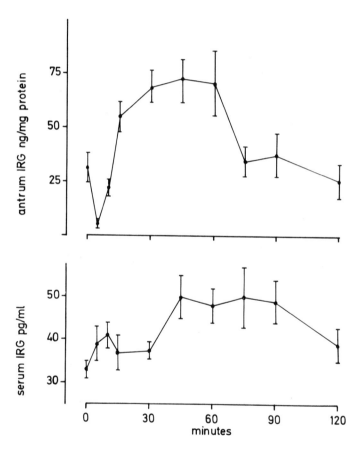

Figure 3. The effect of feeding upon serum (lower
panel) and antral (upper panel) immunoreactive gastrin
(IRG) levels in rats fasted for 48 hours. Each point
represents the result of at least 10 rats (mean ± SEM).

serum response between 45 (50.2±5.3) and 90 (49.2±5.1)
minutes (Fig. 3). There was a moderate increase in
the serum IRG of 5 minutes, at which time a significant *decrease* in the antral IRG was found (fasting:
30.2±5.3 ng/mg; 5 minutes: 4.0±1.2) (Fig. 3). During
the following 25 minutes the antral content increased
dramatically to 70.3±14.1. This high level was maintained until 60 minutes and then it declined gradually.
After only 12 hours fasting, the first serum peak was
even more pronounced. When rats were injected with
cycloheximide (5 mg/kg intraperitoneally) 30 minutes
before feeding, no increase in the antral IRG content
was detected 60 minutes after feeding (Fig. 4).

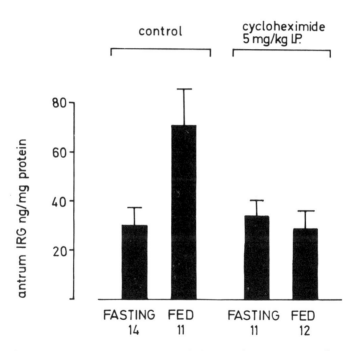

Figure 4. The effect of cycloheximide upon antral
immunoreactive gastrin (IRG) concentration in fasting
and fed rats; 5 mg/kg cycloheximide were injected intraperitoneally 90 minutes before killing. Some of
the rats were fed 60 minutes before killing.

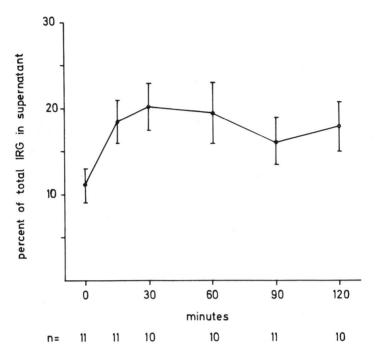

Figure 5. Effect of feeding upon the cellular distribution of immunoreactive gastrin (IRG). The percentage of the total antral IRG present in the 100,000-g supernatant (S-100) was calculated as described in "Methods."

In fasting rats, 11% of the total antral IRG was present in the S-100 (Fig. 5); 15 minutes after feeding, this percentage increased to 18 and remained elevated until 120 minutes.

Ultrastructurally, G-cell granules were characterized as follows: a dark, electron-dense ("full") granule, an intermediate-full, an intermediate-empty (containing only little filamentous material), and a membranous sac ("empty" granule). G-cells from fasting rats contained mainly "full" granules (Fig. 6), whereas 5 minutes after feeding, "empty" granules predominated (Fig. 7). At 60 minutes (Fig. 8) and 120 minutes (Fig. 9), a mixture of the two intermediate and "full" granule types was observed. The calculated G-cell granule density indices for G-cells from fasting, 5-minute, 60-minute and 120-minute rats,

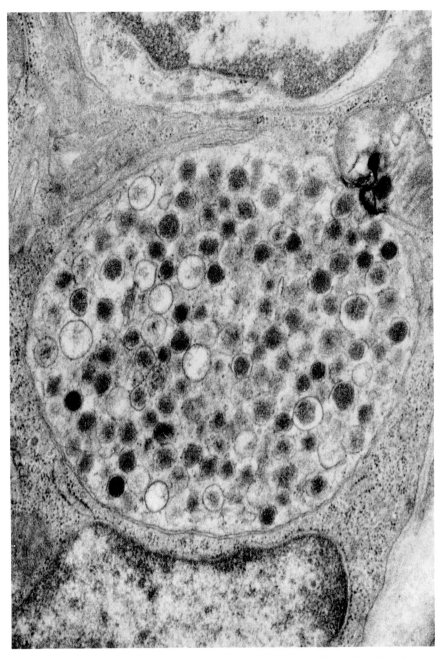

Figure 6. Antral G-cell from a fasting rat. Granules in the basal pole contain electron-opaque or dense material ("full" granules). Few membranous sacs containing filamentous material (×16,800).

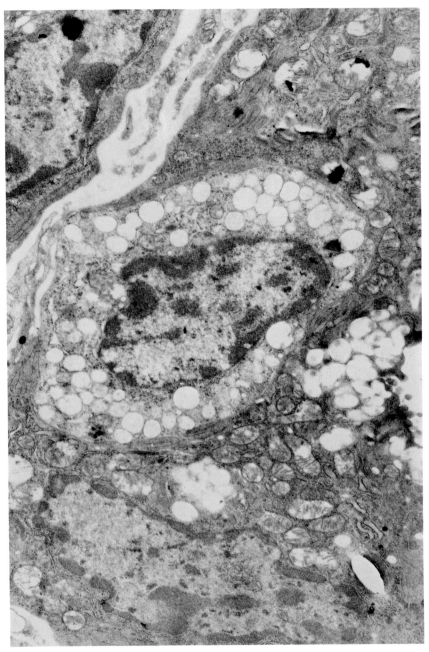

Figure 7. Antral G-cell from a rat five minutes after feeding. Mainly electron-lucent membranous sacs ("empty" granules) in the basal pole orientated towards the capillary (×16,800).

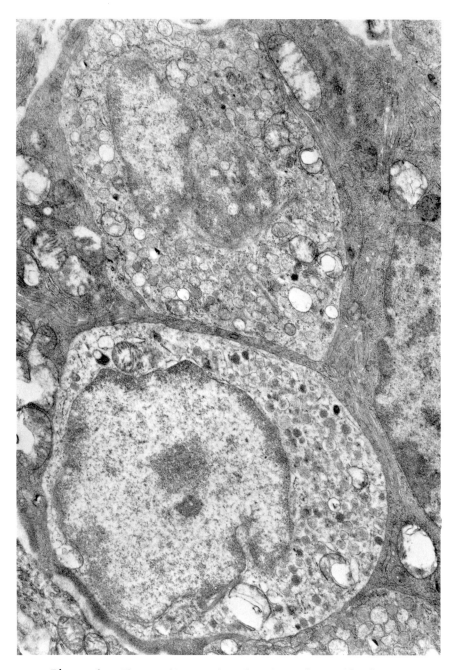

Figure 8. Three adjacent basal poles of G-cells from a
rat 60 minutes after feeding containing granules filled
with electron-opaque material of varying density
(×14,700).

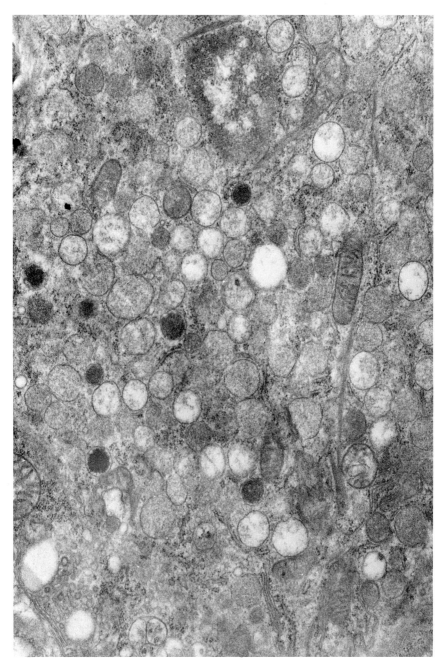

Figure 9. Antral G-cell from a rat 120 minutes after feeding.
Part of the basal pole containing secretory granules of varying
electron density (×20,160).

are depicted in Figure 10. The lower index at five
minutes confirmed the absence of electron-dense granules. The indices at 60 minutes and 120 minutes were
lower than in the fasting state despite significantly
higher IRG concentration (Fig. 3).

DISCUSSION

Five minutes after feeding the striking predominance of "empty" granules occurs concomitantly with
a drastic depletion of the antral IRG concentration.

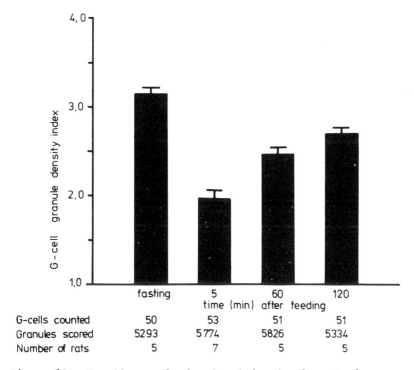

Figure 10. G-cell granule density index in the antral mucosa
of rats after feeding. A high index means many electron-dense
secretory granules, a low index, many electron-lucent membranous sacs. The indices at 5 minutes, 60 minutes, and 120
minutes after feeding are significantly lower than the fasting
index (p <0.001). The indices at 60 and 120 minutes are significantly higher than the 5-minute index (p <0.001).

This finding suggests that these electron-lucent membranous sacs contain very low levels of IRG or none at all. In the ensuing 60 minutes, more electron-dense granules appear, the antral IRG concentration increases 15-fold over the 5-minute value, and 8% more of the total antral IRG is present in the S-100. The suppression of the dramatic antral IRG increase by cycloheximide suggests that this increase is the result of newly synthesized IRG. The higher percentage of IRG in the S-100 from 15 to 120 minutes after feeding, denotes the presence of more cytoplasmic IRG. As a measure of the nongranular IRG, these values may be an underestimation, since during the rapid synthetic phase (10 to 60 minutes), higher IRG levels may be present in the microsomal fraction which would sediment in the 100,000-g pellet with the granules.

Thus, these biochemical and ultrastructural results suggest that the first, minor serum response (10 minutes after feeding) comes from IRG stored in granules and the second, major serum response (45 to 90 minutes after feeding) results mainly from newly synthesized IRG.

The results also suggest that the hormone turnover in the antral G-cells is much faster than in the pancreatic B-cell. Here, newly synthesized insulin is not released before 60 minutes and only in small amounts.[2] Normally, only a small percentage of the insulin stored in secretory granules is released after any stimulus and thereafter the stores are refilled. Insulin is released usually by extrusion of secretory granules (emiocytosis). Only under extreme conditions,[12] and especially in insulinoma cells, nongranular insulin release occurs.[2,3] Gastrin is also stored in secretory granules, but the content of these granules seems to be discharged into the cytoplasm. Emiocytosis has not been observed in cats, rats, or man by Forssmann and Orci[5] or in our studies. Inconsistent occurrence of emiocytosis has been described only by Japanese authors in dogs[7] and man,[11] both after infusion of the antrum with $NaHCO_3$ solution which is a doubtful releaser of gastrin.[8]

The quick change of the antral IRG concentration after feeding, with a 15-fold increase between the 5- and 60-minute values, and the prevention of this increase by cycloheximide, suggest that stimulation of the G-cell induces not only release of stored gastrin but also immediate biosynthesis of the hormone. Possibly, the newly synthesized gastrin can be directly released from the cytoplasm, bypassing the granule-storage stage. This pool seems to be quantitatively more important after stimulation than the hormone stores.

The findings may help to explain the conflicting results published so far on antral gastrin concentration after feeding. Since gastrin release is immediately followed by gastrin synthesis and newly synthesized gastrin contributes a major part to gastrin secretion, antral gastrin concentration is a poor parameter for evaluation of G-cell activity. For the same reason, the ultrastructural evaluation of the G-cell activity using the granule-density index must be done with caution. A low granule-density index indicates always that gastrin has been released recently from granule stores; however, it gives no indication about the total amount of gastrin in the cell. The discrepancy between the elevated IRG content of the antral mucosa together with a low granule-density index found in patients with duodenal ulcer, must be explained by increased amounts of cytoplasmic IRG. The high fasting acidity of DU patients prevents the release of these cytoplasmic gastrin stores. If this inhibitory mechanism is interrupted by feeding or stimulation with concomitant gastric aspiration, however, an exaggerated hormone release occurs. This explains the well-established increased serum IRG response of DU patients to different stimuli.[10]

SUMMARY

1. After fasted rats were fed, they showed a small early increase of serum immunoreactive gastrin (IRG) levels at 10 minutes and a major response between 45 and 90 minutes.
2. IRG concentration of antral mucosa was significantly decreased 5 minutes after feeding and increased 15-fold in the next 25 minutes. This increase of antral IRG concentration could be prevented by intraperitoneal injection of cycloheximide 30 minutes before feeding.
3. The percentage of total IRG in the antral mucosa present in the 100,000-g supernatant increased after feeding.

4. Ultrastructurally, the secretory granules of the
    antral G-cells showed characteristic changes after
    feeding. The granule-density index decreased
    significantly 5 minutes after feeding and in-
    creased again after 60 and 120 minutes without
    reaching the fasting level. Since the IRG con-
    centration at these times was higher than in the
    fasting state, more of their IRG was present in
    a nongranular form in the cytoplasm.
5. These findings suggest that stimulation of the
    G-cell induces release and immediate synthesis
    of IRG and that newly synthesized IRG contributes
    to a major extent to the increase of serum IRG
    levels after feeding.

Acknowledgment

  The authors thank Miss Elisabeth Bothe, Miss Heidi Dörler,
and Miss Jutta Weigt for their expert technical assistance.
This work was supported by the Deutsche Forschungsgemeinschaft,
Bonn-Bad Godesberg, grant Cr 20/7.

References

1. Creutzfeldt W, Creutzfeldt C, Arnold R: Gastrin producing
       cells, in Chey WY and Brooks FP (eds), *Endocrinology
       of the Gut,* Thorofare, NJ: Charles B. Slack, Inc, 1974,
       pp 35-62.
2. Creutzfeldt C, Track NS, Creutzfeldt W: In vitro studies
       of the rate of proinsulin and insulin turnover in seven
       human insulinomas. *Eur J Clin Invest* 3:371-384, 1971.
3. Creutzfeldt W, Arnold R, Creutzfeldt C, Deuticke U, Frerichs
       H, Track NS: Biochemical and morphological investiga-
       tions of 30 human insulinomas: Correlation between the
       tumour content of insulin and proinsulin-like components
       and the histological and ultrastructural appearance.
       Diabetologia 9:217-231, 1973.
4. Evans JC, Reeder DD, Thompson JC: Gastrin concentration
       in gastric mucosa: Effect of food and antrectomy.
       Arch Surg 106:717-718, 1973.
5. Forssmann WG, Orci L: Ultrastructure and secretory cycle
       of the gastrin-producing cell. *Z Zellforsch Mikrosk
       Anat* 101:419-432, 1969.

6. Fyrö B: Effect of feeding on antral and duodenal gastrin
    activity. *Acta Physiol Scand* 74:166-172, 1968.
7. Kobayashi S, Fujita T: Emiocytotic granule release in the
    basal-granulated cells of the dog induced by intra-
    luminal application of adequate stimuli, in Fujita T
    (ed), *Gastro-Entero-Pancreatic Endocrine System*,
    Stuttgart: Georg Thieme Verlag, 1974, pp 49-58.
8. Levant JA, Walsh JH, Isenberg JI: Stimulation of gastric
    secretion and gastrin release by single oral doses of
    calcium carbonate in man. *N Engl J Med* 289:555-558,
    1973.
9. Lichtenberger LM, Castro GA, Copeland EM, Dudrick SJ,
    Johnson LR: The effect of food on rat antral gastrin
    concentration, abstracted. *Gastroenterology* 66:874,
    1974.
10. Mayer G, Arnold R, Feurle G, Fuchs K, Ketterer H, Track NS,
    Creutzfeldt W: Influence of feeding and sham feeding
    upon serum gastrin and gastric acid secretion in
    control subjects and duodenal ulcer patients. *Scand
    J Gastroenterol* 9:703-710, 1974.
11. Osaka M, Sasagawa T, Fujita T: Emiocytotic granule release
    in the human antral endocrine cells, in Fujita T (ed),
    Gastro-Entero-Pancreatic Endocrine System, Stuttgart:
    Georg Thieme Verlag, 1974, pp 59-63.
12. Track NS, Frerichs H, Creutzfeldt W: Release of newly
    synthesized proinsulin and insulin from granulated
    and degranulated isolated rat pancreatic islets. The
    effect of high glucose concentration. *Horm Metab
    Res*, in press.

TROPHIC ACTIONS OF GI HORMONES

TROPHIC ACTION OF GASTROINTESTINAL HORMONES

Leonard R. Johnson

Program in Physiology, University of Texas
Medical School, Houston, Texas

A definition of the word, hormone, will usually
include the phrase, "---a blood-borne regulator of
metabolism and/or secretion." Unfortunately, until
the past few years the possible metabolic effects of
gastrin, cholecystokinin (CCK), and secretin had not
been explored. The reasons for this apparent over-
sight are probably numerous and must certainly include
the fact that the gastrointestinal hormones were discovered because of, and named for, their effects on
secretion or motility, the lack of chemically pure
and synthetic preparations until recent years, and
the lack of interest in the gastrointestinal tract
on the part of endocrinologists and biochemists. As
a result of the work of Gregory and Tracy in England
and Jorpes and Mutt in Sweden, gastrointestinal hormones and active peptides became available in pure
and synthetic preparations in the mid-1960s. Not only
has this led to a clarification of their role in the
regulation of secretion and motility but also to the
realization that the gastrointestinal hormones are
important trophic agents for some tissues of the
gastrointestinal tract.[6]
The first presumptive evidence that gastrointestinal
hormones influenced growth can be found in a number
of reports describing the effects of antrectomy and
vagotomy on the histology of the remaining gastric
mucosa. Lees and Grandjean[14] studied biopsy specimens
of the gastric mucosal remnant in 33 healthy postan-
trectomy patients. They classified only one of these
as normal and 22 as exhibiting moderate to complete
atrophy. Melrose and associates,[18] on the other hand,
found no instances of gastric mucosal atrophy in

biopsy specimens from 41 patients, 1 to 10 years postvagotomy. In another study 56 patients, 81.5% of whom
had had normal preoperative gastric mucosal biopsies,
were subjected to antrectomy for duodenal ulcer.[5]
Twelve months later 70.4% demonstrated atrophic gastri-
tis and decreased thickness of the oxyntic gland mucosa.
Hypotrophy from decreased acid secretion does not
appear to be a factor since vagotomy causes a comparable decrease in acid output.

Hypergastrinemia associated with Zollinger-Ellison
syndrome results in the opposite condition. Gastric
and duodenal mucosal hyperplasia with an increased
parietal cell count are characteristic of this disease.[3] Thus, the overproduction of gastrin is associated with mucosal growth, and the lack of hormone
is associated with atrophy.

These observations led us in 1969 to examine the
effects of pentagastrin on the incorporation *in vitro*
of ^{14}C-leucine into protein of gastric and duodenal
mucosa. These tissues from rats injected with 250
µg/kg pentagastrin showed a 100% to 200% increase in
incorporation of amino acids into protein compared to
saline- or histamine-injected controls. Stimulation
did not occur in either the liver or skeletal muscle.
At that time we hypothesized that gastrin was a trophic
hormone for certain tissues of the gastrointestinal
tract and that this action was independent of its
ability to stimulate acid secretion.[8]

SPECTRUM OF TROPHIC RESPONSES TO GASTRIN

Gastrin has been shown to increase a number of growth-
related parameters and components of the pleiotypic
response (Table 1). Chronic administration of pharmacologic doses of pentagastrin *in vivo* produces parietal cell hyperplasia.[2,20] The hyperplasia, however,
is more general and probably involves most of the
mucosal cell types.[6]

Continuous infusion of pentagastrin for four hours
stimulates mitosis in the oxyntic gland area of the
dog.[21] Increased mitotic activity occurred for approximately 24 hours after the infusion was stopped. Infusion of histamine in a dose that produces comparable
acid secretion had no effect on cell division or DNA
synthesis.

Table 1. Growth-related responses stimulated by gastrin

in vivo	*in vitro*
1. Mucosal hyperplasia	1. Maintain epithelial cell line
2. Mitosis	2. Decrease doubling time
3. DNA synthesis	3. Increase proliferative population
4. Protein synthesis	4. Mitosis
5. RNA synthesis	5. DNA synthesis
	6. Protein synthesis

The synthesis of DNA, RNA, and protein have been studied in detail. Single injections of pentagastrin result in a peak increase in DNA synthesis 16 hours later.[11] The degree of stimulation appears to depend upon the cell turnover time of the tissue involved. For example, the effect on DNA synthesis in duodenal mucosa is usually greater than it is on oxyntic gland mucosa. Protein and RNA synthesis are also stimulated by single injections of pentagastrin, but the peak effect occurs sooner after injection. The proteins whose synthesis is stimulated by gastrin are not se-creted when mucosal specimens are incubated in tissue culture medium.[6] This latter observation indicates that these proteins are probably involved in the syn-thesis of cell components.

Chronic administration of pentagastrin as six injec-tions (250 µg/kg) over a period of 48 hours results in significantly increased levels of DNA, RNA, and pro-tein.[6] These observations rule out the unlikely pos-sibility that increased synthesis is being matched by increased catabolism and cell turnover.

Many of the trophic responses to pentagastrin *in vivo* have been reproduced by adding the pentapeptide *in vitro* to cultures of gastric and duodenal mucosal cells. Pentagastrin inhibited fibroblast growth and promoted the proliferation of epithelial cells in cul-tures of gastric and duodenal mucosa.[16,19] Penta-gastrin-treated cultures of rat duodenal cells had a faster doubling time, 19.5 hours, as compared to 31.5 hours for saline-treated controls.[16] This was due in part to the greater percentage of proliferative cells in the hormone-treated cultures, 73% in comparison to 36% for the controls. The latter determination was done by measuring the incorporation of ^{3}H-thymidine into DNA. The important general conclusion from the cell culture studies *in vitro* is that the trophic effects of gastrin *in vivo* are not mediated by a secondary agent but are direct effects of gastrin itself.

SPECIFICITY OF THE TROPHIC ACTION OF GASTRIN

The tissues trophically stimulated by pentagastrin are listed in Table 2. The action of pentagastrin on the oxyntic gland area of the stomach, duodenum, and pancreas is well documented.[6] In addition, a single injection of pentagastrin resulted in a several-fold increase of DNA synthesis in the ileum.[11] Six injections of pentagastrin over a 48-hour period significantly stimulated DNA synthesis and increased the amounts of DNA and RNA present in the large intestine (unpublished data).

Notable exceptions to the trophic action of gastrin on gastrointestinal tissues are the esophagus and antrum. Gastrin does not increase the incorporation of ^{14}C-leucine into the antrum *in vivo*,[7] nor does it increase DNA synthesis in this tissue or in the esophagus (unpublished data).

The trophic action of gastrin is apparently restricted to the mucosa, at least in the stomach and duodenum. We found no stimulation of protein synthesis in the serosal layer of the stomach[7] and have been unable to demonstrate an effect of pentagastrin on DNA synthesis in the smooth muscle layer of the stomach or

Table 2. Tissue specificity of trophic action of gastrin

Stimulation	No Effect
1. Oxyntic gland area	1. Esophagus
2. Duodenum	2. Antrum
3. Ileum	3. Liver
4. Colon	4. Skeletal muscle
5. Pancreas	5. Kidney

duodenum (unpublished data). In those experiments
DNA synthesis in the mucosa scraped from the same
tissues was doubled by pentagastrin.

To this date, without exception, gastrin has proved
to have no trophic effects on tissues outside the
gastrointestinal tract. Several studies have employed
liver and skeletal muscle as nongastrointestinal tract
control tissues.[8,11] In addition, organs such as the
kidney, spleen, and testis have been examined without
finding increases in size after chronic exposure to
pentagastrin.[13]

MECHANISM OF THE TROPHIC ACTION OF GASTRIN

Gastrin stimulates RNA, protein, and DNA synthesis
in numerous gastrointestinal tract tissues. These are
the most important components of the pleiotypic response to growth-promoting hormones. The effects of gastrin on these biosynthetic processes plus the stimulation of mucosal hyperplasia by chronic doses occur independently of acid secretion.[6] Histamine stimulates
neither hyperplasia[2,6] nor DNA synthesis.[11,21] Injections of the H_2-antagonist, metiamide, which blocked
gastrin-stimulated acid secretion, did not significantly reduce the gastrin effect on DNA synthesis.[12]
The previously mentioned experiments in which gastrin,
administered *in vitro*, stimulated protein and DNA
synthesis and mitosis in cultures of gastric and duodenal cells, prove that the trophic action of this
hormone is a direct one, dependent on neither changes
in the environment of the gut nor on a secondary
trophic agent.

DNA synthesis is often monitored as an index of
trophic stimulation because it actually indicates cell
division. The increase and the peak stimulation of
DNA synthesis in target tissue response to growth hormone, thyroid-stimulating hormone, adrenocorticotrophic
hormone, and other growth-promoting hormones is usually
preceded by increases in both RNA and protein synthesis. As shown in Figure 1, ileal, duodenal, and
oxyntic gland DNA synthesis peak 16 hours after a
single injection of pentagastrin in the rat.[11] The
same amount of time also elapses between stimulation
and peak synthetic rates in the dog gastric mucosa.[21]

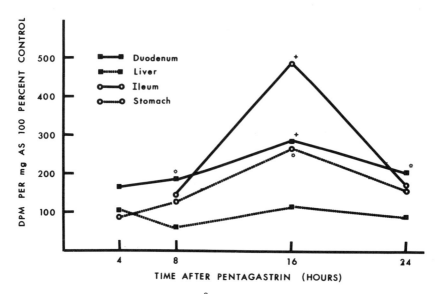

Figure 1. Incorporation of ^{3}H–thymidine into DNA of stomach, liver, duodenum, and ileum at various times after the injection of pentagastrin. * = p <0.01, + = p <0.001. (Reproduced, with permission of *Gastroenterology*.[11])

The incorporation of ^{14}C-leucine into protein of gastric and duodenal mucosa increases approximately four hours after an injection of pentagastrin and reaches peak rate two to three hours later.[4] RNA synthesis, determined by measuring ^{14}C-orotic acid incorporation increases more rapidly and attains maximal rates two or three hours after pentagastrin injection (Enochs and Johnson, unpublished data). The different time patterns for incorporation of labeled material into duodenal mucosal RNA, protein, and DNA after administration of pentagastrin are shown in Figure 2. Whether the increase in protein synthesis is dependent on transcription of RNA is not known at this point. We have examined the different species of RNA, and in preliminary studies pentagastrin increased the synthesis of transfer, messenger and ribosomal RNA. Although these studies are incomplete, it does appear that the RNA, protein, and DNA synthetic responses are similar to those initiated by other trophic hormones. The primary effect of gastrin may well be the stimulation of RNA synthesis, which leads to protein formation and eventually cell division.

220

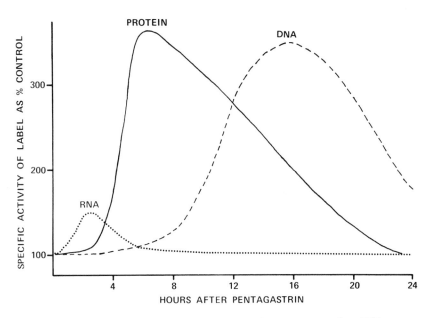

Figure 2. Composite of approximate time courses for RNA, protein, and DNA synthesis in the duodenum following a single injection of pentagastrin.

TROPHIC EFFECTS OF OTHER AGENTS RELATED TO THE GASTROINTESTINAL TRACT

Chronic administration of secretin prevents parietal cell hyperplasia and the increased secretory capacity induced by multiple injections of pentagastrin.[20] Whether this action of secretin could be considered as antitrophic and separate from its ability to inhibit gastric acid secretion, was the subject of a recent study. A single injection of secretin (75 U/kg) inhibited gastrin-stimulated DNA synthesis in both the stomach and duodenum (Fig. 3), indicating that this hormone can also affect biosynthetic processes related to growth.[12] The H_2-receptor antagonist, metiamide, which inhibits gastrin-stimulated acid secretion, did not significantly decrease the stimulation of DNA synthesis promoted by pentagastrin (Fig. 4). Thus, it appears that secretin may act as an antitrophic agent for tissues of the gastrointestinal tract which respond to gastrin.[12] As in the case of gastrin, this action of secretin does not depend upon acid secretion. Whether secretin acts only

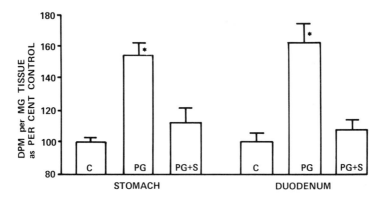

Figure 3. DNA synthesis in oxyntic gland area and duodenum measured as the incorporation of ^{3}H-thymidine. Animals were killed 16 hours after an injection of NaCl (C), pentagastrin (PG) or pentagastrin + secretin (PG + S). Means and standard errors of means for 16 observations. $* = p <0.001$. (Reproduced, with permission of *Gastroenterology.*[12])

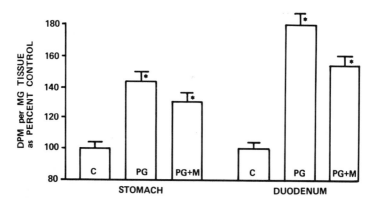

Figure 4. Same as Figure 3 except M = metiamide, 2.0 mg/kg. $* = p <0.001$. (Reproduced, with permission of *Gastroenterology.*[12])

222

to inhibit gastrin-mediated growth or whether it exerts negative effects of its own has not been thoroughly investigated.

Possible trophic actions of CCK have been sought only in the pancreas where it stimulated DNA synthesis and increased the RNA and protein content.[17] Thus, the trophic response to CCK is similar to that caused by gastrin in the same organ and in the other tissues that respond trophically to gastrin.[6] In recently completed experiments, six injections of CCK-octapeptide administered over 48 hours failed to increase DNA synthesis or the RNA and DNA content of the gastric mucosa (Johnson and Guthrie, unpublished data). There were, however, slight, but statistically significant, increases of DNA synthesis and of RNA and DNA content of duodenal mucosa. The C-terminal tetrapeptide of gastrin reproduces all of the biologic actions of the hormone and is identical to the four C-terminal amino acids of CCK. A peptide is more closely related to CCK when its potency for gallbladder contraction and pancreatic enzyme secretion is much greater than for gastric acid secretion. Structurally these peptides differ significantly from the gastrin-related compounds in that the tyrosyl residue is located in the seventh position from the C-terminal end of the molecule and is sulfated. If tyrosine is unsulfated or located in the sixth position, the gastrin pattern predominates. From the foregoing results it appears that peptides possessing the gastrin-like pattern of activity are more potent trophic agents than those related to CCK.

In the same series of studies, prostaglandin E_2 did not stimulate DNA synthesis in the stomach. Since PGE_2 inhibits gastrin-stimulated acid secretion, it was also administered in conjunction with pentagastrin. Unlike secretin, PGE_2 did not alter the trophic response to gastrin. In the duodenum PGE_2 caused a slight increase in DNA synthesis, but the overall amount of DNA was not increased. It is doubtful, therefore, whether PGE_2 is a trophic agent for either the stomach or duodenum.

The trophic responses of the oxyntic gland area and duodenum to the gastrointestinal hormones and related agents are summarized in Table 3.

Table 3. Trophic activity of gut hormones and other agents

	Oxyntic Gland	Duodenum
Gastrin	S	S
CCK	0	S
Secretin	I	I
Histamine	0	0
Metiamide	0a	0a
PGE$_2$	0a	S

S = stimulation
0 = no effect
I = inhibition of gastrin
a = does not inhibit gastrin

SIGNIFICANCE OF THE TROPHIC ACTION OF GASTROINTESTINAL HORMONES

Trophic responses to gastrin have been demonstrated in rats[6] and dogs.[21] The material mentioned at the beginning of this chapter dealing with histologic studies of gastric mucosa from patients who had had gastrectomy or Zollinger-Ellison syndrome, may be interpreted as presumptive evidence of trophic activity in man. Direct studies of the trophic action of gastrin, however, have not been done in man.

The classical method of proving that an effect is due to a particular hormone is to remove the source of the hormone, observe the effect or absence of it, supply the hormone exogenously, and abolish the effect. In rats, antrectomy resulted in approximately 40% decreases in the RNA and DNA content of the duodenum and stomach. A series of pentagastrin injections given to half the antrectomized rats prevented the changes in nucleic acid content.[9] Thus, negative effects on growth of gastrointestinal tissues are caused by removing endogenous gastrin and prevented by supplying the hormone exogenously. This is strong evidence that endogenous gastrin has a physiologic function as a trophic hormone.

Further evidence of the importance of the trophic action of gastrin was derived from studies on newborn rats.[15] Major developmental changes in the structure and physiology of the rat intestine occur during the third week of life when weaning begins. Antral gastrin concentration increased dramatically

at this time from 2 to 18 µg/gm.[15] To test whether
these events were causally related, a group of 14-day-
old rats was prevented from weaning, whereas another
group was allowed to wean normally. The ratios of
gut weight to body weight, gut RNA to body weight,
and gut protein to body weight were significantly
lower in the unweaned rats. Antral gastrin content
also failed to increase substantially in the unweaned
group. In a second series of rats both groups were
prevented from weaning, but one group received injections of pentagastrin. Exogenous pentagastrin significantly increased the ratios of gut to body weight
to values comparable to those seen in weaned rats of
the same age. Thus, some aspects of gut development
are dependent on weaning, and it appears that gastrin
may be the mediator between these two events.[15]

Short periods of food deprivation result in profound
adverse effects on gastrointestinal structure and
function. The factors responsible for the changes in
the gut being more severe than for the remainder of
the body are unknown. In a series of recent studies,
this laboratory has used the intravenously alimented
rat as a model to study gut structure and function in
the well-nourished rat whose gastrointestinal tract
has gone unexposed to food.[1,10,13] Several findings
from those studies are significant to this discussion.
First, ratios of tissue to body weight for the oxyntic
gland area of the stomach, small intestine, and pancreas were significantly reduced in the parenterally
fed rats, whereas the weights of other organs were unaffected. Second, specific and total activities of
the different disaccharidase enzymes were only a fraction of those measured in the orally fed controls.
Third, the parenterally fed rats were nearly depleted
of antral gastrin. Fourth, these results could not
be explained on the basis of food intake, dietary
constituents, enzyme induction, or by the absence of
luminally-derived nutrition in the parenterally fed
rats.

In another set of experiments, one group of intravenously hyperalimented (IVH) rats received a continuous infusion of 60 µg/kg/hr pentagastrin, a dose
less than the D_{50} for acid secretion in this species.
The rats were killed from 10 to 19 days after the
beginning of parenteral feeding and compared to IVH
rats receiving histamine or nothing in addition to the
liquid diet. Serum as well as antral gastrin concentrations decreased significantly in the IVH groups

(Fig. 5). Weights of the oxyntic gland area, small
intestine, and pancreas decreased significantly.
This weight change was, for the most part, prevented
by pentagastrin (Fig. 6). Disaccharidase activities
again decreased precipitously in the IVH rats. Exogenous gastrin completely prevented the change in
disaccharidase activity (Fig. 7). Peroxidase decreased
to 50% of control levels in the IVH rats. This enzyme
probably decreased due to decreased inflammation and
inflammatory cells in the intestines of the parenterally fed rats. As expected, peroxidase activity was
not altered by pentagastrin. These data indicate that
the oral ingestion of food and its presence in the
gastrointestinal tract are necessary to maintain endogenous gastrin levels, and that the trophic action
of endogenous gastrin is essential for the day-to-day

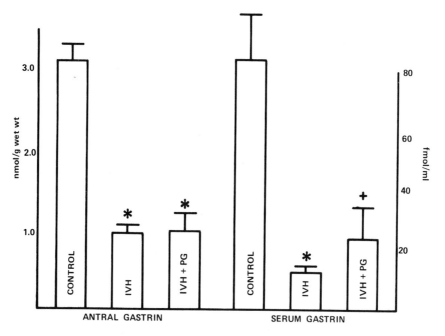

Figure 5. Antral and serum gastrin levels in control, IVH
(intravenously hyperalimented), and IVH rats receiving a continuous infusion of pentagastrin (6.0 µg/kg/hr). Bars and
vertical lines are means and standard errors of the means
for 10 observations. * = p <0.001, + = p <0.005. (Reproduced,
with permission of *Gastroenterology*.[13])

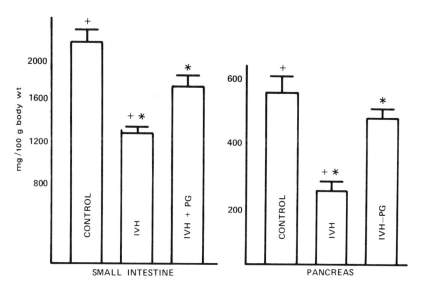

Figure 6. Weights of small intestine and pancreas from rats described in Figure 5. Data are expressed as mg/100 g body weight. + = $p < 0.001$, * = $p < 0.01$. (Reproduced, with permission of *Gastroenterology*.[13])

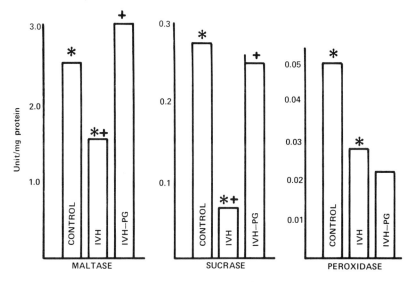

Figure 7. Enzyme activities in unit/mg protein from rats described in Figure 5. Maltase: * = $p < 0.05$, + = $p < 0.01$; Sucrase; * = $p < 0.025$, + = $p < 0.025$; Peroxidase: * = $p < 0.001$. (Reproduced, with permission of *Gastroenterology*.[13])

maintenance of the structural and functional integrity
of the gut.[13]

One may speculate about the possible clinical significance of these data.   As I have already pointed
out, the trophic action of gastrin may be important
in gastrointestinal development and in cases of mal-
nutrition.   The antitrophic action of secretin could
be of use in duodenal ulcer therapy, since secretin
would theoretically decrease the mass of acid-secret-
ing cells as well as inhibit secretion itself.
Gastrin and secretin are also potentially useful
where the primary defect is the under- or overproduction of a tissue dependent on these hormones for
growth.

SUMMARY

The gastrointestinal hormones, and especially
gastrin, have been shown to stimulate growth of the
gastrointestinal mucosa and the pancreas.   This
effect is dependent on the stimulation of RNA and
DNA synthesis and is unrelated to effects on secretion.   Gastrin can exert its trophic action *in vitro,*
and must, therefore, act directly on the biochemical
processes related to growth.   In the absence of
endogenous gastrin, which can be brought about by
surgical antrectomy or by total parenteral feeding,
atrophy occurs in the tissues that are dependent on
gastrin as a growth promoting factor.   Administration
of low doses (less than D_{50}) of exogenous gastrin
largely prevents atrophy in these models.   Thus,
the trophic action of gastrin is a physiologic function of the hormone and is necessary for maintenance
of the structural and functional integrity of the
gastrointestinal tract.

Acknowledgments

Research presented here from the author's laboratory was
supported by National Institutes of Health Grant AM 16505.
Dr. Johnson is the recipient of NIH Research Career Development Award AM 28972.

References

1. Castro GA, Johnson LR, Copeland EM, Dudrick SJ: Decreased
    intestinal disaccharidase and peroxidase activity in
    hyperalimented rats, abstracted. *Fed Proc* 33:692,
    1974.
2. Crean GP, Marshall MW, Rumsey RDE: Parietal cell hyper-
    plasia induced by the administration of pentagastrin
    (ICI 50,123) to rats. *Gastroenterology* 57:147-155,
    1969.
3. Ellison EH, Wilson SD: Further observations on factors
    influencing the symptomatology manifest by patients
    with the Zollinger-Ellison syndrome, in Shnitka TK,
    Gilbert JAL, Harrison RC (eds), *Gastric Secretion:*
    Mechanisms and Control, New York: Pergamon, 1967,
    pp 363-369.
4. Enochs MR, Johnson LR: Pentagastrin stimulates tissue
    growth in stomach and duodenal tissues by stimulating
    protein and nucleic acid synthesis, abstracted.
    Fed Proc 33:309, 1974.
5. Gjeruldsen ST, Myren J, Frethiem B: Alterations of gastric
    mucosa following a graded partial gastrectomy for duo-
    denal ulcer. *Scand J Gastroent* 3:465-470, 1968.
6. Johnson LR: Gut hormones on growth of gastrointestinal
    mucosa, in Chey WY and Brooks FP (eds), *Endocrinology*
    of the Gut, Thorofare, NJ: Charles B. Slack, Inc.,
    1974, pp 163-177.
7. Johnson LR, Aures D, Håkanson R: Effect of gastrin on the
    in vivo incorporation of ^{14}C-leucine into protein of
    the digestive tract. *Proc Soc Exp Biol Med* 132:996-
    998, 1969.
8. Johnson LR, Aures D, Yuen L: Pentagastrin-induced stimula-
    tion of protein synthesis in the gastrointestinal tract.
    Am J Physiol 217:251-254, 1969.
9. Johnson LR, Chandler AM: RNA and DNA of gastric and duodenal
    mucosa in antrectomized and gastrin treated rats.
    Am J Physiol 224:937-940, 1973.
10. Johnson LR, Copeland EM, Dudrick SJ, Lichtenberger L, Castro
    GA: Structural and hormonal alterations in the gastro-
    intestinal tract of parenterally fed rats. *Gastroenter-*
    ology, in press.
11. Johnson LR, Guthrie PD: Mucosal DNA synthesis: A short term
    index of the trophic action of gastrin. *Gastroenterology*
    67:453-459, 1974.
12. Johnson LR, Guthrie PD: Secretin inhibition of gastrin
    stimulated Deoxyribonucleic acid synthesis. *Gastroen-*
    terology 67:601-606, 1974.

13. Johnson LR, Lichtenberger LM, Copeland EM, Dudrick SJ, Castro GA: Physiological significance of the trophic action of gastrin. *Gastroenterology*, in press.
14. Lees F, Grandjean LC: The gastric and jejunal mucosae in healthy patients with partial gastrectomy. *Arch Intern Med* 101:943-951, 1958.
15. Lichtenberger L, Johnson LR: Gastrin in the ontogenic development of the small intestine. *Am J Physiol* 227:390-395, 1974.
16. Lichtenberger LM, Miller LR, Erwin DN, Johnson LR: The effect of pentagastrin on adult rat duodenal cells in culture. *Gastroenterology* 65:242-251, 1973.
17. Mainz DL, Black O, Webster PD: Hormonal influences on pancreatic growth. *Gastroenterology* 64:766, 1973.
18. Melrose AG, Russell RI, Dick A: Gastric mucosal structure and function after vagotomy. *Gut* 5:546-549, 1964.
19. Miller LR, Jacobson ED, Johnson LR: Effect of pentagastrin on gastric mucosal cells grown in tissue culture. *Gastroenterology* 64:254-267, 1973.
20. Stanley MD, Coalson RE, Grossman MI, Johnson LR: Influence of secretin and pentagastrin on acid secretion and parietal cell number in rats. *Gastroenterology* 63:264-269, 1972.
21. Willems G, Vansteenkiste Y, Limbosch JM: Stimulating effect of gastrin on cell proliferation kinetics in canine fundic mucosa. *Gastroenterology* 62:583-589, 1972.

THE TROPHIC EFFECT OF PENTAGASTRIN ON THE PANCREAS

J.A. Barrowman, P.D. Mayston

Department of Physiology, The London Hospital
Medical College, London, England

The gastrointestinal tract responds to a wide variety of stimuli by adaptive changes in both growth and
function. These responses follow physiologic changes,
such as alterations in the quantity and quality of the
diet, and pathophysiologic situations, such as intestinal resection. The mediators of these responses are
not known but neural and humoral mechanisms are likely.
An increasing body of evidence suggests that gastrointestinal hormones exert important trophic influence
on their target tissues both in the mature and developing gut. The best known example of this is the
activity of gastrin and its analogs on gastric parietal cell growth.[7]
In tissues with rapid cell turnover, such as the
mucosa of the small intestine, the mechanisms for
adaptation, either biochemical or structural, would
seem to be readily available. The pancreas, however,
with its low mitotic index, has in the past been considered a relatively stable tissue not liable to much
growth change. Yet, it has long been known that feeding trypsin inhibitors from soybean produces pancreatic hypertrophy in chicks[6] and that after acinar cell
destruction by ethionine, the pancreas is capable of
regeneration.[11]
Until recently, the humoral control of exocrine pancreatic secretion has been considered a function mainly
of secretin and cholecystokinin-pancreozymin (CCK-PZ);
the possible trophic role of these hormones on their
target tissue has been studied by Rothman and Wells.[19]
Their data suggested that CCK-PZ has a trophic effect
on rat pancreas with respect to both structure and
enzyme content, although secretin does not. This

phenomenon has been confirmed by Mainz, Black, and Webster[15] and our own studies.[4] The decapeptide, caerulein, which shares the five C-terminal amino acid sequence of gastrin and CCK-PZ has also been shown, when given as a course of injections, to increase pancreatic weight and enzyme content in rats.[9]

In studies of trophic influences on the pancreas, we chose initially to study pentagastrin (I.C.I. Pharmaceuticals), the synthetic analog of the C-terminal tetrapeptide sequence of CCK-PZ and gastrin: N - t - butyloxycarbonyl - β - alanyl - L tryptophyl - L methionyl - L aspartyl - L phenylalanine - amide.

Our choice was based on the fact that this fragment, which is available as a pure substance, is a secretagogue for both the stomach and the pancreas and has been shown to exert trophic influences both morphologically and biochemically on other tissues of the alimentary tract.[5,7,14]

STUDIES ON NORMAL RATS

Because the relationship between organ weight and body weight in rats was found to depend on the strain of rat, we have confined our studies to male Wistar rats fed on a standard diet. Rats received either pentagastrin, histamine, or 0.9% sodium chloride by subcutaneous injection for 11 days. Pentagastrin was given as 2 mg/100 g body weight in five divided doses daily, and histamine base, 6 mg/100 g body weight/day in doses divided in the same way. At the end of the program the rats were starved for 18 to 21 hours, killed and the pancreata excised *in toto*, weighed and divided into aliquots which were homogenised and, in a first experiment, assayed for soluble protein content, amylase, lipase, and esterase. Tissue was also fixed and prepared by conventional techniques for histologic analysis, and the liver, kidneys, spleen, and a segment of duodenum, from the pylorus to the entry of the common bile duct, were excised and weighed.

In a second experiment the nucleic acid content of the pancreas was studied. Only two groups of rats were studied, that is, a pentagastrin group and a control (0.9% sodium chloride) group. Details of the methods in these two experiments have been described.[17]

Judged both by body weight changes and direct measurements of food intake, the nutrition of the rats in all groups was comparable. No pathologic change was seen in the pancreas of any rat in the groups, either grossly or microscopically, nor were there macroscopic pathologic changes in the stomach or any other tissue excised from the rats. The programme of treatment produced a striking change in pancreatic size in the group receiving pentagastrin (Fig. 1). Tables 1 and 2 summarise the data obtained from the two experiments.

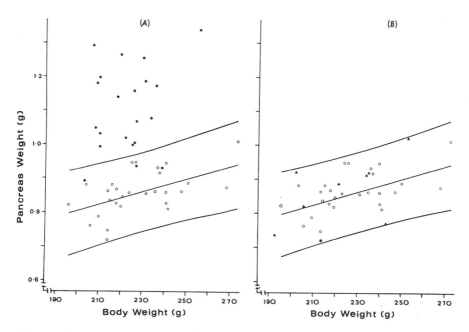

Figure 1. Results of a course of subcutaneous injections of pentagastrin (closed circles, A), histamine (triangles, B) in male Wistar rats. The regression line and 95% confidence limits for individual results of control rats (open circles) are given on both graphs. (Reproduced, with permission of *Quarterly Journal of Experimental Physiology* 56:113–122, 1971.)

Table 1. Results of a course of subcutaneous injections of pentagastrin and histamine in male Wistar rats*

	Histamine	Control (saline injection)	Penta-gastrin	p value (Pentagastrin vs control)
Final body weight	224±8	237±5	222±6	NS
(g)	(8)	(22)	(14)	
Body weight	4.8±1.0	6.8±0.8	4.9±0.9	NS
increase	(8)	(19)	(11)	
Measurements on pancreas:				
Weight	391±13	378±7	496±18	<0.01
(mg/100 g)	(8)	(18)	(10)	
Acinus cell nu-	–	2288±122	1629±42	<0.01
clear count		(6)	(6)	
(30 fields of	1924	1938	–	–
microscope)	(4)	(4)		
Measurements on the pancreatic homogenates				
Soluble protein				
content (mg/100	17.7±0.6	18.7±0.4	18.5±0.6	NS
mg wet weight of	(8)	(22)	(14)	
tissue)				
Amylase (units/mg)	65±4	71±4	54±4	<0.05
	(8)	(22)	(14)	
Lipase (units/mg)	11.9±1.0	10.6±7	8.7±0.9	NS
	(8)	(16)	(8)	
Esterase	5.3±0.5	4.8±0.4	3.2±0.5	<0.05
(μ-equiv/hr/mg)	(8)	(17)	(9)	
Duodenal segment				
weight (mg/100 g)	119±5	103±4	142±7	<0.01
(see text)	(8)	(16)	(8)	
Kidneys weight	907±30	865±13	840±18	NS
(mg/100 g)	(8)	(18)	(10)	
Spleen weight	476±40	387±25	425±63	NS
(mg/100 g)	(8)	(18)	(10)	

* Data are expressed as mean (± SE where five or more observations were made). Figures in parentheses indicate number of observations. Weights are expressed in terms of body weight of the rats at the time of killing. Enzyme measurements in pancreatic homogenates are related to the amount of soluble protein extracted. NS = not significant. None of the data from histamine-injected rats was significantly different from the controls (with the exception of duodenal segment weight, p <0.05).

	Control (saline injections)	Pentagastrin	p value
Final body weight (g)	231±6 (12)	225±6 (12)	NS
Pancreas weight (mg/100 g)	375±9 (11)	493±19 (11)	<0.01
Nucleic acid content of the pancreas			
DNA (μg/100 mg)	460±19 (8)	324±13 (8)	<0.01
RNA ribose (μg/100 mg)	549±22 (8)	647±28 (8)	<0.01
RNA : DNA ratio (μg RNA Ribose/100 μg DNA)	122±7 (8)	201±11 (8)	<0.01
Liver weight (g/100 g)	2.86±0.06 (12)	2.94±0.08 (12)	NS

* Data are expressed as mean ± SE. Figures in parentheses indicate number of observations. Organ weights are expressed in terms of body weight of the rats at the time of killing. Nucleic acid measurements are expressed in terms of the wet weight of pancreatic tissue. NS = not significant.

In our studies pancreatic weights have been related to body weight. The relationship between pancreatic and body weight in our rats could not be distinguished from a simple linear trend. Although the relationships between organ weights and body weight are not linear throughout life, a large study[18] has shown a linear relationship between total body weight and total pancreas wet weight in the range of 100 to 300 g body weight for male Wistar rats. The mean increase in pancreatic weight in the pentagastrin-treated rats was 31% over controls. Histologic studies, soluble protein concentrations, and in a subsequent study, dry weights, show that this weight gain is not due to accumulation of water in the tissue but represents a structural change; there is no evidence of an increase in the endocrine tissue of the pancreas. The changes in acinar cell nuclear count point to a cellular hypertrophy, a conclusion borne out by the nucleic acid data (Tables 2 & 3).

Table 3. Calculated mean content of nucleic acids in the pancreas of control and pentagastrin-treated rats

	Control (saline injections)	Pentagastrin
Total pancreatic RNA (mg)	4.76	7.17
Total pancreatic DNA (mg)	3.99	3.68

From Table 1 it can be seen that the concentration of the enzymes measured in the pancreata tended to be rather lower after pentagastrin treatment than in controls. Calculation of total enzyme content, however (Table 4), shows that there is little change in the total amounts of these enzymes in the gland, although the soluble protein content of the pancreas increased by approximately 20%. Histamine treatment (Table 1) had no significant effect on pancreatic size, soluble protein, or enzyme content.

THE EFFECT OF VARYING THE DOSE AND DURATION OF PENTAGASTRIN TREATMENT

In an experiment in which the effect of duration of pentagastrin treatment was examined, rats received 2 mg/100 g body weight/day and measurements were made after the 5-, 11- and 21-day injections. The mean increases in pancreatic weight, 21%, 31%, and 46%

Table 4. Calculated mean content of enzymes and soluble protein in the pancreas of control and pentagastrin-treated rats

	Control (saline injections)	Pentagastrin
Total amylase	11,900	11,000
Total lipase	1,780	1,775
Total esterase	805	616
Total soluble protein (mg)	168	204

over controls, were approximately linear with time,
and histologic studies of the pancreas after 21 days
of treatment gave results similar in type to those
found with 11 days of treatment.   In five rats receiving pentagastrin, 0.2 mg/100 g body weight/day for 11
days, (one-tenth of our standard dose), no significant
changes were found in pancreatic or duodenal weight or
in soluble protein or enzyme content in the pancreas.

SECRETORY CAPACITY OF THE PANCREAS IN CONTROL AND
PENTAGASTRIN-TREATED RATS

   In an attempt to assess the functional changes induced by pentagastrin treatment, studies were made
of the basal and CCK-PZ-stimulated pancreatic secretion in control and pentagastrin-treated rats.[8]   For
this purpose, rats were anaesthetised with intraperitoneal urethane and at laparotomy a polyethylene
cannula was inserted into the common bile duct close
to the duodenum.   When mixed bile and pancreatic juice
was flowing freely, the bile duct was ligated above
the pancreas and the pylorus was ligated.   After a
three-hour stabilisation period, basal secretion was
assayed over four 10-minute periods, and secretory
responses to CCK-PZ (G.I.H. Research Unit, Karolinska
Institute, Stockholm, 300 Ivy Dog Units per mg, also
containing 24 clinical units of secretin per mg) were
subsequently measured in terms of volume, protein and
amylase.   The response to any dose of hormone was
assessed as the total excess over the basal output
for volume, protein, and amylase.   At the end of the
experiment, the rat was killed, the pancreas was
rapidly excised and weighed, and an aliquot was taken
for DNA measurements.
   Table 5 shows the results of the study of basal
secretion of the pancreas.   Although the basal flow
of pancreatic juice is slightly increased in the
pentagastrin-treated rats, this is not statistically
significant. The flow of protein, however, was significantly greater from the pentagastrin-treated rats
whether expressed as secretion per pancreas or per
milligram of pancreatic DNA.   Amylase output was not
increased, and the nature of the excess protein
secreted is not known.   In response to CCK-PZ, the
output of protein per pancreas or per milligram of

Table 5. Basal secretory activity of the pancreas of control and pentagastrin-treated rats

	Control (saline injections)	Pentagastrin	p value
Number of observations	9	9	
Body weight (g)	252±13	249±9	NS
Pancreas weight (mg)	887±32	1148±42	<0.01
Total DNA content (mg per pancreas)	3.16±0.12	3.04±0.15	NS
Basal secretion per pancreas/10 minutes			
Volume (μl)	5.0±0.4	5.6±0.5	NS
Protein (μg)	370±34	504±50	<0.05
Amylase (U)	48±3	50±5	NS
Basal secretion per mg DNA/10 minutes			
Protein (μg)	121±13	169±11	<0.02
Amylase (U)	15.2±1.0	15.7±1.2	NS
Protein concentration (mg/ml basal secretion)	77±8	94±11	NS
Specific activity of amylase in basal secretion (U/mg protein)	135±10	100±5	<0.02

pancreatic DNA was significantly greater from the pentagastrin-treated rats (Fig. 2), but again no significant differences were seen in volume or amylase output. These results suggest that in terms of protein output there is enhanced 'sensitivity' of the pentagastrin-treated pancreas to CCK-PZ.

STUDIES OF HYPOPHYSECTOMISED RATS

In view of the severe atrophy known to occur in the gastrointestinal tract, in particular the pancreas, after hypophysectomy, we next studied the effect of pentagastrin treatment in such rats. Using the same strain and sex, we divided our rats into four groups; some control rats received injections of 0.9% sodium chloride (saline), hypophysectomised rats received either saline or pentagastrin injections, and other controls remained untreated. The need for the latter group is illustrated in Figure 3 where body weight

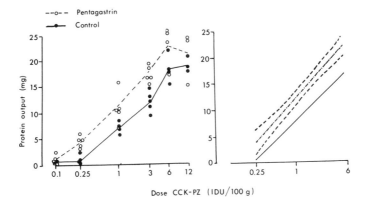

Figure 2. Dose-response curves for control and pentagastrin-treated rats for total protein output in pancreatic secretion *vs* dose of cholecystokinin-pancreozymin. All values have been corrected for basal flow and are therefore independent of the duration of the response. On the left are individual results and in the right hand panel are the regression lines (control rats ———, pentagastrin-treated rats •—•—•—•[together with its 95% confidence limits - - -]). (For details, see text).

changes over the period of treatment are shown for these different groups. The control saline group continued to gain weight following the normal pattern for Wistar rats of this age and body weight. The control untreated group, designated the "starting group," were rats 15 days younger than those of the other groups, which were allowed to attain a body weight of the other groups at the start of the course of injections and could be considered comparable with the other groups. Measurements in this experiment were carried out as in the previous study.[16]

239

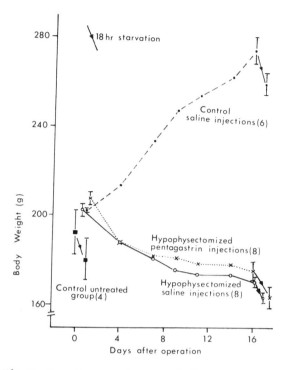

Figure 3. Changes in mean body weight of
each group of rats. All rats were of the
same age (7 weeks) on day 0 of the experiment, the day that two of the groups of
rats were hypophysectomised. For the sake
of clarity, the standard error of the mean
is indicated (vertical lines) only at the
beginning and end of the experiment.
Treatment with pentagastrin or 0.9% NaCl
began on day 1. At the end of the course
of injections the rats were fasted for
18 hours prior to killing, as indicated by
arrows. The untreated group was fasted
for 18 hours from day 0. Figures in
parentheses indicate the number of rats in
each group. (Reproduced, with permission
of *Gastroenterology* 64:391-399, 1973.)

The results of this study are best shown graphically (Figs. 4-7). Hypophysectomy resulted in severe pancreatic atrophy associated with a considerable loss of RNA and a more modest loss of DNA, while cell size decreased. The tissue concentration of DNA increased because of a substantial loss of cytoplasmic constituents. Chronic pentagastrin treatment increased the pancreatic weight in hypophysectomised rats and in our study restored pancreatic weight to a value comparable with that of the "starting group" rats. RNA content was increased, DNA concentration decreased, the RNA:DNA ratio increased towards control measurements. These changes indicate an increase primarily in the cytoplasmic constituents of the tissue. Total pancreatic DNA also increased, however, although to a lesser degree than total RNA, which suggests that pentagastrin treatment had caused both cellular hypertrophy and hyperplasia. This contrasts with the previous conclusions about normal rats where the effect was considered to be primarily cellular hypertrophy. In a further study of pentagastrin treatment in hypophysectomised rats carried out in conjunction with Drs. Crean, Ganguli and Rumsey (M.R.C. Clinical Endocrinology Research Unit, Edinburgh) (unpublished data), essentially similar results were obtained with respect to pancreatic weight, nucleic acids, and cell size. The extractable soluble protein of the pancreas of hypophysectomised rats was found to be 58% less than in control rats, and total pancreatic amylase, trypsinogen and chymotrypsinogen were reduced by 85%, 48%, and 46%, respectively. Pentagastrin treatment increased the total protein content of the pancreas by 24% over control measurements, but no significant changes were recorded in the total amounts of enzyme recovered from the gland.

DISCUSSION

Chronic pentagastrin treatment, acting presumably through receptor sites which recognise the C-terminal tetrapeptide sequence of CCK-PZ, has a pronounced effect on growth in the rat pancreas, which broadly appears to be hypertrophy in the normal adult pancreas, and hypertrophy and hyperplasia in the atrophic pancreas of hypophysectomised rats. The difference in the response of the severely atrophic gland and the

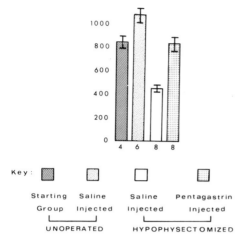

Figure 4. Measurements on the pancreas in hypophysectomy study. Means and standard errors of the mean are shown and the numbers of rats in each group are shown below the columns.

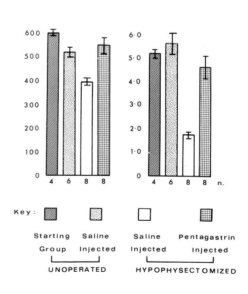

Figure 5. Measurements on the pancreas in hypophysectomy study. Means and standard errors of the mean are shown and the numbers of rats in each group are shown below the columns.

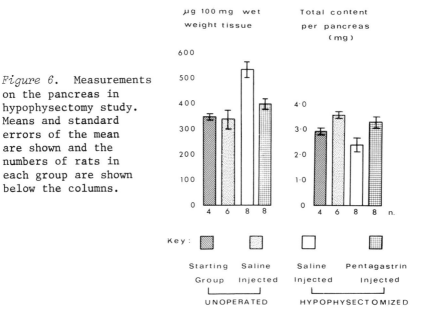

Figure 6. Measurements on the pancreas in hypophysectomy study. Means and standard errors of the mean are shown and the numbers of rats in each group are shown below the columns.

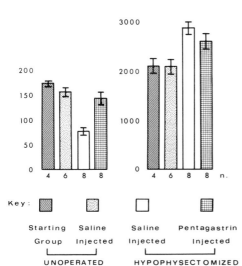

Figure 7. Measurements on the pancreas in hypophysectomy study. Means and standard errors of the mean are shown and the numbers of rats in each group are shown below the columns.

normal pancreas to pentagastrin might be governed by
some intrinsic cell mechanism related to the ratio
of nuclear to cytoplasmic mass.[12] There is some
evidence that a functional change develops in the
hypertrophic pancreas in the form of enhanced sensitivity to CCK-PZ. Pentagastrin did not increase the
enzyme content of the pancreas in any of our experiments, which suggests either that the pentapeptide
has no effect on specific protein synthesis or that
any increase in synthesis is offset by an increased
flow of enzyme from the gland. These results can be
compared with those obtained with CCK-PZ which, weight
for weight, is a much more potent stimulant of pancreatic growth than pentagastrin. In several studies
of chronic CCK-PZ administration to rats, a pronounced
increase was demonstrated in enzyme content in the
pancreas, together with accumulation of RNA and
DNA.[4,15,19,20] Mainz, Black and Webster[15] have proposed on the basis of nucleic acid studies that CCK-
PZ treatment results in hypertrophy and hyperplasia
of the pancreas and our own data in this respect,[4]
using a highly purified CCK-PZ preparation, are in
agreement insofar as there was a substantial accumulation of pancreatic DNA and RNA.

The action of chronic CCK-PZ and pentagastrin on
the pancreas represents an example of the trophic influence of gastrointestinal hormones on their target
tissues. The pancreas is subject to both exogenous
(dietary) and endogenous (endocrine and metabolic)
influences, and CCK-PZ may mediate many of these
effects. The participation of CCK-PZ in changes in
pancreatic size and composition after feeding of
soybean and other trypsin inhibitors has often been
postulated but not proved. Quantitative dietary
changes, hyperphagia, and starvation may also exert
influence on the pancreas through such a mechanism,
and studies are needed to elucidate whether starvation produces its effects on the pancreas[21] through
absence of a stimulus from the gut lumen, through
calorie restriction, or through absence of some specific nutrient.

Endocrine influences on the pancreas are evident
from studies of hypophysectomy and hormone replacement,[2] although it is difficult to distinguish the
effect of reduced dietary intake in this situation.
In addition, the possibility that the pituitary and
its target glands modulate gastrointestinal hormone

levels in the gut mucosa or the responsiveness of the pancreas to these hormones, further complicates the problem. For example, Dorchester and Haist[10] obtained results, which suggest that there are reduced secretin levels in the intestinal mucosa of hypophysectomised rats. In our studies, pentagastrin appears to be capable of stimulating pancreatic growth in the absence of the pituitary. Thus a variety of theoretical mechanisms can be invoked to explain the pancreatic changes (cellular hypertrophy, hyperplasia, and increased sensitivity to CCK-PZ) which we have observed previously in lactating rats.[3] The discovery of new pancreatic secretagogues and chalones such as chymodenin[1] and pancreatone[13] may lead us to appreciate even more complex mechanisms of long-term control of pancreatic structure and function.

SUMMARY

Chronic subcutaneous injection of pentagastrin, an analog of the C-terminal tetrapeptide of gastrin and cholecystokinin-pancreozymin (CCK-PZ), resulted in hypertrophy of the exocrine pancreas of the rat. There was a pronounced accumulation of RNA in the tissue, but total pancreatic DNA was not increased. Total exportable enzyme content of the gland was approximately the same as that of control rats. In response to intravenous injection of CCK-PZ, however, the hypertrophic gland appeared to be more sensitive in terms of protein secretion. Hypophysectomy produced a severe pancreatic atrophy with loss of RNA and DNA. In this situation, a similar course of treatment with pentagastrin resulted in a return of the gland towards control size with accumulation of RNA and DNA. In this case both cellular hypertrophy and hyperplasia occurred. Pentagastrin did not restore exportable enzyme levels from the low levels seen in hypophysectomised rats to normal. These results contrast with the increase in pancreatic hydrolases in the gland after a course of CCK-PZ injections. CCK-PZ and other gastrointestinal hormones probably play a part in the maintenance of structural and functional integrity of the pancreas and may mediate adaptive changes of the pancreas to various environmental stimuli.

Acknowledgment

The authors gratefully acknowledge the financial support of the Wellcome Trust (England) and the generous supplies of pentagastrin provided by Dr. JD Fitzgerald, I.C.I. Ltd., England.

References

1. Adelson JW, Rothman SS: Selective pancreatic enzyme secretion due to a new peptide called chymodenin. *Science* 183:1087-1089, 1974.
2. Baker BL: Restoration of involuted zymogenic cells in hypophysectomized rats by replacement therapy. *Anat Rec* 131:389-403, 1958.
3. Barrowman JA, Mayston PD: Pancreatic secretion in lactating rats. *J Physiol* 229:41P-42P, 1973.
4. Barrowman JA, Mayston PD: The trophic influence of cholecystokinin on the rat pancreas. *J Physiol* 238:73P-75P, 1974.
5. Chandler AM, Johnson LR: Pentagastrin-stimulated incorporation of ^{14}C-orotic acid into RNA of gastric and duodenal mucosa. *Proc Soc Exp Biol Med* 141:110-113, 1972.
6. Chernick SS, Lepkovsky S, Chaikoff IL: A dietary factor regulating the enzyme content of the pancreas: Changes induced in size and proteolytic activity of the chick pancreas by the ingestion of raw soy-bean meal. *Am J Physiol* 155:33-41, 1948.
7. Crean GP, Marshall MW, Rumsey RDE: Parietal cell hyperplasia induced by the administration of pentagastrin (ICI 50,123) to rats. *Gastroenterology* 57:147-155, 1969.
8. Dockray GJ: The action of secretin, cholecystokinin-pancreozymin and caerulein on pancreatic secretion in the rat. *J Physiol* 225:679-692, 1972.
9. De Caro G, Ronconi I, Sporanzi N: Action of caerulein on pancreatic amylase and chymotypsinogen in the rat, in Mantegazza P and Horton EW (eds), *Prostaglandins, Peptides and Amines,* London: Academic Press, 1969, pp 167-179.
10. Dorchester JEC, Haist RE: The secretin content of the intestine in normal and hypophysectomized rats. *J Physiol* 118:188-195, 1952.

11. Fitzgerald PJ, Herman L, Carol B, Roque A, Marsh WH, Rosenstock L, Richards C, Perl D: Pancreatic acinar cell regeneration: I. Cytologic cytochemical and pancreatic weight changes. *Am J Pathol* 52:983-1011, 1968.

12. Goss RJ: *Adaptive Growth*, London: Logos Press, Academic Press, 1964, p. 56.

13. Harper AA, Hood AJC, Mushens J, Smy JR: Inhibition of external pancreatic secretion by extracts of ileal and colonic mucosa. *Proceedings of the meeting of the British Society of Gastroenterology*, September, 1974.

14. Johnson LR, Aures D, Yuen L: Pentagastrin-induced stimulation of protein synthesis in the gastrointestinal tract. *Am J Physiol* 217:251-254, 1969.

15. Mainz DL, Black O, Webster PD: Hormonal control of pancreatic growth. *J Clin Invest* 52:2300-2304, 1973.

16. Mayston PD, Barrowman JA: Influence of chronic administration of pentagastrin on the pancreas in hypophysectomized rats. *Gastroenterology* 64:391-399, 1973.

17. Mayston PD, Barrowman JA: The influence of chronic administration of pentagastrin on the rat pancreas. *Q J Exp Physiol* 56:113-122, 1971.

18. Richards C, Fitzgerald PJ, Carol B, Rosenstock L, Lipkin L: Segmental division of the rat pancreas for experimental procedures. *Lab Invest* 13:1303-1321, 1964.

19. Rothman SS, Wells H: Enhancement of pancreatic enzyme synthesis by pancreozymin. *Am J Physiol* 213:215-218, 1967.

20. Snook JT: Factors in whole-egg protein influencing dietary induction of increases in enzyme and RNA levels in rat pancreas. *J Nutr* 97:286-294, 1969.

21. Webster PD, Singh M, Tucker PC, Black O: Effects of fasting and feeding on the pancreas. *Gastroenterology* 62:600-605, 1972.

NEW RIAs

VALIDATION OF RADIOIMMUNOASSAY

John H. Walsh

Department of Medicine, University of
California, Los Angeles and VA Wadsworth
Hospital Center, Los Angeles, California

GOALS OF RIA

The goals of radioimmunoassay (RIA) of peptide hormones of the gastrointestinal tract can be categorized in several ways. I have chosen to divide them into clinical, biochemical, and physiologic.

Clinical goals include separation of hyper- and hyposecretors of hormones from normal subjects and correlation with disease states. An obvious example of hypersecretion leading to gastrointestinal disease is hypersecretion of gastrin by gastrinoma in the Zollinger-Ellison syndrome. Another example is hypersecretion of VIP in the pancreatic cholera syndrome.[1] Many hormone deficiency states in the endocrine system have been established, but none has yet been identified unequivocally among the classical gastrointestinal hormones.

Hypersecretion of hormones must be distinguished from decreased catabolism. Thus, severe renal failure may cause increased concentrations of hormones that are normally metabolized by the kidneys.

The recognition of heterogeneity of circulating peptide hormones has imposed another complicating factor in clinical interpretation. Greatly increased concentrations of immunoreactive hormone may not be associated with hyperfunction of the target organ if the immunoreactive material is a biologically inactive precursor or fragment of the active hormone. Therefore, in some cases it is necessary to characterize the molecular nature of circulating hormone responsible for increased immunoreactivity in the serum.

251

Radioimmunoassay may be useful in biochemical studies of hormone heterogeneity. Antibodies with appropriate patterns of specificity can be used to identify molecular variants in blood and in tissue extracts. Relative abundance can be quantitated. RIA is a useful tool for monitoring the steps in chemical purification of molecular variants that lead to complete biochemical analysis, and for identification of contamination with structurally similar peptides.

Use of radioimmunoassay for physiologic studies usually requires the ability to measure normal circulating concentrations in basal and stimulated states. In many cases it is necessary to measure with accuracy changes as small as a few picograms per milliliter of serum. For such physiologic purposes, an assay must be both very sensitive and accurate. In addition, it must be specific for physiologically active hormone, or there must be some physical method for separating active from inactive hormone.

Factors that stimulate or inhibit the release of hormone can be measured by RIA, for example, the stimulation of gastrin release by a meal and inhibition of antral acidification, or stimulation of secretin release by intestinal acidification. Many of these factors can be demonstrated independently by other physiologic methods. On the other hand, there are circumstances under which changes in hormone concentration can be measured only by radioimmunoassay. An example is measurement of gastrin during administration of atropine, which masks the physiologic changes by antagonism of the effects of gastrin on its target organ.

Sites of metabolism can be identified by measuring arteriovenous differences across organs responsible for removal or degradation. Whole body clearance rates and disappearance half-times can be measured during and after infusions of pure hormones, and apparent spaces of distribution can be calculated. Knowledge of rates of metabolism makes possible the calculation of hormone secretion rates.

A major physiologic goal of RIA is the correlation of circulating hormone concentrations with biologic function. Inferences can be made concerning the physiologic actions of hormones which have actions on many target organs when administered in large doses. These interpretations must be made with caution, however, because of interactions among different hormones and among hormones and nerves on common target sites. The picture is further complicated when more than one biologically active molecular form of hormone is released by physiologic stimulation.

CONDITIONS FOR SUCCESSFUL RIA

Necessary conditions for successful radioimmunoassay of peptide hormones include development of a working system, minimization of artifacts, and validation.

The first prerequisite condition is the availability of suitable labeled hormone. The labeling process must not destroy immunoreactivity. Some method must be developed to separate labeled hormone from damaged hormone and unreacted iodide. The simplest methods merely separate free iodide from larger molecules. More sophisticated methods, such as ion exchange chromatography, permit isolation of mono- and diiodinated peptides from unlabeled and damaged peptide. The increased specific activity achieved by such purification may offer substantial improvement in assay sensitivity.

Antibodies must have sufficient sensitivity to permit measurement in the desired range of hormone concentration. To measure physiologic changes in circulating peptide hormones may require sensitivity as low as 1 pg/ml in the incubation tube. The pattern of specificity is critical. Intelligent interpretation of RIA results requires knowledge of the pattern of cross-reactivity with naturally-occurring antigenically related proteins and peptides. In some cases, pure hormones are available for this purpose. In many instances, the presence of cross-reacting substances must be determined experimentally by physical fractionation and RIA of tissue extracts and serum.

Standards must be stable under conditions of storage and must be of known potency. Ideally the concentrations of standards should be established independently by chemical analysis and by bioassay. If pure standard of known concentration is not available, it may be necessary to utilize an arbitrary standard obtained from tissue extracts or from serum of a patient with high concentrations. In this circumstance it is essential that the standard be stored under conditions which minimize deterioration.

Stability of reagents is necessary to prevent artifacts, especially during incubation. Enzymes present

in serum may act on labeled hormone or unlabeled
hormone. Inhibition of these enzymes by addition of
inhibitors, dilution of serum, or incubation in the
cold, may be necessary to prevent artifactual results.
   Separation methods also may introduce artifacts.
Nonspecific binding of labeled hormone to serum proteins or anticoagulants can lead to falsely low results unless separation control tubes are included in
the assay. Enzymatic damage of the label may produce
similar results. In double-antibody separation systems, damage to label may be misinterpreted as inhibition of the antigen-antibody reaction and cause
falsely high results. Protein and salt are among
the factors which may interfere with the separation
step. Assays may measure protein concentration rather
than hormone concentration unless conditions are controlled.
   In order to minimize artifacts and variation within
the assay, several steps may be taken. Pipetting and
counting errors can be minimized. Nonspecific incubation effects should be tested systematically and controlled when they are significant. Equilibrium should
be reached before an assay, especially a large one, is
separated. The separation system should be studied
systematically to establish optimal conditions. Deterioration of hormones during storage in serum should
be ruled out by appropriate recovery experiments.
Stability of labeled hormone under conditions of incubation with serum should be demonstrated by measuring binding with excess antibody after incubation.
   Differences in normal values among laboratories
may be due to many of the factors mentioned. It is
of interest that values obtained with early assays
for many hormones are severalfold higher than in
late assays. The papers by Bloom, Chey, Boden, Go,
and Rayford[2-6] are concerned with new assays for
secretin and cholecystokinin. Both of these hormones have offered special problems in labeling and
stability. It is hoped that these new assays can be
used to achieve the goals discussed above.

References

1. Bloom SR, Polak JM: The role of VIP in pancreatic cholera,
       in Thompson JC (ed), *Gastrointestinal Hormones*, Austin:
       University of Texas Press, 1975, pp 635-642.

2. Bloom SR: The development of a radioimmunoassay for secretin, in Thompson JC (ed), *Gastrointestinal Hormones*, Austin: University of Texas Press, 1975, pp 257–268.

3. Chey WY, Tai HH, Rhodes R, Lee KY, Hendricks J: Radioimmunoassay of secretin: Further studies, in Thompson JC (ed), *Gastrointestinal Hormones*, Austin: University of Texas Press, 1975, pp 269–281.

4. Boden G: The secretin radioimmunoassay, in Thompson JC (ed), *Gastrointestinal Hormones*, Austin: University of Texas Press, 1975, pp 283–294.

5. Go VLW, Reilly WM: Problems encountered in the development of the cholecystokinin radioimmunoassay, in Thompson JC (ed), *Gastrointestinal Hormones*, Austin: University of Texas Press, 1975, pp 295–299.

6. Rayford PL, Fender HR, Ramus NI, Reeder DD, Thompson JC: Release and half-life of CCK in man, in Thompson JC (ed), *Gastrointestinal Hormones*, Austin: University of Texas Press, 1975, pp 301–318.

THE DEVELOPMENT OF A RADIOIMMUNOASSAY FOR SECRETIN

S.R. Bloom

The Royal Postgraduate Medical School,
The Hammersmith Hospital, London, England

The role of secretin in digestive physiology has been taken for granted since its discovery, as the first hormone to be identified, more than 70 years ago.[1] A peptide that was purified from the hog duodenum in 1961[9] and subsequently synthesised,[5] clearly had the classical property of stimulating the flow of an alkaline juice from the pancreas. Although it was called "secretin", it was not clear that this peptide was identical to the secretin originally described. To underline the point; another peptide hormone, vasoactive intestinal hormone (VIP),[10] was subsequently found in the small bowel and was indistinguishable from the proposed secretin in its actions on the pancreas.[11] Before the true physiologic role of either substance could be ascertained, it was thus necessary to be able to measure their plasma concentrations. It would then be possible to estimate the amount released after natural stimuli and so to test their individual physiologic actions by means of an exogenous infusion to achieve physiologic levels in the plasma.

The role of secretin in pathologic conditions is no less important. Duodenal ulceration may be caused by an inadequate neutralisation of duodenal acid, consequent on an impairment of secretin release, for example. To study such possibilities properly, it is again necessary to be able to measure plasma secretin levels.

The only technique that has sufficient sensitivity for such plasma measurements is the radioimmunoassay. This technique has proved difficult for secretin, partly because of the shortage of pure hormone, and partly because radioactive labeling of secretin is complicated by the absence of a tyrosine in its amino acid sequence. It is thus only quite recently that reliable secretin assays have been developed.

TECHNICAL PROBLEMS IN THE RADIOIMMUNOASSAY OF SECRETIN

Iodination of Secretin

Several methods have been used to get round the problem of iodinating secretin. First, a synthetic secretin can be used with tyrosine inserted either at position six,[7] replacing phenyalanine, or at position one,[3] replacing histidine. Of course these replacements may affect the molecular configuration and so alter antibody binding, but 6-tyr-secretin apparently has biologic activity[6] and must therefore be very similar in form to natural secretin. A more important practical problem, which attends the use of any synthetic peptide, is the degree of purity of the material used, especially when a solid-phase synthetic procedure is employed.[12] The error peptides present may be impossible to remove and thus significantly bias the assay.

The discovery that iodination of histidine was much easier if the lactoperoxidase technique was used[8] rather than the conventional chloramine T method,[2] has made the use of synthetic secretins unnecessary. A further refinement of the technique is to iodinate only a proportion of the secretin, perhaps 5%, and then to separate the monoiodinated histidinic secretin by ion exchange chromatography. This not only results in a pure monoiodinated secretin of high specific activity (400 µc/µg) but practically eliminates iodination damage. The radioactive secretin so prepared is stable for many months.

Secretin Antisera

The only limitation on raising antisera to secretin is shortage of the hormone. After conjugation to bovine serum albumin by carbodiimide condensation[2] and emulsification in complete Freund's adjuvant, we have found that almost every rabbit injected with secretin produces antibodies. Optimal antibody avidity appears to be achieved by use of relatively small

amounts of antigen given at infrequent intervals, for
example, 25 μg secretin given initially and then in
three and six months, with harvesting after a further
10 days. Secretin appears to be every bit as good an
antigen as insulin, but as the circulating levels of
secretin are perhaps one-fiftieth of those of insulin,
the criteria for useful antisera are much stricter.

In spite of similarities of the amino acid sequence
of secretin with glucagon, VIP, and gastric inhibitory
peptide (GIP),[4] no cross-reaction is seen between
secretin antisera and these hormonal peptides. Studies
with synthetic secretin fragments, suggest that in fact
most secretin antibodies bind preferentially with the
C-terminal end of secretin which has relatively fewer
analogous amino acids.

Secretin Stability

The biologic potency of a secretin solution rapidly
deteriorates on standing, and it was therefore anticipated that there would be considerable problems with
degradation and loss in the radioimmunoassay of secretin. These problems have not materialised. Plasma
samples kept over 18 months apparently still retain
their immunoassayable secretin content if they are
stored at -20C in the presence of 1,000 KIU aprotinin
(Trasylol) per ml. Radioactive secretin label is also
stable for many months and standards are kept as
freeze-dried aliquots at -20C.

Plasma Assay of Secretin

It is a well known fact that any two different laboratories rarely agree on a hormone level measured by
radioimmunoassay. With an established assay, such as
insulin, the disagreements are often minor; perhaps
with luck the results will be within 50% of each other.
With new assays, however, the values found can differ
manyfold. The two most important fundamental weak-
nesses of the technique of radioimmunoassay are first,
that only a variable amino acid conformation is detected and not the whole active hormone, and second,
that many substances can nonspecifically alter antibody binding and so be measured as if they were the
hormone.

The first of these problems, what is being measured, can be minimised by a careful choice of the secretin antisera so that it has the greatest specificity for the whole hormone rather than a possible degradation fragment without biologic activity. Such antisera are further checked by the finding that they have given meaningful results in a defined physiologic situation.

The second problem, the ability of many factors to alter antibody binding nonspecifically, is particularly troublesome in the case of secretin where low circulating concentrations have to be measured and the assay mixture therefore contains either 20% or 40% of the unknown plasma. Again, careful selection of an antiserum relatively insensitive to the influence of plasma will minimise, but not eliminate, such effects. Compensation is achieved by including secretin-free plasma in the standard curve. This is best produced by brief exposure (30 minutes) of fresh plasma to a small volume of well-washed Sepharose beads (500 µl beads to 100 ml plasma), to which a high-titre secretin antisera has been covalently coupled (Cyanogen Bromide Sepharose, Pharmacia AB, Uppsala). Other methods of preparing hormone-free plasma, such as charcoaling, often produce new artifacts. Unfortunately nonspecific plasma effects may differ from plasma to plasma and such differences can be quite large, especially in pathologic conditions, such as uraemia. These problems are circumvented if each individual plasma sample is divided and one portion rendered hormone-free, by use of the Sepharose-bead antibody technique, and then this portion is used to set up a small standard curve from which the untreated portion of plasma is read off.

THE MEASUREMENT OF FASTING LEVELS OF SECRETIN IN MAN

The assay system used for estimating fasting levels of secretin in man is shown in Table 1. Conditions were chosen so that with secretin-free plasma, there was a 50% binding of the secretin label. When plasma containing 45 pg/ml was used, binding decreased to 40%, and thus with adjacent single samples a difference of 9 pg/ml could be detected with 95% confidence. As fasting secretin levels appeared possibly to be below 9 pg/ml, the problems of plasma-nonspecific effects became highly significant. Fifteen plasma samples

Table 1. Protocol for the secretin radioimmunoassay (standards are added in secretin-free plasma)

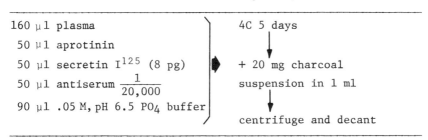

160 µl plasma	4C 5 days
50 µl aprotinin	↓
50 µl secretin I^{125} (8 pg)	+ 20 mg charcoal
50 µl antiserum $\frac{1}{20,000}$	suspension in 1 ml
90 µl .05 M, pH 6.5 PO$_4$ buffer	↓
	centrifuge and decant

from healthy fasting subjects were therefore measured in which 15 standard curves were set up in their own plasma which had been rendered secretin-free (40 µl antisecretin Sepharose beads per 4 ml plasma for 30 minutes). Total secretin extraction was tested by confirming that extra added secretin was completely removed. The mean fasting secretin level was 0.6± 0.7 pg/ml. Nonspecific plasma effects caused an apparent variation between plasmas of about 25 pg/ml, which was not extractable, however, by the Sepharose-bound secretin antisera. Our routine assay has therefore been set up so that the plasma used in the standard curve was chosen to have relatively low nonspecific effects to avoid a reading of less than zero for some unknown plasmas. It would be preferable, of course, to extract each individual plasma on every occasion, but shortage of both time and secretin antisera preclude this.

SECRETIN RELEASE IN PIGS

As porcine secretin was used to raise the antibodies, and is employed for label and for standards, it seemed most appropriate to avoid any possibility of problems due to species differences and therefore to study secretin physiology in pigs. In conjunction with Dr. Julia Polak and Mr. S.N. Joffe at The Hammersmith Hospital, the changes in flow of pancreatic juice, hormone levels, mucosal hormone content and immunocytochemical appearance of the S-cells have been correlated. Pigs were studied under nitrous oxide anaesthesia, after having been induced with halothane alone.

Any pig that showed a sign of surgical stress, for
example, a mean blood pressure below 70 mm Hg, was
immediately discarded. The pyloric sphincter was
tied and a tube was introduced into the duodenum.
The jejunum was drained at 20 cm distal to its origin
and was tied off distal to the drain. The bile duct
and pancreatic duct were also cut and cannulated, and
the secretions were collected over 5-minute intervals.
Acid was introduced at the rate of 1.1 mEq per minute
(11 ml 0.1 N HCl) over a 30-minute period. The rise
of plasma secretin and resulting release of pancreatic
bicarbonate are shown in Figure 1. There was a consistent portosystemic gradient of secretin concentration in each pig, which was most pronounced in the
earlier part of the response. A brisk response of
pancreatic juice flow occurred, which closely followed
the rise of plasma secretin, but after acid withdrawal
the decline of flow was slightly delayed by comparison
with the fall in plasma hormone levels. A small mucosal biopsy was taken 5 cm below the duodenal acid

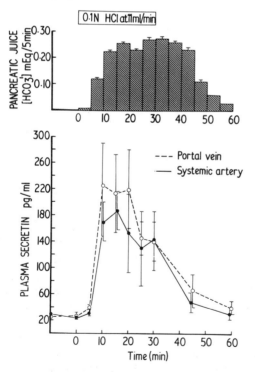

Figure 1. Pancreatic
bicarbonate output and
plasma secretin levels
during a 30-minute acid
infusion in the duodenum
and upper jejunum of the
anaesthetised pig. Means
and SEM of four pigs are
shown.

inlet tube before stimulation, and at a parallel, but
separate, site at the end of stimulation. A part of
each biopsy was extracted for the measurement of total
secretin content and a part was studied immunohisto-
chemically by Dr. Julia Polak. The mean reduction in
the radioimmunoassayable secretin content per mg wet
tissue was 43±7%. Using a TV Image Analyser to quantitate the hormone content of the S cells, Dr. Polak
found a 51±10% reduction (Fig. 2). No change in
hormone content of other duodenal endocrine cells was
observed nor was there any change in the gross appearance of the mucosa. The close correlation of functional and morphologic changes represents a significant
advance in the study of gastrointestinal endocrinology.

SECRETIN RELEASE IN SUBJECTS WITH A DUODENAL ULCER

Twelve healthy volunteers (mean age 38 years) and
23 subjects with duodenal ulcer (mean age 42 years)

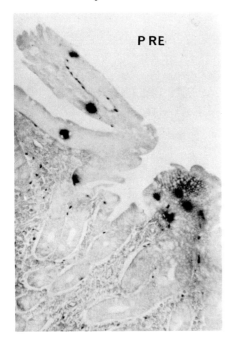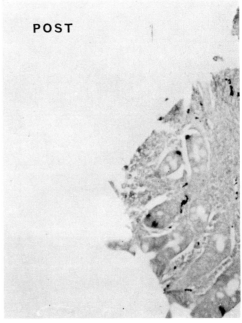

Figure 2. Immunoperoxidase staining of porcine secretin cells
from the duodenum. The section on the left was taken before
acid stimulation and on the right after a 30-minute intraduodenal infusion of 1.1 mEq acid/min (×130).

were studied in conjunction with Mr. A.S. Ward,
Sheffield Royal Infirmary. Tubes were passed into
the stomach and duodenum and a steady acid secretory
plateau was maintained by a continuous intravenous
infusion of pentagastrin (6 μg/kg/hr) throughout the
test. Gastric acid was collected by continuous gastric suction. Duodenal loss, checked by a phenol red
recovery method, was not significantly different between the two groups and was about 10%.[13] Secretin
release was stimulated by the intraduodenal infusion
of 4 mEq of 0.1 N HCl over 5 minutes (Fig. 3). The
mean integrated secretin release, for the 10 minutes
after initiating the intraduodenal acid infusion, was
413±29 pg/ml/min in the normal subjects and 273±23
pg/ml/min in the subjects with duodenal ulceration
(p <0.001). Gastric acid production in the controls
dropped 37±10% from a mean preintraduodenal acid
plateau of 4.8±0.6 mEq/10 min and in duodenal ulcer
subjects dropped 23±5%, from 7.4±0.5 mEq/10 min.
There was no correlation between secretin release and

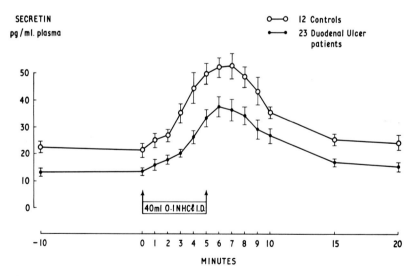

Figure 3. Plasma secretin concentrations after a 0.8 mEq/min
intraduodenal acid infusion in 35 recumbent subjects. (Mean
and SEM shown).

acid inhibition (r = 0.054). To try to ascertain
whether this impaired secretin release in duodenal
ulcer subjects was a direct result of their condition,
the group was divided into long history patients
(mean 16.4 years, n = 15) and short history (mean
3.3 years, n = 7) but the secretin release was identical in the two groups (273±31 and 274±38 pg/ml/
min). It is at least possible, therefore, that this
secretin abnormality might antedate the onset of the
ulcer.

PHYSIOLOGIC ROLE OF SECRETIN IN MAN

Six subjects studied in the same experimental protocol as above received an infusion of exogenous secretin of 0.125 CU/kg over six minutes instead of intraduodenal acid. The plasma secretin levels achieved are
shown in Figure 4 and are compared with the levels

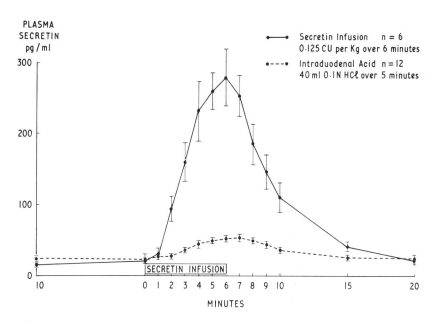

Figure 4. Comparison of exogenous and endogenously produced
elevations in secretin levels in recumbent subjects. The
dotted line is the same response reproduced from the control
subjects shown in Figure 3. (Mean and SEM shown).

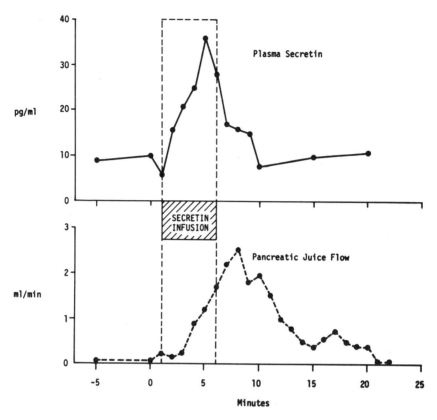

Figure 5. Plasma secretin concentration and pancreatic juice flow, collected through a pancreatic duct cannula previously introduced during duodenoscopy, following a six-minute infusion of 1.25 ng/kg/min of pure porcine secretin in a normal subject.

seen in the normal subjects after the intraduodenal acid infusion. Although plasma secretin was far higher after the exogenous infusion, very little inhibition of gastric acid production occurred in these subjects (mean reduction 16±11%) compared with that following the intraduodenal acid (mean reduction 37±10%). Thus it seems likely that secretin is not an important mediator of the gastric acid inhibition seen after duodenal acidification.[13]

Cannulation of the human pancreatic duct during duodenoscopy allows direct and sensitive measurement of pancreatic juice output. In conjunction with Dr.

Peter Cotton at The Middlesex Hospital, we have studied the effect of secretin infusions designed to produce blood levels in the physiologic range. One
such experiment is shown in Figure 5. We have consistently found that a 20 pg/ml elevation of plasma secretin can produce a substantial flow of alkaline
pancreatic juice.

SUMMARY

We therefore conclude that secretin is physiologically active in controlling duodenal acid neutralisation and that its impaired release in subjects with
duodenal ulceration may be of considerable consequence.

Acknowledgments

I would like particularly to acknowledge the considerable
part played in these studies by Mr. M.G. Bryant and the other
technicians of the Cobbold Laboratory of the Middlesex Hospital.
Synthetic secretin and secretin fragments were very generously
supplied by Dr. Rolf Geiger of Farbwerke Hoechst AG and pure
porcine secretin by Professor V. Mutt of the Karolinska Institute,
Stockholm.

References

1. Bayliss WM, Starling EH: The mechanism of pancreatic secre-
       tion. *J Physiol* 28:325-353, 1902.
2. Bloom SR: Hormones of the gastrointestinal tract. *Brit Med
       Bull* 30:62-67, 1974.
3. Bloom SR, Ogawa O: Radioimmunoassay of human peripheral
       plasma secretin. *J Endocrinol* 58:24-25, 1973.
4. Bodanszky M, Klausner YS, Said SI: Biological activities of
       synthetic peptides corresponding to fragments of and to
       the entire sequence of the vasoactive intestinal peptide.
       Proc Natl Acad Sci USA 70:382-384, 1973.
5. Bodanszky M, Ondetti MA, Levine SD, Narayanan VL, von Saltza
       M, Sheehan JT, Williams NJ, Sabo EF: Synthesis of a
       heptacosapeptide amide with the normal activity of
       secretin. *Chem Industr* 42:1757-1758, 1966.

6. Chey WY, Hendricks J: Biological actions of a synthetic
    secretin and 6 tyrosyl secretin in rats and dogs, in
    Chey WY, Brooks FP (eds), *Endocrinology of the Gut,*
    Thorofare NJ: Charles B. Slack, Inc., 1974, pp 107-115.
7. Guiducci M: Solid phase synthesis of porcine secretin and
    6 tyrosyl secretin, in Chey WY, Brooks FP (eds),
    Endocrinology of the Gut, Thorofare NJ: Charles B. Slack,
    Inc., 1974, pp 103-106.
8. Holohan KN, Murphy RF, Flanagan RWJ, Buchanan KD, Elmore DT:
    Enzymic iodination of the histidyl residue of secretin:
    A radioimmunoassay of the hormone. *Biochim Biophys Acta*
    332:178-180, 1973.
9. Jorpes E, Mutt V: On the biological activity and amino acid
    composition of secretin. *Acta Chem Scand* 15:1790-1791,
    1961.
10. Said SI, Mutt V: Polypeptide with broad biological activity:
    Isolation from small intestine. *Science* 169:1217-1218,
    1970.
11. Said SI, Mutt V: Isolation from porcine intestinal wall of
    a vasoactive octacosapeptide related to secretin and
    to glucagon. *Eur J Biochem* 28:199-204, 1972.
12. Tregear GW, Reitschoten JV, Greene E, Keutmann HT, Niall HD,
    Parsons JA, Potts JT: Principles and recent applications
    in solid-phase synthesis of peptide hormones, in Chey WY,
    Brooks FP (eds), *Endocrinology of the Gut,* Thorofare NJ:
    Charles B. Slack, Inc., 1974, pp 1-15.
13. Ward AS, Bloom SR: The role of secretin in the inhibition
    of gastric secretion by intraduodenal acid. *Gut* 15:
    889-897, 1974.

RADIOIMMUNOASSAY OF SECRETIN: FURTHER STUDIES

William Y. Chey, Hsin-Hsiung Tai,
Ross Rhodes, K.Y. Lee, J. Hendricks

The Isaac Gordon Center for Digestive Diseases,
The Genesee Hospital and Department of Medicine,
University of Rochester School of Medicine and
Dentistry, Rochester, New York

In 1969 we produced successfully an antisecretin
sera of very high titer in New Zealand rabbits[1-3,5]
with use of a pure synthetic porcine secretin supplied
generously by Dr. Ondetti and his associates at the
Squibb Institute for Medical Research. Recently we
again confirmed the high specificity of these antisera
to porcine secretin. The sera did not cross-react
with other gut hormones, including pancreatic glucagon, gastric inhibitory polypeptide, vasoactive intestinal polypeptide, motilin, synthetic human gastrin I
and pure cholecystokinin.

The availability of these antisera and the successful
preparation of ^{125}I-labeled synthetic porcine secretin
of high specific activity,[14] made it possible to develop a simple and rapid radioimmunoassay (RIA) method
for secretin.[13] In addition, with availability of
highly specific antigastrin sera obtained from New
Zealand rabbits, with human synthetic gastrin I used
as an immunogen, we can now assay both secretin and
gastrin simultaneously.[13] The assay results are re-
liably reproducible. As little as 2-3 pg/ml of plasma
secretin as well as gastrin can be measured (Fig. 1),
and the coefficients of variation of these two hormone
assays are minimal (Table 1). Our recent investigations have involved radioimmunoassay of both secretin
and gastrin.

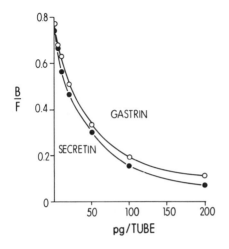

Figure 1. Standard curves of radioimmunoassay (RIA) of secretin and gastrin.

Table 1. Precision of simultaneous measurements of plasma secretin and gastrin

Sample No.		1	2	3	4	5	6
Plasma A	Secretin	58.2	63.0	69.9	60.7	56.0	60.9
(pg/ml)	Gastrin	83.3	87.2	78.7	89.9	80.8	84.6
Plasma B	Secretin	91.7	98.9	99.8	95.2	99.3	99.5
(pg/ml)	Gastrin	228.4	215.7	238.3	241.0	221.4	231.4

7	8	9	10	Mean ± SEM (pg/ml)	Coefficient of variation %
64.8	69.5	64.0	68.1	63.5±1.5	7.4
81.9	85.6	87.2	84.9	84.5±1.0	3.7
97.2	97.1	80.7	97.6	95.7±1.8	6.1
236.3	219.3	234.8	213.6	228.0±3.1	4.3

FASTING PLASMA RADIOIMMUNOREACTIVE SECRETIN AND GASTRIN

We have measured fasting plasma secretin and gastrin levels of various species including man, and dogs, sheep, goats, cats, rabbits, and rats, as shown in Figure 2. The fasting plasma levels of secretin were surprisingly low in all species except for cats and were similar in values among those species studied (Fig. 2). Furthermore, the fasting secretin levels are comparable to those of gastrin measured in our laboratory. One exception was the levels of rabbit gastrin which were higher than those of other animal species.

PLASMA RIA SECRETIN AND GASTRIN RESPONSES TO A MEAT MEAL AND HYDROCHLORIC ACID

In order to study RIA secretin levels in plasma, dogs were prepared with gastric fistulae and two duodenal cannulae with an inner diameter of 0.5 cm, one placed

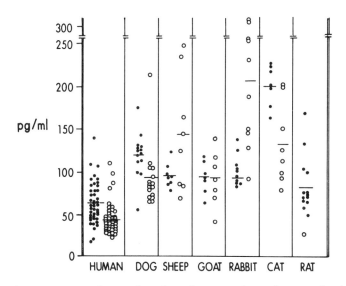

Figure 2. Fasting plasma levels of secretin and gastrin in man and in dogs, sheep, goats, rabbits, cats,and rats. Solid circles represent plasma secretin levels and open circles, plasma gastrin levels.

in the upper duodenum, 1½ inches distal to the pyloroduodenal junction and the other in the mid-duodenum
2½ inches distal to the proximal fistula. After a
full recovery from the surgery, peripheral venous
blood plasma secretin and gastrin responses were
studied after ingestion of a commercial meat meal,
Ken-L-Burger, 750 grams, and the acidity of the
duodenal contents aspirated from the proximal cannula
was determined.[9] As shown in Figure 3, a pronounced
increase was observed in the plasma gastrin levels in
response to the meat meal, but the secretin levels
did not change significantly. Serial determinations
of pH of the duodenal contents fluctuated between
5.0 and 6.0.

Recently we have studied the effects of duodenal
acidification on the peripheral venous blood plasma
secretin levels in conscious dogs.[9] In a fasting
dog, 0.1 N HCl was infused into the proximal duodenal
fistula while the acidity of the duodenal contents
obtained from the distal duodenal fistula was determined (Fig. 4). The plasma secretin levels increased
dramatically from 124 to 262 pg/ml, an 111% increase,
as duodenal contents were acidified. The results of

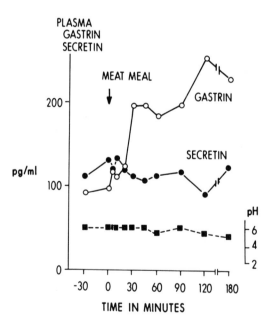

Figure 3. Plasma
secretin and gastrin
levels and pH of duo-
denal contents of a
conscious dog with
duodenal cannulae, in
response to ingestion
of a meat meal.

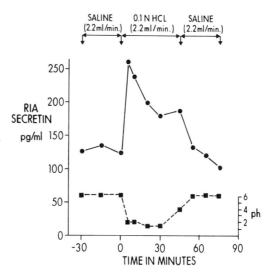

Figure 4. Plasma secretin levels and pH of duodenal contents in a conscious dog with duodenal cannulae, in response to intraduodenal infusion of 0.1 N HCl solution at a rate of 2.2 ml/min.

the same experiment performed in the same dog at one week intervals were almost identical. A similar experiment was performed in conscious dogs after the dogs had been fed with the same meat meal. Acidification of the duodenal contents by the infusion of 0.1 N HCl through the proximal duodenal cannula, 45 minutes after the ingestion of a meal, resulted again in a dramatic increase in the secretin levels (Fig. 5).

Similar studies were carried out in man also to determine the secretin responses in peripheral venous plasma to ingestion of a meat meal and intraduodenal infusion of 0.1 N HCl solution.[15] The results of studies in healthy human subjects were comparable to those in dogs. Ingestion of a ground beef steak in an amount of 250 grams resulted in no significant change in the secretin levels (Fig. 6), whereas the levels of gastrin increased greatly. Duodenal pH ranged from 6.6 to 4.5 during the entire experimental period of three hours. In the same man in a fasting state, a 0.1 N HCl solution was infused to acidify duodenal contents (Fig. 7). In order to maintain the pH of duodenal contents below 3.0 in this subject, an irrigation rate of 8.6 ml/min was required. As the pH decreased below 3.0, the plasma secretin levels increased from a range of 80-90 pg/ml to that of 140 pg/ml (Fig. 7). Similar observations were made in five human subjects.[15] The plasma gastrin levels, however, did not change as expected.

273

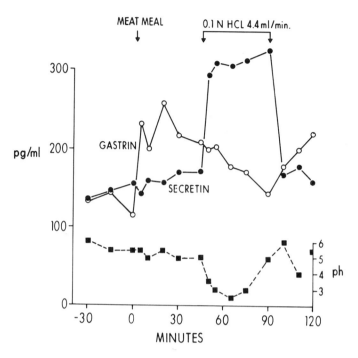

Figure 5. The effect of duodenal acidification on plasma secretin and gastrin levels in a dog with duodenal cannulae, following ingestion of a meat meal.

CORRELATION BETWEEN EXOCRINE PANCREATIC SECRETION AND
PLASMA SECRETIN LEVELS IN CONSCIOUS DOGS

In order to perform this investigation, an external pancreatic fistula was made and a special duodenal cannula was placed in such a manner that a testing substance could be introduced into the duodenum or duodenal contents could be obtained through the cannula, while exocrine pancreatic juice could be collected.[4] As the dog ingested a meat meal, there was a pronounced increase in bicarbonate secretion (Fig. 8) which coincided with pronounced increases in volume of pancreatic juice. The pH of the duodenal contents ranged from 5.0 to 6.8 in this particular dog. Again no discernible change was observed in the plasma secretin levels. In the same dog, 0.1 N HCl solution was introduced into the duodenum at rates of 0.2, 0.4, 0.8 and 1.6 ml/min for 30 minutes.

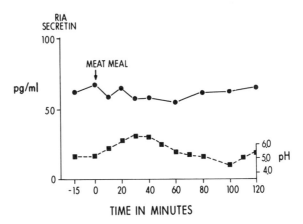

Figure 6. Plasma secretin levels and pH of the duodenal contents in a healthy man after ingestion of a meat meal.

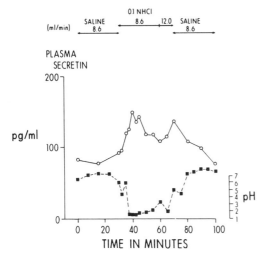

Figure 7. Plasma secretin levels and pH of the duodenal contents in a healthy man in response to intraduodenal infusion of 0.1 N HCl solution.

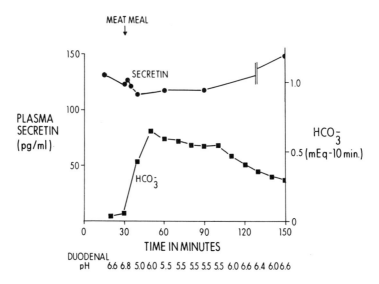

Figure 8. Plasma secretin levels, pancreatic secretion of bicarbonate and pH of the duodenal contents in a dog with external pancreatic fistula in response to ingestion of a meat meal.

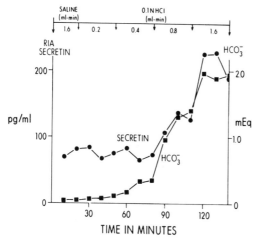

Figure 9. Plasma secretin levels, pancreatic secretion of bicarbonate, and pH of the duodenal contents in a dog with external pancreatic fistula, in response to intraduodenal infusion of 0.1 N HCl solution.

276

When the pH decreased below 2.5, exocrine pancreatic
secretion of bicarbonate was stimulated (Fig. 9). As
the rate of acid infusion was increased, the bicarbonate secretion increased proportionally and at the
rate of 1.6 ml/min, the degree of bicarbonate secretion was comparable to that observed after ingestion
of a meat meal in the same dog. In contrast to observations made after the dog was fed a meat meal, the
plasma RIA secretin levels increased concomitantly as
external pancreatic secretion of bicarbonate increased.
No change was observed in plasma gastrin levels. We
have confirmed again in our conscious dogs that intraduodenal infusion of 10% or 20% glucose solution at a
rate of 2.2 ml/min caused no change in either exocrine
pancreatic secretion or plasma secretin levels (Fig. 10).
The infusion of 0.1 N HCl, however, resulted in pronounced increases in both the plasma secretin levels
and pancreatic secretion of bicarbonate.

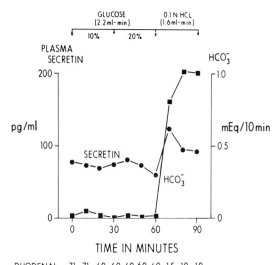

Figure 10. Plasma secretin levels, pancreatic secretion of
bicarbonate and pH of the duodenal contents in a dog with
external pancreatic fistula, in response to intraduodenal
infusion of glucose solution followed by the infusion of
0.1 N HCl solution.

DISCUSSION

The development of a satisfactory radioimmunoassay method of secretin has been difficult because the porcine secretin used for iodination lacks a tyrosyl residue. A simple and rapid method of preparing ^{125}I-labeled secretin of high specific activity has been developed in our laboratory.[14] Moreover, this method now allows us to maintain the labeled hormone in a stable condition for 30 days or more. It is found that the fasting concentrations of secretin in peripheral venous plasma are remarkably low in most species studied, and are comparable to those of gastrin. The relatively high concentrations of secretin in fasting cats, and of gastrin in fasting rabbits, are difficult to explain at this time.

Although we confirmed our previous observation[15] that duodenal acidification by hydrochloric acid causes a significant increase in the concentration of secretin in peripheral venous plasma in both conscious man and dogs, the observation that no significant increase in the RIA secretin levels followed ingestion of a meat meal in both man and dogs puzzled us temporarily. Serial studies of duodenal contents, however, showed that pH rarely reached below 4.0 after ingestion of the meal. A pronounced increase in the secretin levels after the acidification of the duodenal contents (even after ingestion of a meat meal) convinced us that endogenous release of secretin is indeed dependent on H^+ ion in the duodenal contents as claimed by Grossman.[6] Certainly, intraduodenal administration of glucose has not influenced either exocrine secretion of bicarbonate or plasma secretin levels in man[5] and in dogs (as shown in the present study), although it has been reported by Young and associates[16] that glucose solution increases the secretin level. The specificity of antisecretin sera used by Young and associates[16] might not be comparable to that of the antisera used in our laboratory.

Although no significant increase occurred in the plasma secretin levels after ingestion of a meat meal in either man or dogs, a pronounced increase in bicarbonate secretion was observed in the dogs with pancreatic fistula. These observations lead us to consider two hypotheses. As has been reported by Henriksen,[8] Henriksen and Worning,[7] and Meyer and his colleagues,[11] cholecystokinin-pancreozymin (CCK-PZ)

in its exogenous form[7,8] or endogenous form[11] augments
the response to exogenous secretin. Moreover, it has
been stated recently by Said and Makhlouf[12] that vasoactive intestinal polypeptide (VIP) stimulates electro-
lytes and water secretion by the pancreas in cats, and
that in dogs, it acts as a partial agonist to secretin.
Thus during normal alimentation, it is possible that
exocrine pancreatic secretion of water and bicarbonate
may occur as a consequence of the interactions between
a small amount of secretin released from the upper
segment of duodenum and CCK-PZ (as well as VIP) released from the small intestinal mucosa. If this
assumption is correct, further studies are needed to
demonstrate (by RIA of plasma secretin) that a minute
but substantial amount of endogenous secretin is
released during the alimentation.

An alternative hypothesis is that there may be another unknown hormone or hormones that stimulate water
and bicarbonate secretion by the pancreas which are
not dependent upon acid pH of the duodenal contents.
In this regard it is interesting to note the recent
work by Meyer and Jones[10] that fatty acid soaps
stimulate a pancreatic juice characteristic of neither
exogenous secretin nor exogenous CCK-PZ alone. Although their actions could be explained by the release
of both hormones in varying amounts, as they stated,
it is also possible that fatty acids may indeed
stimulate endogenous release of another hormone yet
to be discovered.

SUMMARY

Plasma secretin and gastrin levels were measured
simultaneously by use of simple and sensitive radioimmunoassay (RIA) methods for secretin and gastrin.
As small an amount as 2-3 pg/ml of plasma secretin
or gastrin can be measured. Plasma secretin levels
ranged mostly from 15 to 150 pg/ml in fasting healthy
human subjects, and in dogs, sheep, goats, rabbits,
and rats. They were comparable with the corresponding levels of gastrin in each species. In both man
and dogs, the plasma secretin levels increased significantly when the duodenal pH was decreased below
4.0 by infusion of 0.1 N HCl solution, but did not
change significantly after ingestion of a meat meal,
although plasma RIA gastrin levels increased significantly. Serial determinations of duodenal pH

ranged from 4.5 to 7.4. Glucose solutions of various concentrations failed to influence the secretin levels in conscious dogs, which confirmed our previous observations in man. In the dogs with an exocrine pancreatic fistula, duodenal acidification by infusion of 0.1 N HCl caused concomitant increases in both RIA secretin levels and bicarbonate secretion of the pancreas. After ingestion of a meal, bicarbonate output increased significantly, but RIA secretin levels did not. These observations indicate that plasma RIA secretin levels are raised by duodenal acidification only. The studies suggest strongly that the increase in bicarbonate output after a meal is attributed to either an interaction between a small quantity of endogenously released secretin and other hormone, such as cholecystokinin-pancreozymin or vasoactive intestinal polypeptide. Another alternative suggestion is that there may be another hormonal agent (or agents) playing an important role in stimulating exocrine pancreatic secretion of bicarbonate.

Acknowledgment

This work was supported in part by NIAMDD 16939 and NIAA00192-03.

References

1. Boden G, Chey WY: Preparation and specificity of antiserum to synthetic secretin and its use in a radioimmunoassay (RIA). *Endocrinology* 92:1617-1624, 1973.
2. Boehm M, Lee Y, Chey WY: Radioimmunoassay of secretin: I. Production of secretin antibodies and development of the radioimmunoassay, in Chey WY, Brooks FP (eds), *Endocrinology of the Gut,* Thorofare NJ: Charles B. Slack, Inc., 1974, pp 310-319.
3. Chey WY, Hendricks J: Biological actions of a synthetic secretin and 6-tyrosyl-secretin in rats and dogs, in Chey WY, Brooks FP (eds), *Endocrinology of the Gut,* Thorofare NJ: Charles B. Slack, Inc., 1974, pp 107-115.
4. Chey WY, Hendricks J, Tai HH: Observations on plasma RIA secretin and gastrin levels and exocrine pancreatic secretion in response to a meat meal and duodenal acidification in dogs, in preparation.

5. Chey WY, Oliai A, Boehm M: Radioimmunoassay of secretin: II. Studies on correlation between RIA secretin levels and biological investigations, in Chey WY, Brooks FP (eds), *Endocrinology of the Gut*, Thorofare NJ: Charles B. Slack, Inc., 1974, pp 319–326.

6. Grossman MI: Control of pancreatic secretion, in Beck IT, Sinclair DG (eds), *The Exocrine Pancreas*, Proceedings of a Symposium held at Queen's University, Kingston, Ontario, June, 1969. London: Churchill, 1969, pp 59–73.

7. Henriksen FW: Effect of pancreozymin on the canine pancreatic secretion of fluid and bicarbonate. *Scand J Gastroenterol* 3:637–640, 1968.

8. Henriksen FW, Worning H: The interaction of secretin and pancreozymin on the external pancreatic secretion in dogs. *Acta Physiol Scand* 70:241–249, 1967.

9. Lee KY, Tai HH, Chey WY: Plasma RIA secretin and gastrin responses to a meat meal and duodenal acidification, in preparation.

10. Meyer JH, Jones RS: Canine pancreatic responses to intestinally perfused fat and products of fat digestion. *Am J Physiol* 226:1178–1187, 1974.

11. Meyer JH, Spingola LJ, Grossman MI: Endogenous cholecystokinin potentiates exogenous secretin on pancreas of dog. *Am J Physiol* 221:742–747, 1971.

12. Said SI, Makhlouf GM: Vasoactive intestinal polypeptide: Spectrum of biological activity, in Chey WY, Brooks FP (eds), *Endocrinology of the Gut*, Thorofare NJ: Charles B. Slack, Inc., 1974, pp 83–87.

13. Tai HH, Korsch B: Simultaneous radioimmunoassay of secretin and gastrin, in preparation.

14. Tai HH, Korsch B, Chey WY: Preparation of ^{125}I-labeled secretin of high specific radioactivity, submitted.

15. Tai HH, Rhodes R, Chey WY: Plasma RIA secretin and gastrin responses to a meat meal and duodenal acidification in man, in preparation.

16. Young JD, Lazarus L, Chisholm DJ, Atkinson FFV: Radioimmunoassay of secretin in human serum. *J Nucl Med* 9:641–642, 1968.

SECRETIN RADIOIMMUNOASSAY

Guenther Boden

Department of Medicine, Section of Metabolism
and the General Clinical Research Center,
Temple University Health Sciences Center,
Philadelphia, Pennsylvania

Until recently, secretin could be measured only by
bioassay. As is true for most bioassays, the secretin
bioassay is both nonspecific and not sufficiently
sensitive to measure the hormone in biologic fluids.
The availability of highly purified natural and synthetic secretin during the past few years has made it
possible to develop specific and sensitive radioimmunologic methods for its determination. In 1972
we first reported a workable, sensitive and specific
secretin radioimmunoassay,[4] and later published the
details.[2,3] The following is a presentation of some
of the essential aspects of this assay and includes
some of the data obtained with its use.

METHODS

Preparation of Radiolabeled Secretin

Iodination of secretin, which lacks tyrosine residues, has been considered difficult,[1] but it has been
found that secretin can be successfully iodinated
with either chloramine-T[3,13] or lactoperoxidase[10] used
as oxidizing agents (Table 1).

Purification of Radiolabeled Secretin

The radiolabeled secretin was purified from non-
reactive ^{125}I and damaged ^{125}I secretin in a two-step
procedure with talc tablets and cellulose used

283

Table 1. Iodination of secretin

0.5M phosphate buffer pH 7.5	0.025 ml
Add secretin in 1/10 N HCl (conc. 1 µg/1 µl)	0.003
Add Na ^{125}I (1 mCi)	0.003
Add chloramine-T* (12 µg in 0.05M phosphate buffer). Shake gently for about 1 minute	0.020
Add Na metabisulfite (192 µg in 0.05M phosphate buffer).	0.080
Add normal human serum	0.100

* For the enzymatic iodination:

Add lactoperoxidase (50 µg in 0.05M phosphate buffer adjusted to pH 6.0)	0.010
Add H_2O_2 (6 µmols)	0.010
Shake gently for 15 minutes	

Table 2. Purification of ^{125}I secretin

Add 100 µl of the original iodination mixture to ½ talc tablet
(50 mg)

Wash with 1.5 ml serum
discard supernatant

Wash residue with 1.5 ml distilled H_2O
discard supernatant

Elute ^{125}I secretin with 2 ml acetic acid acetone

Transfer eluate to cellulose column (10 x 7 cm)

Wash twice with 0.05 PO_4 buffer containing 0.5% BSA

Elute ^{125}I secretin with 2 ml of 0.1 N HCl

Discard first 1.0 ml (fraction 1)
Collect remainder (fraction 2)

Additional elution with 1.0 ml of 0.1 N HCl
Collect entire eluate (fraction 3)

284

according to the method of Rosselin and associates (Table 2).[12] The chloramine-T technique as used in our laboratory usually resulted in specific activities of about 150 mci/mg (Fig. 1). Slightly higher specific activities were obtained using lactoperoxidase. This was probably due to the much longer time allowed between the addition of the oxidizing agent and the addition of sodium metabisulfite (1 minute for chloramine-T, 15 minutes for lactoperoxidase). On chromatoelectrophoresis, between 90% and 98% of the radioactivity remained at the origin of the cellulose paper and was considered to be pure, intact ^{125}I-labeled secretin. Binding to excess antibody ranged from 85% to 95% by either method.

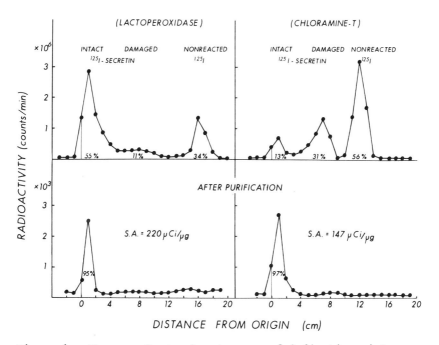

Figure 1. Chromatoelectrophoretograms of iodination mixtures before purification (upper panel) and after purification with talc and cellulose (lower panel). The iodinations were performed with lactoperoxidase (left side of the figure) or with chloramine-T (right side of the figure).

Stability of Secretin

Secretin, both labeled and unlabeled, was not stable in solution. We have found that ^{125}I-labeled secretin remained relatively intact for at least four days when kept in 0.1 N HCl, but was degraded progressively in the presence of dilute serum.[3] The addition of the kallikrein inhibitor, Trasylol, sufficiently stabilized the ^{125}I secretin for the duration of the incubation period.[3] Similarly, nonlabeled secretin lost approximately 50% of its immuno- and bioactivity during one month of storage in solution.[6] Cystein HCl which is present in the purified secretin obtained from the gastrointestinal hormone research laboratory, Stockholm, greatly prolonged immuno- and bioactivity of the hormone.[6]

Production and Characteristics of Antibodies

Antibodies to pure synthetic secretin coupled with carbodiimide to bovine serum albumin, were produced in random-bred New Zealand white rabbits. The specificity of the antisera obtained is depicted in Figure 2. Human insulin, human growth hormone, porcine ACTH, human LH and FSH, bovine-porcine glucagon and human gastrin I in doses far exceeding the physiologic range did not cross-react with this antiserum. The very weak cross-reaction observed with porcine cholecystokinin (CCK - the 10% pure preparation) was almost certainly caused by contamination with secretin. The same antiserum was evaluated with respect to its binding affinity to several synthetic secretin fragments. The antiserum reacted equally with the complete secretin molecule (S 1-27) and the C-terminal tricosapeptide (S 5-27) (Fig. 3). Its affinity to the C-terminal tetradecapeptide (S 14-27) was approximately 50% of that of the complete secretin molecule. By comparison, the amino terminal tetradecapeptide (S 1-14) exhibited only minimal cross-reaction. These observations indicated that the binding sites of this antiserum recognize predominantly the C-terminal end of the secretin molecule. This conclusion was supported by the observed lack of cross-reaction with glucagon, which with the sole exception of a glutamine residue in position 3, has the identical N-terminal 8-amino acid sequence as secretin.

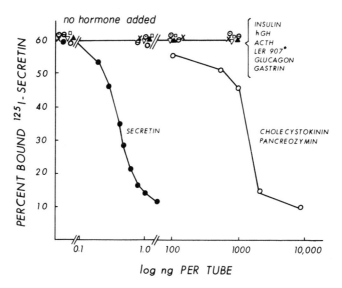

Figure 2. Immunoreactivity of several polypeptide and glycoprotein hormones with the antiserum used for the radioimmunoassay. All values represent means of triplicate determinations.
(Reproduced, with permission of *Endocrinology*.[3])

Assay Procedure

The reactants and volumes of the radioimmunoassay
are listed on Table 3. Figure 4 shows the mean of
12 consecutive standard curves obtained using this
technique. The sensitivity of the radioimmunoassay
was 200 μU/ml serum equivalent to approximately 50
pg/ml.[5] Intra-assay variation was 9% and interassay
variation was 17%. The mean of the recoveries of
known amounts of secretin in diluted human sera was
87%.[3]

RESULTS

Normal Values

Fasting secretin concentrations were found to range
from less than 50 pg to 150 pg/ml serum. The higher
values, reported earlier,[3] were caused by factors in
some human sera as yet unidentified, which interfered
with the radioimmunoassay. This problem, however,

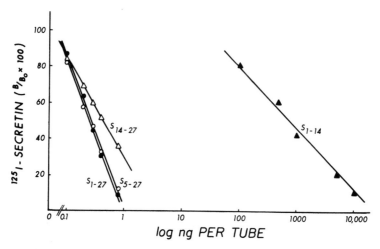

Figure 3. Immunoreactivity of synthetic secretin and three synthetic secretin fragments with the antiserum. Shown are the means of triplicate determinations and the calculated lines of regression. B, precipitated radioactivity in presence of unlabeled secretin. B_o, precipitated radioactivity in absence of unlabeled secretin. (Reproduced, with permission of *Endocrinology*.[3])

Table 3. Reactants and volumes of the radioimmunoassay for secretin

Secretin standard containing 0.25 ml of secretin-free serum or the unknown serum sample diluted with buffer	1.25 ml
Addition of antisecretin serum	0.10
Addition of Trasylol (1000 KIU)	0.10
Incubation for 3 days at 4C	
Addition of secretin ^{125}I	0.05
Incubation for 2 days at 4C	
Addition of sheep antirabbit γ-globulin serum (1:20)	0.10
and normal guinea pig serum (1:200)	0.10
Incubation for 12 hours at 4C	
Centrifugation, decantation, counting	

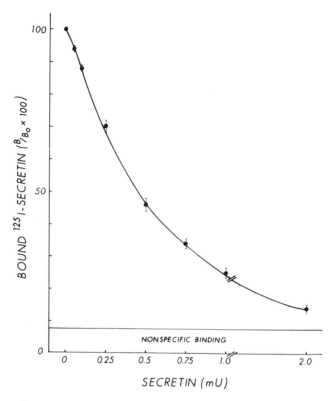

Figure 4. Means (±SEM) of 12 consecutive standard
curves with pure secretin. B, precipitated radioactivity in presence of unlabeled secretin.
B_O, precipitated radioactivity in absence of unlabeled secretin. (Reproduced, with permission
of Academic Press.[2])

could be circumvented by methanol extraction of the
sera.[2] Fasting concentrations of immunoreactive
secretin (IRS) were generally between 10% and 30%
higher in portal venous blood than in femoral venous
blood, which indicates continuous basal secretion of
secretin into the portal system during fasting.

Stimulation of Secretin Release

Following a protein-rich meal, IRS concentrations
rose two- or threefold in dogs (Boden, unpublished
observation). When the major components of such a
meal, amino acids, free fatty acids, and different
sugars, were administered intraduodenally to anesthetized dogs, however, it was found that none of these
substrates had an effect on circulating IRS concentrations.[8] Similarly, hypo-, iso-, or hypertonic
saline or glucose solutions, had no effect on secretin release.[7,8] In contrast, when HCl (21 mEq/30 min)
was infused intraduodenally, IRS rose almost instan-
taneously in the portal circulation, and after a short
delay, in the peripheral circulation (Fig. 5).[7] From
these results it would appear that intestinal acidification by gastric contents represents the major
stimulus for IRS release and that amino acids, fatty
acids, and sugars have no major stimulatory effects.
Nevertheless, it is possible that fatty acids, for
instance, stimulate the release of secretin in quantities too small to be detected in our assay. Meyer
and Jones[11] have estimated that release of as little
as 0.125 U/kg/hr of secretin would be sufficient to
explain the enhanced bicarbonate excretion that they
have observed in dog experiments after infusion of

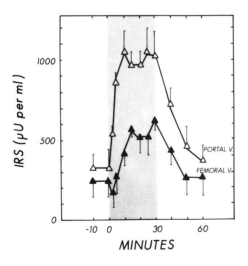

Figure 5. Effects of
intraduodenal infusion
of HCl (21 mEq/ 30 min)
on portal venous (open
triangles) and femoral
venous (closed triangles)
serum IRS concentrations.
Shown are mean ± SEM of
six experiments on anes-
thetized dogs.

fatty acids. Release of 0.125 U/kg/hr of secretin into the peripheral circulation would increase venous IRS concentration by about 57 μU/ml, which would be undetectable at the present sensitivity of our assay.

Half-life of Secretin

The volume of distribution for secretin was determined in experiments in which unlabeled secretin was infused intravenously into dogs.[7] The volume of distribution was found to be 17% of body weight, which indicates that the hormone was distributed throughout the extracellular space. After discontinuation of the secretin infusion, IRS disappeared from the peripheral blood with a half-time of three minutes (Fig. 6).

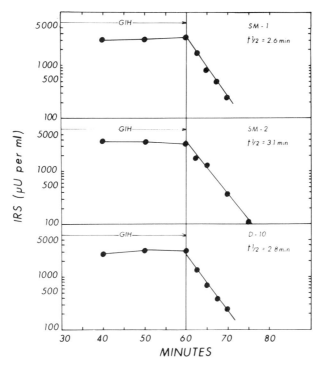

Figure 6. IRS concentrations during and after infusion of exogenous secretin at a constant rate. Shown are the results of three individual experiments. (Reproduced, with permission of the *Journal of Clinical Investigation.*[8])

The metabolic clearance rate was calculated to be
730 ml/min.[7] From these data we have calculated that
intraduodenal administration of HCl in dogs resulted
in delivery of about 1.4 U/kg/hr of secretin into the
peripheral circulation.[7]

Organ Distribution of Radiolabeled Secretin

In the study of organ distribution, metabolism, and
excretion of ^{125}I-labeled secretin in rats, it was
found that ^{125}I secretin bound specifically to plasma
membrane fractions obtained from pancreas and stomach
(Sivitz and Boden, unpublished observations). Other
experiments suggested that labeled secretin is degraded by liver and kidney and is excreted through urine
and feces.[9]

SUMMARY

A double-antibody radioimmunoassay for secretin is
described. This method uses a specific antiserum
produced in rabbits to synthetic secretin which was
coupled to bovine serum albumin. This antiserum
recognizes the complete secretin molecule as well as
large carboxy-terminal secretin fragments. Synthetic
secretin is labeled with ^{125}I, with either chloramine-
T or lactoperoxidase used as oxidizing agent. The
sensitivity of the assay is 50 pg/ml of serum. Fasting secretin concentrations ranged from less than
50 pg/ml to 150 pg/ml of serum. Immunoreactive secretin (IRS) concentration rises severalfold following
intraduodenal administration of HCl or ingestion of
a protein meal. In contrast, intraduodenal administration of amino acids, oleic acid or glucose, fruc-
tose, and sucrose in hypo-, iso-, or hypertonic solutions has no effect on circulating IRS concentration
in anesthetized dogs. The half-life of disappearance
of exogenously administered secretin is approximately
three minutes. The secretin distribution space is
17% of the body weight and the metabolic clearance
rate is 730 ml/min. Approximately 1.4 U/kg/hr of
secretin is released into the periphery after maximal
stimulation with intraduodenal HCl.

Acknowledgments

This work was supported in part by U.S. Public Health Service Grants 1 R01 AM 16348-01 MET and 5 M01 RR 349, NIH, General Clinical Research Centers Branch, National Institutes of Health.

References

1. Berson SA, Yalow RS: Radioimmunoassay in gastroenterology. *Gastroenterology* 62:1061-1084, 1972.
2. Boden G: Secretin, in *Methods of Hormone Radioimmunoassay*, New York: Academic Press, 1974, pp 275-288.
3. Boden G, Chey WY: Preparation and specificity of antiserum to synthetic secretin and its use in a radioimmunoassay (RIA). *Endocrinology* 92:1617-1624, 1973.
4. Boden G, Chey WY, Dinoso VP: A sensitive and specific radio-immunoassay (RIA) for secretin, abstracted, in *4th International Congress of Endocrinology. Abstracts of Short Communications*, International Congress Series 256. Amsterdam: Excerpta Medica, 1972, p 70.
5. Boden G, Dinoso VP, Owen OE: Immunological comparison of natural and synthetic secretins. *Horm Metab Res* 5: 237-240, 1973.
6. Boden G, Dinoso VP, Owen OE: Immunological potency and stability of native and synthetic secretins. *Gastro-enterology* 67:1119-1125, 1974.
7. Boden G, Essa N, Owen OE, Reichle FA: Effects of intra-duodenal administration of HCl and glucose on circu-lating immunoreactive secretin and insulin concentra-tions. *J Clin Invest* 53:1185-1193, 1974.
8. Boden G, Essa N, Owen OE: Effects of intraduodenal amino acids, fatty acids and sugars on secretin concentrations. *Gastroenterology*, in press.
9. Gulati SC, Boden G: Organ distribution and excretion of radioactivity after injection of ^{125}I secretin in rats, abstracted. *Clin Res* 20:869, 1972.
10. Holohan KN, Murphy RF, Flanagan RWJ, Buchanan KD, Elmore DT: Enzymic iodination of the histidyl residue of secretin: A radioimmunoassay of the hormone. *Biochim Biophys Acta* 322:178-180, 1973.
11. Meyer JH, Jones RS: Canine pancreatic responses to intes-tinally perfused fat and products of fat digestion. *Am J Physiol* 226:1178-1187, 1974.
12. Rosselin G, Assan R, Yalow RS, Berson SA: Separation of antibody bound and unbound peptide hormones labelled

with iodine-131 by talc powder and precipitated silica. *Nature* 212:355-358, 1966.

13. Young JD, Lazarus L, Chisholm DJ, Atkinson FFV: Radio-immunoassay of secretin in human serum. *J Nucl Med* 9:641-642, 1968.

PROBLEMS ENCOUNTERED IN THE DEVELOPMENT
OF THE CHOLECYSTOKININ RADIOIMMUNOASSAY

Vay L.W. Go, William M. Reilly

Gastroenterology Unit, Mayo Foundation,
Rochester, Minnesota

Several radioimmunoassays for cholecystokinin (CCK) have now been described.[1-5,7-9] None has succeeded in giving a reasonable value for CCK concentration in human blood, however, and the problems encountered in setting up the assay are by no means solved. Several factors have contributed to some of the problems, including the nonavailability of pure human CCK, the difficulty of iodinating (the only tyrosine residue in the porcine CCK molecule is sulfated), the lack of a reference preparation for use as a working standard, and the relatively low immunogenic potency of CCK. Because of these factors, the laboratories performing these studies have used different preparations of CCK for labeling, for production of antisera, and for working standards in setting up the assay (Table 1). This multiplicity has resulted in the lack of agreement among reported values for CCK in the peripheral circulation.

This report will explore three areas: various techniques used in the radioiodination of CCK, the development of antisera, and the standard used in the different assay systems.

PREPARATION AND PURIFICATION OF RADIOLABELED CCK

CCK has been labeled with ^{125}I or ^{131}I by the chloramine-T method of Hunter and Greenwood.[6] Batches of porcine CCK varied from 10% to 99% in purity. When a 10% or 20% pure preparation of porcine CCK is used, considerable difficulty is usually encountered in

Table 1. Radioimmunoassays of CCK

Development of antibodies -- immunogens used

   Jorpes porcine CCK
      8.5% pure (Reeder)
     10.0% pure (Englert, Go)
     20.0% pure (Go)
     99.0% pure (Go)

   Boot's porcine CCK
     0.05% pure (Young, Harvey)

   Squibb's CCK octapeptide (Go)

Radioiodination of CCK*

   Jorpes porcine CCK
     10% pure (Young)
     16% pure (Reeder)
     20% pure (Englert)
     99% pure (Harvey, Go)

   Boot's porcine CCK

   Squibb's CCK octapeptide (Go)
     (sulfated or unsulfated)

Standards

   Jorpes porcine CCK
     10% pure (Englert)
     17% pure (Reeder)
     20% pure (Englert)
     99% pure (Harvey, Go)

   Boot's porcine CCK (Young)

---

* Specific activities: 99% pure CCK-PZ = 127 ± 7 µci/µg;
                  sulfated octapeptide = 73 ± 11 µci/µg;
                  unsulfated octapeptide = 204 ± 10 µci/µg.

---

purifying the radiolabeled CCK by the gel filtration technique. Because the antisera have all been produced against crude preparations of CCK, a highly purified radiolabeled CCK (preferably greater than 95% purity) is essential for accuracy and specificity in the measurement of CCK.

Recently, Dr. V Mutt of the Karolinska Institute, Stockholm, Sweden, has made available a 99% pure preparation of porcine CCK for radiolabeling purposes.

The specific activities obtained are much lower, however, than those obtained with other gastrointestinal hormones, such as gastrin I or glucagon, in which the tyrosine residue is not sulfated. Our laboratory had the same experience in radiolabeling the octapeptide of CCK (Squibb Laboratory; kindly supplied by Dr. Miguel Ondetti). A threefold increase in specific activity can be obtained with radiolabeling the unsulfated octapeptide of CCK as compared to the sulfated octapeptide (Table 1).

PRODUCTION OF ANTISERA

CCK appears to be a relatively nonimmunogenic antigen. Antisera have been produced in chickens, guinea pigs, and rabbits. Various preparations of porcine CCK, either conjugated to albumin or unconjugated, have been used as immunogens (Table 1). The antisera obtained are of low titer and, surprisingly, show no (or only slight) cross-reactivity with gastrin, despite the similarity of the biologically active COOH-terminal portion. This suggests that the antisera that are available to date from all laboratories, recognize the nonbiologically active portion of CCK. Therefore, the immunologic activity that is measured may or may not correlate with the biologic activity that one wishes to measure in biologic fluids, including blood. We found further that, with porcine CCK as immunogen, some of the antisera did not cross-react with human CCK.[3] In order to raise an antibody that can measure the biologically active COOH-terminal portion of CCK, we conjugated CCK octapeptide to albumin and used this compound to immunize rabbits. Unfortunately, the antisera that we obtained cross-reacted with gastrin I equally in molar ratio. Although these antisera to CCK octapeptide recognized the biologically active end of the CCK molecule, they lack the specificity one hopes to attain (unpublished data).

CCK STANDARD

Currently, there is no standard reference preparation. Different laboratories (Table 1) used different preparations of porcine CCK as a laboratory working standard. The crude CCK (<99% pure preparation) from Karolinska Institute or Boot's preparation is not satisfactory for repeated use as standard in the assay system because of variation in the quoted potency per unit weight or the presence of a biologically potent fragment of CCK in various preparations. Even though biologic potencies are the same in different crude preparations of CCK, different immunologic activities have been detected.[2] This variability of immunologic activity of various porcine CCK preparations may explain the discrepancies in values obtained by the various published radioimmunoassay systems. Ideally, therefore, 99% pure porcine CCK with a biologic activity of 3,000 Ivy dog units/mg should be used for the reference standard.

SUMMARY

Until pure human CCK is available, the porcine CCK preparation will continue to be used in the development of radioimmunoassays for the measurement of CCK in biologic fluids including human blood. It is advisable, from our experience and that of others, that the radiolabeled CCK and the CCK working standard should be 99% pure. Because not all reported assay systems have used the 99% pure preparation of CCK for these purposes, the reported values for CCK concentration should be considered as preliminary.

Acknowledgments

This study was supported in part by grant AM 6908 from the National Institute of Arthritis, Metabolism and Digestive Diseases.

References

1. Englert E Jr: Radioimmunoassay (RIA) of cholecystokinin (CCK), abstracted. *Clin Res* 21:207, 1973.
2. Go VLW, Cataland S, Reilly W: Radioimmunoassay (RIA) of cholecystokinin-pancreozymin (CCK-PZ) in human serum, abstracted. *Gastroenterology* 66:700, 1974.

3. Go VLW, Ryan RJ, Summerskill WHJ: Radioimmunoassay of porcine cholecystokinin pancreozymin. *J Lab Clin Med* 77:684-689, 1971.
4. Harvey RF, Dowsett L, Hartog M, Read AE: A radioimmunoassay for cholecystokinin-pancreozymin. *Lancet* 2: 826-828, 1973.
5. Harvey RF, Mathur MS, Dowsett L, Read AE: Measurement of cholecystokinin-pancreozymin levels in peripheral venous blood in man, abstracted. *Gastroenterology* 66:707, 1974.
6. Hunter WM, Greenwood FC: Preparation of iodine[131] labeled human growth hormone of high specific activity. *Nature* 194:495-496, 1962.
7. Reeder DD, Becker HD, Smith NJ, Rayford PL, Thompson JC: Radioimmunoassay of cholecystokinin. *Surg Forum* 23:361-362, 1972.
8. Reeder DD, Becker HD, Smith NJ, Rayford PL, Thompson JC: Measurement of endogenous release of cholecystokinin by radioimmunoassay. *Ann Surg* 178:304-310, 1973.
9. Young JD, Lazarus L, Chisholm DJ, Atkinson FFV: Radioimmunoassay of pancreozymin cholecystokinin in human serum. *J Nucl Med* 12:743-745, 1969.

RELEASE AND HALF-LIFE OF CCK IN MAN

Phillip L. Rayford, H. Roberts Fender,
N. Ian Ramus, David D. Reeder,
James C. Thompson

Department of Surgery, The University of Texas
Medical Branch, Galveston, Texas

Several investigators[4,5,7,8,13,22] have reported the development and validation of specific radioimmunoassays which are sensitive enough to measure concentrations of cholecystokinin (CCK) in serum. There was generally good agreement among these investigators concerning increased levels of CCK in healthy normal subjects after the ingestion of a meal. Harvey[7] reported "very considerably raised" fasting serum CCK concentrations in patients with pancreatic exocrine deficiency. Studies have not been conducted, however, to determine the temporal pattern of food-stimulated release of CCK in man during both physiologic and pathologic conditions.

We have used a specific anti-CCK rabbit serum and 99% pure cholecystokinin as both a labeled antigen and as a reference preparation to validate a sensitive, specific and accurate CCK radioimmunoassay (RIA). This radioimmunoassay has been employed to measure endogenous release of cholecystokinin in normal man, and in patients with diabetes, duodenal ulcer disease, and the Zollinger-Ellison syndrome. We have also determined the disappearance half-time of exogenously administered cholecystokinin from the circulation of normal man. The results of these studies are the subject of this report.

MATERIALS AND METHODS

Food Study

Fifteen normal subjects, 10 patients with diabetes, 15 patients with duodenal ulcer disease (eight preoperative and seven postoperative), and eight patients with Zollinger-Ellison syndrome (postoperative) participated in the study. All fasted for at least 14 hours before the study. Blood samples were collected twice during fasting and at regular time intervals after eating.

Disappearance Half-time of Cholecystokinin

Four normal human subjects participated in this study. Two blood samples were collected before intravenous infusion, for five minutes, of 1 IDU/kg/min (IDU = Ivy dog unit) of 16% pure CCK (500 IDU), obtained from the Gastrointestinal Hormone (GIH) Laboratory, Karolinska Institute, Stockholm. Blood samples were collected at three minutes, at the end of the five-minute infusion, and after the infusion at one-minute intervals for 10 minutes and at two-minute intervals for an additional 10 minutes. All blood specimens were centrifuged at 500 G for 20 minutes in a refrigerated centrifuge at 5C. Serum samples were collected and stored frozen until assayed for cholecystokinin concentrations.

Radioimmunoassay (RIA)

The concentration of CCK in test samples was measured by radioimmunoassay. The principles and basic techniques for developing an RIA have been previously described.[2] The technical procedures used, (buffers, incubation times, counting techniques) have been reported.[10,13]

Generation of Antiserum

The method used to generate antisera has been previously described by Vaitukaitis and colleagues.[20] Purified CCK (500 IDU/mg)was used as an immunogen to generate an anti-CCK serum in New Zealand white rabbits. Thirty micrograms of the immunogen were emulsified in 1 ml of 0.0. M phosphate buffered saline at pH 7.8 and an equal volume of complete Freund's adjuvant. The emulsion was injected, intradermally, into 30 to 50 sites along the limbs and backs of the rabbits. In addition, 0.5 ml of crude *Bordetella pertussis* (Eli Lilly Corp., Indianapolis, Ind.) was injected subcutaneously. Booster injections were administered biweekly and the rabbits were bled on alternate weeks. An antiserum (UT-122) that bound 25% to 35% of labeled antigen at final dilution of 1:2500 was used to develop the CCK radioimmunoassay.

Iodination

Cholecystokinin was iodinated with carrier-free [125]I (Amersham/Searle Corp, Arlington, Ill.) to specific activities of 30 to 50 µci/µg by the method of Greenwood, Hunter, and Glover.[6] Separation of labeled polypeptide from free iodine was achieved by gel filtration through Sephadex G10 (Pharmacia Fine Chemicals Inc., Piscataway, NJ).

Statistical Method

For each CCK radioimmunoassay, 99% pure CCK (3000 IDU/mg, GIH Laboratory) was used as a reference standard. The logit transformation method of Rodbard[16] was used to generate dose-response curves for dose interpolations of amounts of CCK in test samples, and CCK was calculated as picograms per milliliter (pg/ml) of serum. Mean CCK concentrations were analyzed for significance using the paired "t" test.[18] Differences with a *p* value of less than 0.05 were considered significant.

Calculation of Disappearance Half-time of Cholecystokinin

The linear regression method described by Walsh and colleagues[21] was used to calculate the disappearance half-time of exogenous cholecystokinin. The mean basal CCK concentration was subtracted from all other values for each person in the study. Peak CCK

concentrations (time 0) were assigned a value of 100%
and the percent for each time period was calculated
by dividing each CCK concentration by the peak CCK
value. Percent values were then converted to natural
logarithms and the data were analyzed by linear regression analysis with time used as the independent
variable and natural logarithms of percent peak CCK
concentration as the dependent variable. This analysis resulted in equation of the regression line:

$$y = a + bx$$

where: $y = \log_n$ percent peak CCK concentration;
             a = value of y when $x = 0$;
             b = slope of the regression line;
    and x = time in minutes.

The disappearance half-time was calculated by dividing 0.693, the natural logarithm of 2, by the
slope of the regression line.

RESULTS

Specificity of Cholecystokinin Radioimmunoassay

Sixteen percent pure CCK and 99% pure CCK, whose
bioassay potencies were 500 IDU/mg and 3000 IDU/mg
respectively, were radioiodinated and each was used
as a labeled antigen. Graded amounts of unlabeled
99% pure CCK or 16% pure CCK were tested in the RIA
system to determine their ability to displace each
of the labeled CCK preparations from combination with
CCK antibody (UT-122, 1:2500 final dilution). When
16% pure CCK was used as a labeled tracer, 2 to 120 ng
of 16% pure CCK produced a linear dose-response
curve; however, amounts of 99% pure CCK up to 50 ng
did not compete with the labeled hormone for CCK
antibody (Fig. 1). In contrast to our findings with
labeled 16% pure CCK, linear inhibition lines were
produced by graded amounts of both 99% pure CCK
(0.04 to 2 ng) and 16% pure CCK (1.5 to 20 ng) when
99% pure CCK was employed as a labeled antigen in
the RIA system (Fig. 1). The immunopotency ratio of
the two CCK preparations could then be calculated,
and on a mass basis, 99% pure CCK was approximately
25 times more immunoreactive than 16% pure CCK.
Based on these observations, 99% pure CCK was used

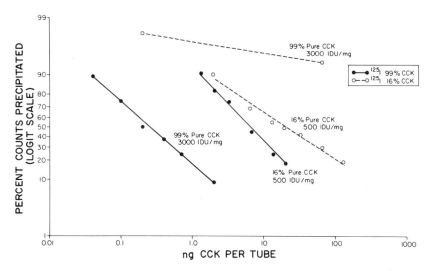

Figure 1. Inhibition lines generated by graded amounts of 99% pure CCK and by 16% pure CCK, with either 99% pure CCK or 16% pure CCK used as a labeled antigen.

as both a labeled antigen and as a reference standard in all subsequent assays.

The ability of unlabeled purified hormones, some whose molecular structure was similar to CCK, to displace labeled CCK from combination with antiserum was tested in the radioimmunoassay system. Insulin, secretin, glucagon, pentagastrin, caerulein, and human growth hormone did not compete with ^{125}I cholecystokinin for antibody sites in quantities ranging from 4 to 1000 ng per tube (counts bound >93%) (Fig. 2). The C-terminal octapeptide of CCK (Op-CCK) and synthetic human gastrin (SHG I) did displace labeled CCK from CCK antibody, but inhibition lines generated by these preparations were not parallel to the dose-response curve of 99% pure CCK (Fig. 2). The mass of Op-CCK, however, was approximately 25 times greater and, more importantly, the mass of SHG I was 400-500 times greater than the mass of purified CCK required for an equivalent displacement of ^{125}I cholecystokinin from combination with antibody.

In order to test the ability of the radioimmunoassay system to quantify CCK in serum, graded

305

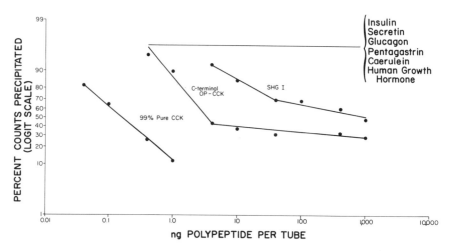

Figure 2. Inhibition lines generated by graded amounts of 99% pure CCK and other polypeptides in the CCK radioimmunoassay, with 99% pure CCK used as a labeled antigen.

volumes (50 to 500 µl) of serum from a patient with the Zollinger-Ellison syndrome were analyzed in the cholecystokinin radioimmunoassay. The serum dose-response curve and the dose-response curve generated by 99% pure CCK were parallel (Fig. 3). The data indicate that the concentration of CCK in volumes of serum up to 500 µl can be measured in the radioimmuno-assay system.

Concentrations of CCK in Man

Normal man. Mean basal CCK serum concentrations in 15 normal subjects were 731±87 pg/ml and 702±92 pg/ml. Fifteen minutes after food, serum CCK levels increased to 912 pg/ml and were significantly elevated above basal at 30, 60, 90, 180, and 240 minutes postpran-dially (Fig. 4).

Diabetics. Mean basal serum CCK concentrations in ten diabetic patients were 578±113 pg/ml and 584±124 pg/ml (Fig. 5). Five minutes after the ingestion of food, the mean serum CCK concentration was 894 pg/ml, sig-nificantly greater than basal. Mean CCK levels rose to 1550 pg/ml 15 minutes after food, but this value was not significantly different from mean basal CCK

306

concentration. At 30 and 60 minutes, CCK concentrations dropped to 969 and 823 pg/ml and remained relatively constant, but greater than basal, throughout the remainder of the test period (Fig. 5).

Duodenal Ulcer Patients (Preoperative). Basal serum CCK concentrations were 643±74 pg/ml and 654±64 pg/ml. Cholecystokinin levels were significantly increased at 5, 10, 15, and 30 minutes after eating (Fig. 6). Although CCK concentrations were consistently greater than basal levels at 45, 90, 120, 150, and 180 minutes after eating, these concentrations were not significantly different from basal (Fig. 6).

Duodenal Ulcer Patients (Postoperative). Serum CCK concentrations increased from basal values of 765±93 pg/ml and 733±109 pg/ml to 935, 984, 1116, and 1444 pg/ml at 5, 10, 15, and 30 minutes after food (Fig. 7). Significant elevations of CCK were found at the 15- and 30-minute time periods. CCK dropped at 45 minutes and continued to decline to basal values and below at 90, 120, 150, and 180 minutes after eating.

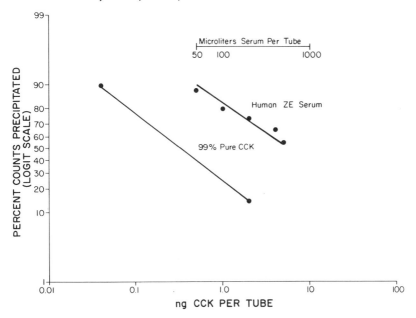

Figure 3. Dose-response curves generated by graded quantities of 99% pure CCK and serum from a patient with the Zollinger-Ellison syndrome (ZE) in the CCK radioimmunoassay.

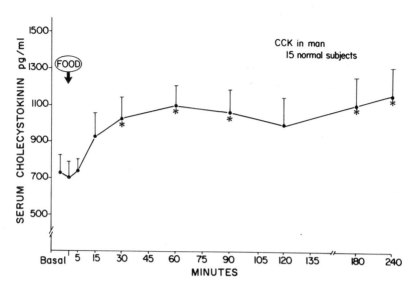

Figure 4. Cholecystokinin concentrations (pg/ml ± SE) in the serum of 15 normal subjects before and at different time periods after the ingestion of a high-protein and high-carbohydrate meal. Asterisk identifies values significantly elevated above basal.

Zollinger-Ellison Patients (Postoperative). Mean cholecystokinin concentrations in the serum of eight patients with Zollinger-Ellison syndrome, postoperatively, were 2075±320 pg/ml and 1800±266 pg/ml (Fig. 8). Serum cholecystokinin attained a peak value of 2787 pg/ml at 15 minutes and declined steadily, reaching basal levels 150 minutes after food. There was no significant elevation of CCK levels due to food.

Disappearance Half-time of Exogenous CCK. Mean serum CCK concentrations (pg/ml) were plotted against time in minutes (Fig. 9). Mean basal CCK concentrations were 921±193 pg/ml and 812±169 pg/ml. The level increased to 5604±1780 pg/ml at three minutes and was 9600±2207 pg/ml at the end of the five-minute infusion. After the infusion, cholecystokinin levels declined rapidly to 3300±667 pg/ml at five minutes, 1605±126 pg/ml at 14 minutes and 1062±57 pg/ml at 25 minutes. Analysis of the data by linear regression method resulted in a correlation coefficient (r)

308

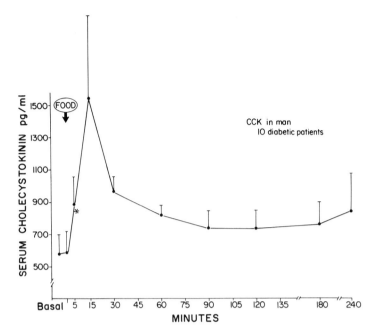

Figure 5. Cholecystokinin concentrations (pg/ml ± SE) in the serum of 10 diabetic patients before and at different time periods after the ingestion of a high-protein and high-carbo-hydrate meal. Asterisk identifies values significantly elevated above basal.

of -0.96, a slope of 0.28 and the disappearance half-time of 2.4 minutes. A plot of the results is shown in Figure 10.

DISCUSSION

The antiserum employed to develop the cholecysto-kinin radioimmunoassay was generated in rabbits with 16% pure CCK used as an immunogen.[13] This antiserum, at a final dilution of 1:2500, bound approximately 30% of both 16% pure and 99% pure radioiodinated CCK. Since our antiserum bound both 16% pure and 99% pure CCK with approximately the same degree of affinity, we conducted experiments to test the suitability of each of the CCK preparations for use as labeled tracer in the cholecystokinin radioimmunoassay.

309

Amounts of unlabeled 99% pure CCK ranging up to
50 ng did not displace significant quantities of
radioiodinated 16% pure CCK from combination with
our antiserum. Perhaps the less pure CCK preparation
contains substances, other than CCK, that hamper the
ability of 99% pure CCK to compete effectively with
it for antibody sites. It has previously been reported[11] that a labeled porcine follicle-stimulating
hormone (PFSH), contained contaminant that interfered
with the ability of serum to displace the labeled
compound in a quantitative fashion from combination
with a specific PFSH antiserum. Purification of the
labeled PFSH by column chromatography on an anion-
exchange resin (AG 1x10 chloride form) resulted in a
labeled preparation that proved suitable for quantitatively determining amounts of PFSH in serum.

When 16% pure cholecystokinin was employed as both
a labeled and an unlabeled antigen in combination
with our antiserum, the resultant dose-response curve
did not depart from linearity. The range of the
dose-response curve was 2 to 120 ng of 16% pure CCK;

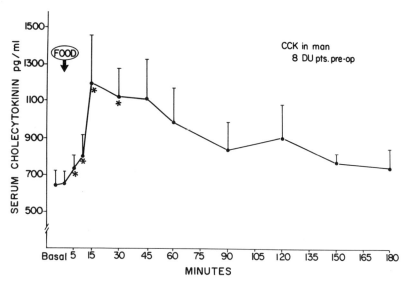

Figure 6. Cholecystokinin concentrations (pg/ml ± SE) in the
serum of eight duodenal ulcer preoperative patients before and
at different time periods after the ingestion of a high-protein
and high-carbohydrate meal. Asterisk identifies values significantly elevated above basal.

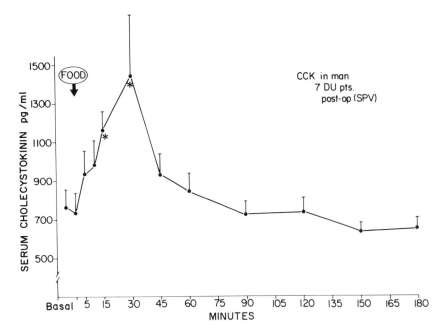

Figure 7. Cholecystokinin concentrations (pg/ml ± SE) in the serum of seven duodenal ulcer patients postoperatively (after selective proximal vagotomy [SPV]), before and at different time periods after the ingestion of a high-protein and high-carbohydrate meal. Asterisk identifies values significantly elevated above basal.

therefore, its use for dose interpolation would result in extremely high estimates of the concentration of CCK in test samples. The results suggested that this combination of antigens was not optimal for measuring cholecystokinin concentrations in test samples. Reeder and associates,[13] however, used a different cholecystokinin antiserum, and 16% pure CCK as a labeled antigen and as a reference standard, to develop a specific CCK radioimmunoassay. This RIA was capable of detecting changes in endogenous levels of CCK during different physiologic and stimulated states.

When 99% pure CCK was used as a labeled tracer with a 1:2500 dilution of our CCK antiserum, linear dose-response lines were generated by both 1.5 to 20 ng of 16% pure CCK and by 0.04 to 2 ng of 99% pure CCK.

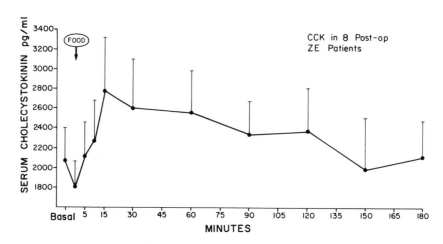

Figure 8. Cholecystokinin concentrations (pg/ml ± SE) in the serum of eight postoperative ZE patients before and at different time periods after the ingestion of a high-protein and high-carbohydrate meal.

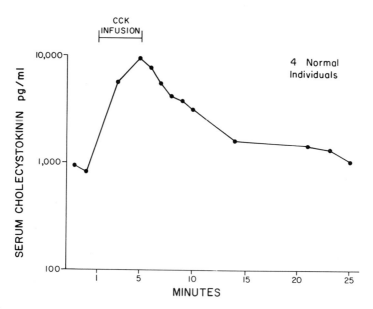

Figure 9. Serum cholecystokinin concentrations in four normal subjects before, during, and after a five-minute infusion of 16% pure CCK (1 IDU/kg).

312

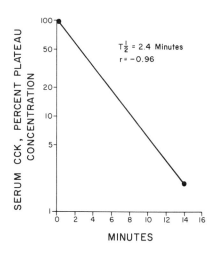

Figure 10. The semilogarithmic plot of the disappearance half-time of exogenous CCK from the circulation of four normal subjects after a five-minute infusion of 16% pure CCK (1 IDU/kg). The slope and correlation coefficient (r) were calculated by unweighted linear regression analysis.

Since 99% pure CCK was approximately 25 times more immunopotent than 16% pure CCK, use of the less pure cholecystokinin preparation for dose interpolation would result in higher estimates of the concentration of CCK in test samples. On the other hand, potency estimates obtained using the homologous antigen system (99% pure CCK) were more consistent with expected physiologic serum levels of cholecystokinin. Based upon these studies, we have employed 99% pure CCK as a labeled antigen to develop and validate the RIA, and, in addition, we have used 99% pure CCK as a reference standard for dose interpolation.

Neither insulin, secretin, glucagon, pentagastrin, caerulein nor growth hormone displaced significant amounts of labeled CCK from combination with CCK antibody. Synthetic human gastrin I and OP-CCK did cross-react in the assay system, but the inhibition lines generated by these preparations were not parallel to the dose-response curve generated by 99% pure CCK. If these data were used, however, to calculate the immunopotency ratios of the compounds (on a mass basis), unlabeled CCK was 25 times more effective than the C-terminal octapeptide of CCK and 400-500 times more effective than synthetic human gastrin I in competing with ^{125}I CCK for antibody. The amount of cross-reactivity observed with gastrin should not adversely affect the determination of CCK in the serum of humans during most physiologic and pharmacologic states. Use of this immunologic assay, however, for determination of serum CCK levels in patients with

313

the Zollinger-Ellison syndrome (whose serum gastrin levels are extremely elevated) should be interpreted with caution.

Mean fasting levels of cholecystokinin were 731 and 765 pg/ml in normal subjects, 578 and 594 pg/ml in diabetics, 643 and 654 pg/ml in preoperative duodenal ulcer patients, and 765 and 733 pg/ml in postoperative duodenal ulcer patients. These serum concentrations are probably near the upper limit of that expected during the resting state. Rubin and Engel[17] gave a rapid intravenous injection of 0.25 IDU (85 ng)/kg of 99% pure CCK to anesthetized dogs and found that this stimulated minimal pancreatic secretion. This dose of CCK would represent a serum concentration of approximately 2 ng/ml if the exogenously administered CCK was equally distributed throughout the circulation. If these results were applied to man, then serum concentrations of cholecystokinin up to 2000 pg/ml would not exceed expected physiologic levels during fasting. In normal subjects CCK levels increased steadily and significantly at 30, 60, 90, 180, and 240 minutes after food and were relatively constant from 30 minutes to the end of the 240-minute test period. These data concerning the time-related peak of CCK after the ingestion of the test meal, are consistent with those reported by Harvey and colleagues.[7] They measured cholecystokinin-pancreozymin levels in five healthy subjects after the ingestion of one pint of milk. They reported that cholecystokinin levels increased from basal values of less than 100 pg/ml to levels of 8 to 16 ng/ml within 35 minutes and thereafter declined rapidly, approaching basal value within 45 minutes. In our normal subjects, serum cholecystokinin concentrations peaked at 30 minutes and remained consistently elevated above basal for 240 minutes after the food stimulus. Since our subjects received a high-protein and high-carbohydrate diet with higher osmolarity than the pint of milk fed by Harvey and associates,[7] the observed difference in the temporal pattern of release of CCK could be due to retention of the hyperosmolar meal in the stomach.

In diabetic patients, mean serum CCK concentration was significantly greater than basal five minutes after the ingestion of the test meal and attained a peak value of 1550 pg/ml 15 minutes after eating. This value was not significantly greater than basal because one diabetic subject was included whose serum

CCK concentration was considerably greater than all the others at this time period. In both groups of duodenal ulcer patients, as with diabetics, CCK levels increased more rapidly and declined more rapidly when these temporal patterns of release are compared with those determined for our normal subjects. Perhaps a rapid increase and precipitous decrease in serum CCK levels after eating might be characteristic of patients with diabetes or duodenal ulcer disease. Since cholecystokinin is released when food is in the duodenum, the rapid rise and fall of serum CCK in diabetic and duodenal ulcer patients may reflect increased rates of gastric emptying in these subjects.

The greatest concentration of CCK was found in the serum of postoperative patients with Zollinger-Ellison syndrome. Mean fasting serum CCK concentrations were 2075±320 pg/ml and 1800±266 pg/ml. These levels were increased to 2787±540 pg/ml at 15 minutes and declined slowly reaching basal levels 150 minutes after eating. There was no significant increase above basal in serum CCK concentrations at the different time periods after the ingestion of food. This lack of significance may be attributed to the considerable variation of CCK levels during fasting and to variations of CCK levels in Zollinger-Ellison syndrome patients in response to the test meal. Although gastrin does cross-react slightly with our CCK antibody, we found no correlation between high levels of gastrin and high levels of CCK in patients with the Zollinger-Ellison syndrome (e.g., one patient had a serum gastrin level of 26,000 pg/ml and CCK of 1200 pg/ml; another patient had a serum gastrin of 4000 pg/ml and CCK of 1800 pg/ml). This suggests absolute hypercholecystokininemia in these patients.

The disappearance half-time of exogenous cholecystokinin from the circulation of four normal subjects was determined by infusion of 1 IDU/kg of 16% pure CCK for five minutes and determining serum CCK concentrations at regular time intervals. By linear regression analysis, we calculated a half-time of 2.44 minutes. These results were in good agreement with the half-time of 2.59 minutes for exogenous CCK in dogs as reported by Reeder and colleagues[15] and were also consistent with the disappearance half-time of approximately two minutes that has been reported for exogenous 17-amino acid gastrin.[12] Berry and Flowers[1] estimated that the half-life of exogenous CCK in two cats was 10 to 15 minutes. They used a less sensitive bioassay, however, to measure serum concentrations of CCK. Harvey and associates[7] suggested that the half-life of endogenous cholecystokinin in man was five to seven minutes. Since cholecystokinin has been reported to exist in two related forms[3,9] physiologically released CCK is, in all probability, a mixture of these molecular forms and a disappearance half-time of five to seven minutes is consistent with the half-time of 8.62 minutes that has been reported for endogenous mixed molecular gastrin in dogs.[19] The results indicate that cholecystokinin is removed rapidly from the circulation of both man and dogs.

SUMMARY

A radioimmunoassay (RIA) for cholecystokinin (CCK) has been developed and validated. The antiserum used was generated in rabbits using 16% pure (500 IDU/ml) cholecystokinin as an immunogen. Results of studies using 16% pure CCK and 99% pure (3000 IDU/mg) CCK as both a labeled antigen and as reference preparations, indicated that 99% pure CCK was more suitable for developing the RIA and for determining concentrations of cholecystokinin in test samples. In this homologous assay system, no cross-reactivity was observed with insulin, secretin, glucagon, pentagastrin, caerulein, or human growth hormone. The C-terminal octapeptide of CCK and synthetic human gastrin I did cross-react in the RIA system but the degree of cross-reactivity of these compounds did not adversely affect the ability of the RIA to quantify cholecystokinin in test samples. Basal serum CCK concentrations were 731±87 pg/ml in normal subjects, 578±113 pg/ml in diabetic patients, 643±74 pg/ml in preoperative duodenal ulcer patients, 765±93 pg/ml in postoperative duodenal ulcer patients and 2075±320 pg/ml in postoperative ZE patients. Serum CCK levels were significantly increased above basal in all subjects except in the Zollinger-Ellison syndrome patients, but both release and disappearance rates of CCK were more rapid in diabetic and duodenal ulcer patients than in normal subjects. The disappearance half-time of exogenous (16% pure) CCK in normal subjects was 2.44 minutes.

Acknowledgments

This work is supported by grants from the National Institutes of Health (AM 15241) and General Clinical Research Centers Branch, DHEW Grant (RR 00073), and by a grant from the John A. Hartford Foundation, Inc. N.I. Ramus is the recipient of a Wellcome Research Travel Grant.

References

1. Berry H, Flower RJ: The assay of endogenous cholecystokinin and factors influencing its release in the dog and cat. *Gastroenterology* 60:409–420, 1971.
2. Berson SA, Yalow RS: Immunoassay of protein hormones, in Pincus G, Thimann KV, Astwood EB (eds), *The Hormones*, New York: Academic Press, 1964, pp 557–630.
3. Debas HT, Grossman MI: Pure cholecystokinin: Pancreatic protein and bicarbonate response. *Digestion* 9:469–481, 1973.
4. Englert E Jr: Radioimmunoassay (RIA) of cholecystokinin (CCK), abstracted. *Clin Res* 21:207, 1973.
5. Go VLW, Ryan RJ, Summerskill WHJ: Radioimmunoassay of porcine cholecystokinin-pancreozymin. *J Lab Clin Med* 77:684–689, 1971.
6. Greenwood FC, Hunter WM, Glover JS: Preparation of ^{131}I-labelled human growth hormone of high specific radioactivity. *Biochem J* 89:114–123, 1963.
7. Harvey RF, Dowsett L, Hartog M, Read AE: A radioimmunoassay for cholecystokinin-pancreozymin. *Lancet* 2:826–828, 1973.
8. Harvey RF, Dowsett L, Hartog M, Read AE: Radioimmunoassay of cholecystokinin-pancreozymin. *Gut* 15:690–699, 1974.
9. Mutt V, Jorpes JE: Structure of porcine cholecystokinin-pancreozymin: 1. Cleavage with thrombin and with trypsin. *Eur J Biochem* 6:156–162, 1968.
10. Odell WD, Rayford PL, Ross GT: Simplified, partially automated method for radioimmunoassay of human thyroid-stimulating, growth, luteinizing and follicle stimulating hormones. *J Lab Clin Med* 70:973–980, 1967.
11. Rayford PL, Brinkley HJ, Young EP, Reichert LE, Jr: Radioimmunoassay of porcine FSH. *J Anim Sci* 39:348–354, 1974.
12. Reeder DD, Jackson BM, Brandt EN, Jr, Thompson JC: Rate and pattern of disappearance of exogenous gastrin in dogs. *Am J Physiol* 222:1571–1574, 1972.

13. Reeder DD, Becker HD, Smith NJ, Rayford PL, Thompson JC:
    Measurement of endogenous release of cholecystokinin
    by radioimmunoassay. *Ann Surg* 178:304-310, 1973.
14. Reeder DD, Becker HD, Rayford PL, Thompson JC: Cholecysto-
    kinin: Measurements by radioimmunoassay, in Chey WY,
    Brooks FP (eds), *Endocrinology of the Gut,* Thorofare NJ:
    Charles B. Slack, Inc, 1974, pp 327-336.
15. Reeder DD, Villar HV, Brandt EN, Jr, Rayford PL, Thompson
    JC: Radioimmunoassay measurements of the disappearance
    half-time of exogenous cholecystokinin, abstracted.
    Physiologist 17:319, 1974.
16. Rodbard D: Statistical aspects of radioimmunoassay, in
    Odell WD, Daughaday WH (eds), *Principles of Competitive
    Protein Binding Assays,* Philadelphia: JB Lippincott and
    Co, 1971, pp 204-259.
17. Rubin B, Engel SL: Some biological characteristics of
    cholecystokinin (CCK-PZ) and synthetic analogues, in
    Andersson S (ed), *Nobel Symposium 16. Frontiers in
    Gastrointestinal Hormone Research,* Stockholm: Almquist
    and Wiksell, 1973, pp 41-56.
18. Steel RGD, Torie JH: *Principles and Procedures of Statistics,*
    New York: McGraw-Hill Book Company Inc, 1960, pp 67-87.
19. Thompson JC, Rayford PL, Ramus NI, Fender HR, Villar HV:
    Patterns of release and uptake of heterogeneous forms
    of gastrin, in Thompson JC (ed), *Gastrointestinal
    Hormones,* Austin: University of Texas Press, 1975,
    pp 125-151.
20. Vaitukaitis JL, Robbins JB, Nieschlag E, Ross GT: A method
    for producing specific antisera with small doses of
    immunogen. *J Clin Endocrinol Metabol* 33:988-995, 1971.
21. Walsh JH, Debas HT, Grossman MI: Pure human big gastrin:
    Immunochemical properties, disappearance half-time, and
    acid-stimulating action in dogs. *J Clin Invest* 54:
    477-485, 1974.
22. Young JD, Lazarus I, Chisholm DJ: Radioimmunoassay of
    pancreozymin cholecystokinin in human serum. *J Nucl
    Med* 10:743-745, 1969.

BINDING SITES AND ACTIONS OF GI HORMONES

EFFECTS OF GASTROINTESTINAL HORMONES ON ADENYLATE CYCLASE ACTIVITY IN PANCREATIC EXOCRINE CELLS

Hayden L. Klaeveman, Thomas P. Conlon,
Jerry D. Gardner

Section on Gastroenterology, Digestive Diseases
Branch, National Institute of Arthritis, Metabolism,
and Digestive Diseases, National Institutes of Health,
Bethesda, Maryland

The first step in the mechanism of action of polypeptide hormones is generally agreed to be an interaction of the hormone with the plasma membrane. This combination initiates (by a mechanism whose details at the molecular level are not known) a sequence of changes in cellular function, the last of which is usually referred to as the "hormone response."

In the present study we have explored the interaction of two structurally distinct classes of polypeptide hormones with plasma membranes prepared from homogenous suspensions of isolated pancreatic exocrine cells. The interaction was monitored by measuring the change in activity in adenylate cyclase, an enzyme whose activation (and consequent increase in cellular adenosine 3',5'-cyclic monophosphate [cyclic AMP]) is thought to mediate the effect of several polypeptide hormones on their target tissues.[25] One class of hormones tested was that containing cholecystokinin and gastrin; the other contains secretin, vasoactive intestinal peptide (VIP), glucagon, and gastric inhibitory peptide (GIP).

MATERIALS AND METHODS

$[\alpha^{32}P]$ATP (10-20 ci/mM), $[\alpha^{32}P]$GTP (10-20 ci/M) and $[^3H]$cyclic AMP (22 ci/mM) were purchased from New England Nuclear Corp., Boston, Mass. Synthetic C-terminal octapeptide of porcine cholecystokinin

(SQ 19844, CCK-octapeptide) was kindly provided by
Dr. M Ondetti, Squibb Institute of Medical Research.
Natural porcine secretin and porcine VIP were gifts
from Prof. Viktor Mutt, GIH Research Unit, Karolinska
Institutet, Stockholm, Sweden. Prostaglandin E$_1$ (PGE$_1$)
was a gift from Dr. John Pike, Upjohn Co., Kalamazoo,
Mich. Pentagastrin (Peptavalon) was obtained from
Ayerst Laboratories, New York, N.Y.; synthetic human
gastrin I from Imperial Chemical Industries, London,
England; porcine glucagon from Eli Lilly, Indianapo-
lis, Ind.; and synthetic porcine secretin from Schwarz/
Mann, Rockville, Md. All other chemicals and reagents
were of the highest grade commercially obtainable.

Tissue Preparation

Male Hartley strain albino guinea pigs, 350-400 g,
were obtained from the Small Animals Section, Veteri-
nary Resources Branch, N.I.H. Following an overnight
fast the guinea pigs were killed by cervical dislocation. The pancreas was dissected free of fat and
mesentery, and isolated pancreatic exocrine cells
were prepared by the procedure of Amsterdam and
Jamieson.[3] Cells were isolated by incubating 0.8 g
of tissue in a Krebs-Ringer-bicarbonate solution
equilibrated with 95% O_2 and 5% CO_2 (pH 7.4), and
containing 1-amino acid supplement, 0.1 mg/ml soybean
trypsin inhibitor, and 14 mM glucose. Crude collagenase and hyaluronidase, $MgCl_2$, $CaCl_2$, and EDTA were
added as previously described.[3] The tissue was incubated at 37C in a Dubnoff shaking metabolic incu-
bator (130 oscillations/min). The entire isolation
procedure required approximately 90 minutes from the
time the guinea pigs were sacrificed. At the end of
the incubation, cells were liberated by passage
through a Pasteur pipet five times. They were then
layered over Krebs-Ringer-bicarbonate solution containing 4% albumin, 1.0 mM $CaCl_2$, 1.2 mM $MgCl_2$, and
centrifuged at 50 × g for 5 minutes at 4C. More than
95% of the cells were zymogen-containing exocrine
cells when examined by light and electron microscopy.
Viability of these cells was demonstrated by their
ability to exclude trypan blue, to incorporate ^{3}H-L-
leucine into cellular protein, and to maintain their
cellular concentrations of sodium and potassium for
up to four hours.

Adenylate Cyclase Assay

Isolated cells, which had been washed free of excess extracellular calcium, were lysed at 4C by adding 10 volumes of a solution containing 10 mM dithiothreitol, 3 $MgCl_2$, and 20 mM Tris-HCl (pH 7.4) and vortexing for 30 seconds. The mixture was then spun at 1000 x G for three minutes at 4C in an International centrifuge. The supernatant, containing the plasma membranes, was assayed immediately for adenylate cyclase.

Adenylate cyclase activity was determined by measuring the formation of ^{32}P-labeled cyclic AMP from $[\alpha^{32}P]ATP$. The final reaction mixture (70 µl) contained: Tris-HCl, 50 mM, pH 7.4; 5.0 mM $MgCl_2$; 9 mM theophylline; 10 mM KCl; 0.125 mM $[\alpha^{32}P]ATP$; ATP regenerating system (14 µg of creatine phosphokinase; 10 mM creatine phosphate; membranes; hormones or as otherwise stated). Incubation was carried out in a Dubnoff metabolic shaker at 37C. The reaction was stopped by adding 100 µl of "stopping solution" containing 2.5% sodium dodecyl sulfate, 40 mM ATP and 1.25 mM [^3H]cyclic AMP (approximately 20,000 cpm). Assay blanks were prepared by omitting membranes or by adding membranes after the stopping solution (both methods gave equivalent blank values). Isolation and detection of cyclic [^{32}P]AMP were performed with the procedure described by Salomon, Londos, and Rodbell.[36] After adding 0.8 ml H_2O to each reaction tube, the tubes were mixed and decanted into· columns (0.4x15 cm) containing 1 ml of Dowex 50 AG WX4. The eluate from this and two successive 1-ml H_2O washes were discarded. Three milliliters H_2O were then added to each column and the eluate was collected; 0.2 ml of 1.5 M imidazole-HCl, pH 7.2, was added to the 3-ml fraction, and the contents were mixed and decanted into columns (0.4x15 cm) containing 0.6 g neutral alumina previously washed with 8 ml of 0.1 M imidazole-HCl, pH 7.05. The eluate was collected directly into scintillation vials containing 15 ml Aquasol. After the columns were drained completely, an additional 2 ml of 0.1 M imidazole-HCl, pH 7.5, were added to the columns and collected in the scintillation vials. Liquid scintillation counting was performed with a Packard model 3320 liquid scintillation counter. Results were corrected for recovery of [^3H] cyclic AMP which was 70% to 80%. Blank values for ^{32}P were usually 4-7 cpm above machine background.

Adenylate cyclase activity in the membrane preparation remained constant at 37C for at least 10 minutes
in the presence or absence of agents which increase
enzyme activity. Protein concentration was determined by the method of Lowry and colleagues[22] with
bovine serum albumin as a standard. Adenylate cyclase activity remained constant between 75 and
300 μg protein per incubation tube. All assays were
performed with protein concentrations used in this
range and with enzyme activity expressed as picomoles
of cyclic AMP formed per milligram of protein per
10 minutes.

RESULTS

Table 1 lists those hormones that were tested for
an effect on pancreatic adenylate cyclase. Of the

Table 1. Adenylate cyclase activity in guinea pig pancreas
exocrine cell membranes -- Effect of hormones

Hormone (conc.)	Adenylate cyclase*
	(pmols cAMP formed/ mg/10 min)
None	15.0±0.6 (8)
CCK-octapeptide (10^{-6} M)	22.5±2.8 (8)†
VIP (2.5x10^{-6} M)	20.9±1.5 (12)†
Natural secretin (3x10^{-6} M)	17.1±0.7 (8)†
Synthetic secretin (3x10^{-6} M)	17.4±0.9 (6)†
Gastrin I (10^{-5} M)	15.5±0.6 (10)
Gastrin II (10^{-5} M)	15.3±0.6 (4)
Pentagastrin (10^{-5} M)	15.2±0.9 (6)
Glucagon (3x10^{-6} M)	14.4±0.4 (4)
PGE_1 (10^{-5} M)	17.1±0.7 (8)†
Carbamylcholine (10^{-5} M)	15.3±0.6 (6)
Sodium fluoride (10^{-3} M)	67.7±1.29 (16)†

* Results represent the mean ± 1 SD. The number in parenthesis is the number of experiments. Values for each experiment were determined in duplicate.
† Significantly greater than control using Student's t-test
(p <0.01).

hormones tested, CCK-octapeptide and VIP produced the greatest stimulation. Prostaglandin E_1 and natural and synthetic secretin each produced a small but significant increase in enzyme activity. Neither gastrin I, gastrin II, nor pentagastrin, which are structurally similar to CCK-octapeptide,[23] nor glucagon, which is structurally similar to VIP and secretin[23] stimulated pancreatic adenylate cyclase. Carbamylcholine, which, like cholecystokinin, stimulates amylase release by isolated pancreatic cells,[3] did not activate adenylate cyclase. As has been observed in other mammalian tissues,[25] sodium fluoride produced maximal stimulation of adenylate cyclase. None of the agents listed in Table 1 altered guanylate cyclase activity (assayed according to the method of Thompson and associates.[39])

An effect of CCK-octapeptide on pancreatic adenylate cyclase activity was detectable at 2×10^{-8} M and half-maximal activation of adenylate cyclase by CCK-octapeptide occurred at 2×10^{-7} M (Fig. 1). A double reciprocal plot of the increase in adenylate cyclase activity as a function of CCK-octapeptide concentration gave a straight line with the y-intercept significantly different from zero. Stimulation of pancreatic adenylate cyclase by CCK-octapeptide was enhanced by increasing the magnesium concentration (Fig. 2). Increasing the calcium concentration substantially reduced basal enzyme activity as well as the stimulation produced by CCK-octapeptide, VIP, or sodium fluoride (Fig. 3). Adding EDTA (5 mM) to the assay did not alter basal adenylate cyclase activity (results not shown).

Gastrin I (5×10^{-5} M), which alone did not alter adenylate cyclase activity, inhibited the stimulation produced by CCK-octapeptide (Fig. 1). A double-reciprocal plot of CCK-octapeptide stimulation in the presence of gastrin, produced a straight line with a y-intercept which was the same as that for CCK-octapeptide alone but with a significantly greater slope. Gastrin II and pentagastrin gave similar results, but neither VIP, secretin, nor glucagon altered the stimulation of adenylate cyclase activity produced by CCK-octapeptide (results not shown). Stimulation of adenylate cyclase by VIP was detectable at 10^{-7} M, and half-maximal at 10^{-6} M (Fig. 4). A double-reciprocal plot of VIP stimulation gave a straight line with the y-intercept significantly different from zero.

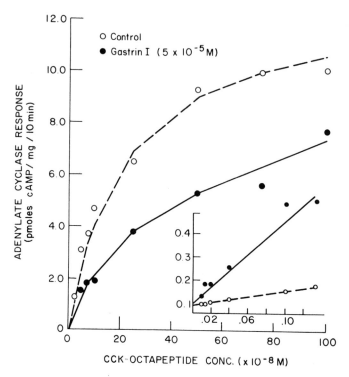

Figure 1. Stimulation of adenylate cyclase activity
in guinea pig pancreas exocrine cell membranes by
CCK-octapeptide. Values are expressed as activity
with, minus activity without, the indicated hormones.
Results given are the means for four separate experiments and each point was determined in duplicate.
Basal adenylate cyclase activity was 14.0±0.8 pmols
cAMP formed/mg/10 min   (mean ±1 SD). The *insert* is a
double-reciprocal plot of the values in the main
figure.

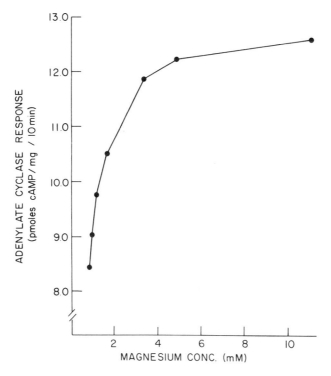

Figure 2. Effect of magnesium on CCK–octapeptide stimulation of adenylate cyclase activity in guinea pig pancreas exocrine cell membranes. Values are expressed as activity with, minus activity without, CCK-octapeptide (2×10^{-6} M). Results given are the means of three separate experiments and each point was determined in duplicate.

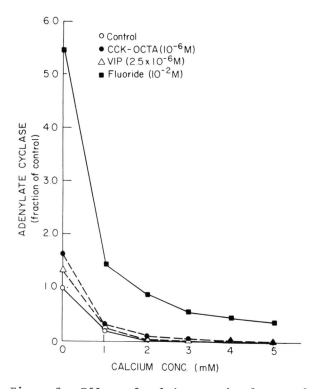

Figure 3. Effect of calcium on adenylate cyclase activity in guinea pig pancreas exocrine cell membranes. Values are expressed as the fraction of control activity (control activity is measured without added calcium, hormones, or sodium fluoride). Results given are the means of three experiments and each point was determined in duplicate.

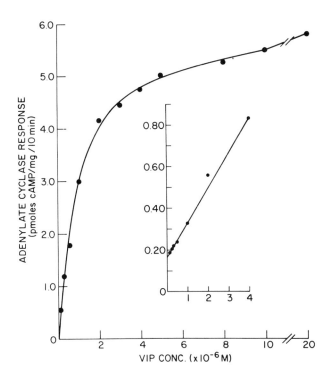

Figure 4. Stimulation of adenylate cyclase
activity in guinea pig pancreas exocrine cell
membranes by VIP. Values are expressed as activity with, minus activity without, VIP. Results
given are the means of four separate experiments
and each point was determined in duplicate.
The *insert* is a double reciprocal plot of the
values in the main figure.

Gastrin I (5×10^{-5} M) did not alter the stimulation of adenylate cyclase by VIP or secretin (Table 2). Glucagon (3×10^{-6} M) did not alter the stimulation of adenylate cyclase by VIP (Table 2), secretin, or CCK-octapeptide (results not shown). Stimulation of adenylate cyclase activity by maximally effective concentrations of VIP and CCK-octapeptide together, was the same as the sum of the stimulatory effects of each agent alone (Table 2). In contrast, stimulation of adenylate cyclase activity by VIP plus secretin was the same as with VIP alone (Table 2).

In other tissues guanyl, as well as other nucleotides, may alter both basal and hormone-stimulated adenylate cyclase activity.[6,7,13,14,19-21,29,30,40] Table 3 lists those nucleotides (as well as guanosine) that were tested for an effect on adenylate cyclase. Of these compounds, only 5'-guanylyl imidodiphosphate (GMPPNP), a nonmetabolizable analog of GTP,[14] increased basal adenylate cyclase. Stimulation of adenylate cyclase was detectable at concentrations above 10^{-6} M GMPPNP (Fig. 5) and was still increasing at 10^{-3} M.

Table 2. Adenylate cyclase activity in guinea pig pancreas exocrine cell membranes -- Hormone interactions

Hormone (conc)	Stimulation of adenylate cyclase* (pmols cAMP/mg/10 min)		
	Alone	Plus gastrin I (5×10^{-5} M)	Plus VIP (5×10^{-6} M)
CCK-octapeptide (10^{-6} M)	7.6±0.6	4.9±0.4	12.8±1.1
Gastrin I (5×10^{-5} M)	0.1±0.3	---	5.6±0.4
VIP (5×10^{-6} M)	5.8±0.6	5.6±0.5	---
Synthetic secretin (3×10^{-6} M)	2.4±0.5	2.5±0.4	5.7±0.4
Glucagon (3×10^{-6} M)	-0.2±0.4	0.1±0.3	5.9±0.3

* Results expressed as adenylate cyclase activity with, minus activity without, the indicated hormones. Each value represents the mean of three experiments ± 1 SD. Values for each experiment were determined in duplicate.

Table 3. Effect of nucleotides on pancreatic adenylate cyclase

Agent	Adenylate cyclase (pmols cAMP/mg/10 min)
None	14.9±0.8
GTP	14.1±0.4
GDP	14.8±0.8
GMP	14.7±1.5
Guanosine	14.7±1.8
GMPPNP	21.6±1.6*
GDP	15.5±0.6
XTP	14.7±0.9
ITP	15.5±1.4
UTP	14.6±0.3
CTP	14.9±0.2

Each value represents the mean ± 1 SD of three experiments. The concentration of all agents was 10^{-5} M.

* Significantly greater than control (p <0.01).

GMPPNP (10^{-5} M) significantly increased the stimulation of adenylate cyclase produced by CCK-octapeptide (Fig. 6). A double-reciprocal plot of cyclase stimulation as a function of CCK-octapeptide concentration indicated that GMPPNP increased the maximal stimulation produced by the hormone (significant increase in y-intercept) but did not alter the concentration of CCK-octapeptide required for half-maximal stimulation (no change in x-intercept) (Fig.6--insert). GMPPNP also potentiated the stimulation of adenylate cyclase produced by VIP (Fig. 7). In contrast to the effect of the guanyl nucleotide on stimulation of adenylate cyclase by CCK-octapeptide, GMPPNP increased both the maximal stimulation produced by VIP and the hormone concentration required for half-maximal stimulation. None of the agents which alone failed to stimulate adenylate cyclase (gastrin I, gastrin II, pentagastrin, glucagon and carbamylcholine) were found to be capable of stimulating the enzyme in the presence of GMPPNP.

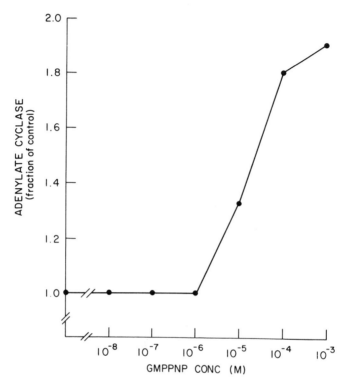

Figure 5. Effect of GMPPNP on adenylate cyclase
activity in guinea pig pancreas exocrine cell membranes. Values are expressed as the fraction of
adenylate cyclase activity obtained without GMPPNP.
Results given are the means of four separate experiments and each point was determined in duplicate.

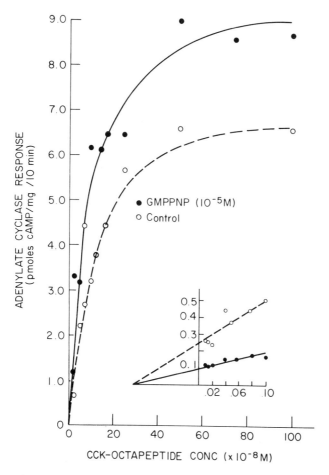

Figure 6. Effect of GMPPNP on CCK–octapeptide
stimulation of adenylate cyclase activity in
guinea pig pancreas exocrine cell membranes.
Values are expressed as activity with, minus
activity without, CCK-octapeptide. Results given
are the means of three separate experiments and
each point was determined in duplicate. The
insert is a double-reciprocal plot of the values
in the main figure.

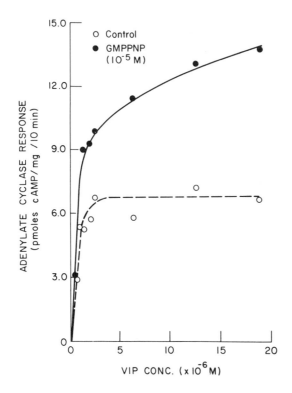

Figure 7. Effect of GMPPNP on VIP stimulation of adenylate cyclase activity in guinea pig pancreas exocrine cell membranes. Values are expressed as activity with, minus activity without, VIP. Results given are the means of four separate experiments and each point was determined in duplicate.

DISCUSSION

For polypeptide hormones it is generally agreed that the first step in the production of a biologic effect is the interaction of the hormone with its plasma "membrane receptor."[31] ("Membrane receptor" is used in the functional sense to refer to that portion of the plasma membrane with which a hormone interacts to produce a biologic effect. This definition is more restrictive than that for a "membrane binding site" in that the former requires the production of a biologic effect.) It would be ideal to examine this interaction directly, by examining binding of radiolabeled hormones to the plasma membrane and the relation between hormone binding and the production of a biologic effect. On many occasions we have prepared iodinated CCK-octapeptide using either chloramine-T[16] or lactoperoxidase;[11,38] however, we have been uniformly unsuccessful in producing a biologically active, iodinated hormone. This

is probably attributable to oxidation of either or
both of the methionine residues which are important
for biologic activity (ref 32 plus unpublished data) or
alteration of the microenvironment in the region of
the sulfate on the tyrosine residue by the introduction of the iodide atom.[32]

Information can be obtained, albeit indirectly,
about hormone-receptor interaction by examining the
biologic response produced by a hormone. The assumption made here is that a biologic response cannot occur
without the receptor being occupied by a hormone. The
converse, however, does not necessarily follow, that
is, occupation of a receptor site by a hormone may
occur without the production of a biologic response.[26]
In the present study we have investigated the interaction of several hormones with their receptors on
plasma membranes prepared from a homogeneous population
of isolated pancreatic exocrine cells as reflected by
changes in the activity of the membrane-associated
enzyme adenylate cyclase. Although activation of this
enzyme appears to be the mechanism through which many
hormones exert their effects on target tissues,[25] it
should be kept in mind that alteration of adenylate
cyclase activity in a particular membrane preparation
by a particular hormone does not necessarily indicate
that the biologic effects of the hormone are mediated
by the adenylate cyclase-cyclic AMP system. Instead,
the change in enzyme activity may occur indirectly as
a consequence of direct effects of the hormone on other
membrane functions, such as magnesium binding, calcium
binding, guanyl nucleotide metabolism.

CCK-octapeptide, gastrin I, gastrin II and pentagastrin possess the same common C-terminal tetrapeptide.[23] These agents also produce similar biologic
effects in various gastrointestinal tissues, although
their relative potencies vary depending on the particular function and species being studied.[23] In the
present experiments, CCK-octapeptide increased adenylate cyclase activity in pancreatic exocrine cell
membranes. A double-reciprocal plot of the increase
in enzyme activity versus concentration of CCK-octapeptide resulted in a straight line, which indicated
that in terms of the biologic response, CCK-octapeptide interacts with a single class of receptors and
that half-maximal stimulation (50% receptor occupancy?) occurs at a hormone concentration of 2×10^{-7} M.

Gastrin I, gastrin II and pentagastrin at concentrations as high as 10^{-4} M failed to alter adenylate
cyclase activity. Each of these peptides, however,
could inhibit, in a dose-dependent fashion, the
stimulation of adenylate cyclase produced by CCK-
octapeptide. On a double-reciprocal graph of the
increase in adenylate cyclase activity versus concentration of CCK-octapeptide, addition of gastrin I
(5×10^{-5} M) increased the slope but did not alter the
intercept on the x-axis. In particular, this concentration of gastrin increased by fivefold the concentration of CCK-octapeptide required for half-maximal
stimulation of adenylate cyclase activity but did
not alter the magnitude by which the enzyme could be
maximally stimulated. That is, gastrin is a competitive inhibitor of CCK-octapeptide in this system and
occupation of the CCK-octapeptide receptor by gastrin
does not result in stimulation of adenylate cyclase.

From the results given in Figure 1, the concentration of gastrin required for it to occupy 50% of the
receptor sites may be calculated to be 2×10^{-5} M (that
is, 100 times greater than the concentration of CCK-
octapeptide required for the same rate of occupancy
of receptor sites). We interpret these results to
indicate that the C-terminal pentapeptide of the CCK-
octapeptide molecule has sufficient molecular specificity to permit binding of the peptide to the receptor. The additional three amino acids not only increase the affinity with which CCK-octapeptide binds
to the receptor (by 100-fold) but also enable CCK-
octapeptide to stimulate adenylate cyclase. Our
finding that gastrin was unable to stimulate adenylate cyclase at concentrations at which it was able
to inhibit the effect of CCK-octapeptide, appears to
exclude the possibility that the C-terminal pentapeptide portion of the molecule is responsible for
the stimulation of adenylate cyclase and that the
additional three amino acids function to increase
the affinity with which the molecule binds to the
receptor.

VIP, secretin, and glucagon are similar both in
their chemical structure and in their spectrum of
biologic activities. VIP has six amino acids in the
same position as does glucagon and nine amino acids
in the same position as does secretin.[23] All three
hormones can increase adenylate cyclase activity in
plasma membranes from fat cells[10] and from

hepatocytes,[10] can inhibit gastric secretion,[4,17] and can produce intestinal secretion.[4,5,12,15,37] Both VIP and glucagon stimulate hepatic glycogenolysis[18] and myocardial contraction,[34] whereas both VIP and secretin stimulate pancreatic exocrine secretion.[35] Studies with iodinated glucagon and iodinated VIP indicate that secretin and VIP interact with the same membrane receptor in liver and fat and that in both tissues this receptor is functionally distinct from the membrane receptor for glucagon.[10]

In plasma membranes from isolated guinea pig pancreatic exocrine cells, VIP and secretin but not glucagon stimulated adenylate cyclase activity. A double-reciprocal plot of the increase in enzyme activity as a function of VIP concentration gave a straight line, which indicates that in terms of the biologic response, VIP interacts with a single class of receptors and that half-maximal stimulation occurs at a hormone concentration of 1×10^{-6} M. Secretin also stimulated adenylate cyclase activity; however, the magnitude of this stimulation, although statistically significant, was small and prevented us from establishing a precise dose-response relation. Glucagon (5×10^{-6} M), which alone failed to alter adenylate cyclase activity, also failed to alter stimulation produced by VIP or secretin. Stimulation of adenylate cyclase activity produced by VIP plus secretin was the same as produced by VIP alone. These results indicate that isolated pancreatic exocrine cells have a plasma membrane receptor which interacts with VIP and secretin but not with glucagon.

Gastrin failed to inhibit stimulation of adenylate cyclase by VIP or secretin, and stimulation of enzyme activity by VIP plus CCK-octapeptide was the same as the sum of the stimulation produced by each agent individually. These results indicate that the membrane receptor for CCK-octapeptide (which also interacts with gastrin I, gastrin II, and pentagastrin) is functionally distinct from the membrane receptor with which VIP and secretin interact.

Using the intact cat pancreas, Case and associates[9] found that both secretin and cholecystokinin stimulated cellular concentrations of cyclic AMP but that the time-course of the response differed for the two hormones. Rutten, DePont and Bonting[33] reported that secretin and cholecystokinin each stimulated adenylate cyclase activity in homogenates from rat pancreas and that calcium inhibited (and magnesium potentiated) the hormone response. Other agents that were tested by these investigators and found to be inactive were glucagon, pentagastrin, α- and β-adrenergic catecholamine, carbamylcholine, and acetylcholine. Secretin and cholecystokinin each appeared to be interacting with a single order of sites in producing activation of adenylate cyclase. In contrast to the findings in the present study, Rutten and associates[33] found that the effect of cholecystokinin overlapped with that of secretin.

The present studies indicate that in plasma membranes from isolated guinea pig pancreatic exocrine cells, the receptor that interacts with CCK-octapeptide and gastrin is functionally distinct from the receptor that interacts with VIP and secretin, even though both receptors produce an equivalent biologic response (activation of adenylate cyclase). One possibility which the present studies cannot exclude is that cells possessing receptors for CCK-octapeptide do not possess receptors for secretin and VIP and *vice versa*. In intact cell systems, however, the effect of these two classes of hormones on pancreatic function is different. Secretin is a strong stimulant of water and ion secretion and a weak stimulus of enzyme secretion; cholecystokinin is a strong stimulus of enzyme secretion and a weak stimulus of water and ion secretion.[23] The results in the present studies should *not* be taken as evidence that CCK-octapeptide or secretin produce their alteration of pancreatic function by activating adenylate cyclase and increasing cellular cyclic AMP. It is possible, for example, that the ability of cholecystokinin to cause calcium efflux from the isolated pancreas *in vitro*[8] as well as from pancreas slices[24] might reflect mobilization of membrane-bound calcium. It is conceivable (but by no means demonstrated) that in our membrane preparation release of bound calcium might result in increased adenylate cyclase activity or, alternatively, that this effect might not occur in intact cells. This type of mechanism might also account for the finding by Amer[1,2] that CCK-octapeptide and gastrin stimulate cyclic nucleotide phosphodiesterase activity partially purified from rabbit gallbladder but do not alter cellular concentrations of cyclic AMP.

In vivo cholecystokinin potentiates secretin stimulation of pancreatic water and ion secretion, and secretin potentiates cholecystokinin stimulation of pancreatic enzyme secretion.[23] The present studies indicate that not only is the receptor for CCK-octapeptide and gastrin functionally distinct from that from VIP and secretin, but that in terms of their effect on adenylate cyclase there is no interaction between these two receptors. In particular, the stimulation produced by CCK-octapeptide plus VIP was the same as the sum of the stimulation observed with each agent alone. We did not observe the mutual potentiation which occurs *in vivo*. There are a number of possible explanations for this apparent discrepancy and obviously additional studies will be required to clarify the mechanism by which cholecystokinin and secretin enhance the effect of each other *in vivo*.

Purine and, in particular, guanyl nucleotides have been found to alter hormone-sensitive adenylate cyclase in various tissues[6,7,13,14,19-21,29,30,40] and thus constitute a potential system for regulating the biologic effects of hormones on their target tissues. Of the nucleotides tested in the present study, only 5'-guanylyl imidodiphosphate (GMPPNP), a nonmetabolizable analog of GTP,[14] altered adenylate cyclase activity in plasma membranes from isolated pancreatic exocrine cells. The absence of an effect of GTP as well as other nucleotides may reflect their degradation by tissue nucleotidases during the course of the assay;[14] however, additional studies will be required to confirm this point directly. This ability of the guanyl nucleotide alone to activate adenylate cyclase offers a potential alternative mechanism by which a particular agent might *indirectly* stimulate adenylate cyclase and increase cellular cyclic AMP. That is, a hormone might increase adenylate cyclase and cellular cyclic AMP by virtue of its ability to increase cellular concentrations of GTP.

The present studies also illustrate the potential role of guanyl nucleotides in regulating the biologic effect which occurs as a consequence of hormone-receptor interaction. In particular, GMPPNP potentiated the stimulation of adenylate cyclase by CCK-octapeptide as well as by VIP. In the case of CCK-octapeptide, the guanyl nucleotide did not alter the hormone concentration required for half-maximal stimulation.

In the context of hormone-receptor interaction, adding
GMPPNP did not alter the occupation of receptor sites
by CCK-octapeptide but amplified the response produced
as a consequence of this interaction.   In the case of
VIP, the guanyl nucleotide increased both the stimulation of adenylate cyclase produced by VIP and the hormone concentration required for half-maximal stimulation.   In the context of hormone-receptor interaction
GMPPNP reduced the apparent affinity of the membrane-
receptor for VIP but as with CCK-octapeptide the guanyl
nucleotide amplified the response produced as a result
of receptor occupation by the hormone.
   The observations noted in previous studies[25] as well
as in the present one that calcium decreases and that
magnesium increases adenylate cyclase activity, illustrate two other potential mechanisms by which a hormone might *indirectly* alter adenylate cyclase activity,
that is, by altering either the calcium or magnesium
(or both) that is available in the region of the membrane containing the enzyme molecule.   We also found
that magnesium stimulated and that calcium inhibited
CCK-octapeptide activation of adenylate cyclase.
Thus, in addition to guanyl nucleotides, the concentrations of divalent cations can modulate the response
produced as a consequence of hormone-receptor interaction.   Rasmussen and associates[27,28] have elaborated
in some detail on the potential role of calcium in
the mechanism of hormone action.   It should also be
kept in mind that these interpretations of the effects
of guanyl nucleotides and divalent cations in terms of
hormone-receptor interaction are quite tentative and
cannot be interpreted unequivocally until direct observations of hormone-receptor interactions are made.

SUMMARY

   Adenylate cyclase activity in plasma membranes from
isolated pancreatic exocrine cells is stimulated by
low concentrations of CCK-octapeptide, VIP or secretin.
Gastrin which at concentrations as high as 10^{-4} M
failed to alter adenylate cyclase activity, inhibited
the stimulation of enzyme activity produced by CCK-
octapeptide but not that produced by VIP or secretin.
Glucagon, which is structurally similar to VIP and
secretin, did not stimulate adenylate cyclase activity or alter the stimulation produced by VIP or

secretin. The stimulation of adenylate cyclase
activity by CCK-octapeptide was additive with that
produced by VIP.

The guanyl nucleotide GMPPNP potentiated the stimulation of adenylate cyclase produced by CCK-octapeptide and that produced by VIP. GMPPNP increased the
magnitude by which adenylate cyclase could be maximally stimulated by CCK-octapeptide but did not alter
the hormone concentration required for half-maximal
stimulation of enzyme activity. GMPPNP increased
the magnitude by which adenylate cyclase could be
maximally stimulated by VIP and increased the hormone
concentration required for half-maximal stimulation.

These results indicate that the membrane receptor
for CCK-octapeptide (which also interacts with gastrin)
is functionally distinct from the membrane receptor
with which VIP and secretin interact.

References

1. Amer MS: Studies with cholecystokinin *in vitro*: III. Mech-
     anism of the effect on the isolated rabbit gall bladder
     strips. *J Pharmacol Exp Ther* 183:527-534, 1972.
2. Amer MS, McKinney GR: Studies with cholecystokinin *in vitro*:
     IV. Effects of cholecystokinin and related peptides on
     phosphodiesterase. *J Pharmacol Exp Ther* 183:535-548,
     1972.
3. Amsterdam A, Jamieson JD: Structural and functional
     characterization of isolated pancreatic exocrine
     cells. *Proc Natl Acad Sci USA* 69:3028-3032, 1972.
4. Barbezat GO, Grossman MI: Intestinal secretion: Stimula-
     tion by peptides. *Science* 174:422-424, 1971.
5. Barbezat GO, Grossman MI: Glucagon stimulates intestinal
     secretion. *Lancet* 1:918, 1971.
6. Bilezikian JP, Aurbach GD: The effects of nucleotides on
     the expression of β-adrenergic adenylate cyclase
     activity in membranes from turkey erythrocytes.
     J Biol Chem 249:157-161, 1974.
7. Bockaert J, Roy C, Jard S: Oxytocin-sensitive adenylate
     cyclase in frog bladder epithelial cells: Role of
     calcium, nucleotides, and other factors in hormonal
     stimulation. *J Biol Chem* 247:7073-7081, 1972.
8. Case RM, Clausen T: The relationship between calcium ex-
     change and enzyme secretion in the isolated rat
     pancreas. *J Physiol* 235:75-102, 1973.

9. Case RM, Johnson M, Scratcherd T, Sherratt HSA: Cyclic adenosine 3',5'-monophosphate concentration in the pancreas following stimulation by secretin, cholecysto-kinin-pancreozymin and acetylcholine. *J Physiol* 223: 669-684, 1972.

10. Desbuquois B, Laudat MH, Laudat P: Vasoactive intestinal polypeptide and glucagon: Stimulation of adenylate cyclase activity via distinct receptors in liver and fat cell membranes. *Biochem Biophys Res Commun* 53: 1187-1194, 1973.

11. Frantz WL, Turkington RW: Formation of biologically active ^{125}I-prolactin by enzymatic radioiodination. *Endocrinology* 91:1545-1548, 1972.

12. Gardner JD, Peskin GW, Cerda JJ, Brooks FP: Alterations of *in vitro* fluid and electrolyte absorption by gastro-intestinal hormones. *Am J Surg* 113:57-64, 1967.

13. Goldfine ID, Roth J, Birnbaumer L: Glucagon receptors in β-cells. Binding of ^{125}I-glucagon and activation of adenylate cyclase. *J Biol Chem* 247:1211-1218, 1972.

14. Harwood JP, Löw H, Rodbell M: Stimulatory and inhibitory effects of guanyl nucleotides on fat cell adenylate cyclase. *J Biol Chem* 248:6239-6245, 1973.

15. Hicks T, Turnberg LA: The influence of secretin on ion transport in the human jejunum. *Gut* 14:485-490, 1973.

16. Hunter WM, Greenwood FC: Preparation of iodine-131 labelled human growth hormone of high specific activity. *Nature* 194:495-496, 1962.

17. Johnson LR, Grossman MI: Secretin: The enterogastrone released by acid in the duodenum. *Am J Physiol* 215:885-888, 1968.

18. Kerins C, Said SI: Hyperglycemic and glycogenolytic effects of vasoactive intestinal polypeptide. *Proc Soc Exp Biol Med* 142:1014-1017, 1973.

19. Krishna G, Harwood JP, Barber AJ, Jamieson GA: Requirement for guanosine triphosphate in the prostaglandin acti-vation of adenylate cyclase of platelet membrane. *J Biol Chem* 247:2253-2254, 1972.

20. Kuo WN, Hodgins DS, Kuo JF: Adenylate cyclase in islets of Langerhans: Isolation of islets and regulation of adenylate cyclase activity by various hormones and agents. *J Biol Chem* 248:2705-2711, 1973.

21. Leray F, Chambaut AM, Hanoune J: Role of GTP in epinephrine and glucagon activation of adenyl cyclase of liver plasma membrane. *Biochem Biophys Res Commun* 48: 1385-1391, 1972.

22. Lowry OH, Rosebrough NJ, Farr AL, Randall RJ: Protein measurement with the Folin phenol reagent. *J Biol Chem* 193:265-275, 1951.

23. Makhlouf GM: The neuroendocrine design of the gut: The play
    of chemicals in a chemical playground. *Gastroenterology*
    67:159–184, 1974.
24. Matthews EK, Petersen OH, Williams JA: Pancreatic acinar
    cells: Acetylcholine-induced membrane depolarization,
    calcium efflux and amylase release. *J Physiol* 234:
    689–701, 1973.
25. Perkins JP: Adenyl cyclase, in Greengard P, Robison GA (eds),
    Advances in Cyclic Nucleotide Research, New York: Raven
    Press, 1973, pp 1–64.
26. Pohl SL, Krans HMJ, Birnbaumer L, Rodbell M: Inactivation
    of glucagon by plasma membranes of rat liver. *J Biol
    Chem* 247:2295–2301, 1972.
27. Rasmussen H: Cell communication, calcium ion, and cyclic
    adenosine monophosphate. *Science* 170:404–412, 1970.
28. Rasmussen H, Tenenhouse A: Cyclic adenosine monophosphate,
    Ca^{++}, and membranes. *Proc Natl Acad Sci USA* 59:1364–
    1370, 1968.
29. Rodbell M, Birnbaumer L, Pohl SL, Krans HMJ: The glucagon-
    sensitive adenyl cyclase system in plasma membranes of
    rat liver: V. An obligatory role of guanyl nucleotides
    in glucagon action. *J Biol Chem* 246:1877–1882, 1971.
30. Rodbell M, Karns HMJ, Pohl SL, Birnbaumer L: The glucagon-
    sensitive adenyl cyclase system in plasma membranes of
    rat liver: IV. Effects of guanyl nucleotides on bind-
    ing of ^{125}I-glucagon. *J Biol Chem* 246:1872–1876, 1971.
31. Roth J: Peptide hormone binding to receptors: A review
    of direct studies in vitro. *Metabolism* 22:1059–1073,
    1973.
32. Rubin B, Engel SL: Some biological characteristics of
    cholecystokinin (CCK-PZ) and synthetic analogues, in
    Andersson S (ed), *Nobel Symposium 16. Frontiers in
    Gastrointestinal Hormone Research,* Stockholm: Almquist
    and Wiksell, 1972, pp 41–55.
33. Rutten WJ, DePont JJHHM, Bonting SL: Adenylate cyclase in
    the rat pancreas. Properties and stimulation by hor-
    mones. *Biochim Biophys Acta* 274:201–213, 1972.
34. Said SI, Bosher LP, Spath JA, Kontos HA: Positive inotropic
    action of newly isolated vasoactive intestinal polypep-
    tide (VIP), abstracted. *Clin Res* 20:29, 1972.
35. Said SI, Mutt V: Isolation from porcine-intestinal wall of
    a vasoactive octacosapeptide related to secretin and
    to glucagon. *Eur J Biochem* 28:199–204, 1972.
36. Salomon Y, Londos C, Rodbell M: A highly sensitive
    adenylate cyclase assay. *Anal Biochem* 58:541–548,
    1974.

37. Sanzenbacher LJ, Mekhjian HS, King DR, Zollinger RM: Studies
    on the potential role of secretin in the islet cell
    tumor diarrheogenic syndrome. *Ann Surg* 176:394-402,
    1972.
38. Shiu RPC, Kelly PA, Friesen HG: Radioreceptor assay for
    prolactin and other lactogenic hormones. *Science*
    180:968-971, 1973.
39. Thompson WJ, Williams RH, Little SA: Activation of guanyl
    cyclase and adenyl cyclase by secretin. *Biochim
    Biophys Acta* 302:329-337, 1973.
40. Wolff J, Cook GH: Activation of thyroid membrane adenylate
    cyclase by purine nucleotides. *J Biol Chem* 248:350-
    355, 1973.

PHOTOAFFINITY LABELING OF SECRETAGOGUE RECEPTORS IN THE PANCREATIC EXOCRINE CELL

Richard E. Galardy, James D. Jamieson

Section of Cell Biology, Yale University
School of Medicine, New Haven, Connecticut

Peptide Hormone Receptors

The first step in a hormone-mediated biologic response is the binding of the hormone to a cell or cell constituent. Only by the direct interaction of the hormone with its receptor can the information carried by the hormone be translated into a physiologically significant response. In the case of peptide hormones it is becoming clear that the receptor, or at least the hormone-binding component of the receptor, is located on the plasma membrane of the cell. The binding of radiolabeled hormone to target cell plasma membranes, for example, has been shown for glucagon in liver and fat cells,[30] and in the β-cells of the pancreatic islets,[14] for ACTH[10] and for angiotensin[15] in adrenocortical membranes, for insulin in liver and fat cell membranes,[6,23] for vasopressin in kidney membranes[2,39] and for thyrotropin in thyroid plasma membranes.[43] This binding is frequently accompanied by the activation (or inhibition) of a nucleotide cyclase system, which is thought to mediate the response of the cell to the hormone. In addition, several peptide hormones have been shown to trigger target cell activity without entering the cell, which lends strong support to the supposition that peptide hormone receptors are located on the plasma membrane. For instance, insulin,[4] ACTH,[38] and prolactin,[41] coupled to large inert polymers, are biologically active yet clearly cannot penetrate the plasmalemma. In a few cases, protein complexes have been isolated from target cell plasma

345

membranes which retain the ability to bind the peptide hormone and are thus presumed to be components of the peptide hormone receptor site. These include binding complexes for insulin from liver and fat cell plasma membranes[6] and for human chorionic gonadotropin from corpora lutea.[17]

More detailed biochemical and chemical information about peptide hormone receptors is extremely scarce. Cuatrecasas[7] gives a molecular weight of about 300,000 for the insulin receptor complex, and Haour and Saxena[17] estimate a molecular weight of from 30,000 to 70,000 for the peptide binding component of the human chorionic gonadotropin receptor. In addition, the insulin receptor may be a glycoprotein.[7]

Almost nothing is known about pancreozymin (=cholecystokinin) receptors. The biologic activity of pancreozymin includes the stimulation of gallbladder contraction, the stimulation of the secretion of pancreatic juice high in enzyme and proenzyme content, and the stimulation of the secretion of insulin from pancreatic islets.[37] In the pancreatic acinar cell, pancreozymin directly stimulates secretory protein release, appears to possess a receptor separate from that for cholinergic stimuli (ref 15 plus JD Jamieson, unpublished data), and does not act via the release of endogenous cholinergic agents.[27] There is some evidence that the stimulation of the secretion of exportable protein by pancreozymin may be mediated by cyclic AMP.[22,25,27,34] In all but one case, however, this conclusion is based only on the observation that high concentrations of cyclic AMP (or a derivative of cyclic AMP) and theophylline acted to stimulate secretion. Only Johnson and associates[22] demonstrated an increase of cyclic AMP levels in direct response to pancreozymin infusion (*in vivo* and *in vitro* in the cat pancreas) and interpreted their experiments as suggesting that the rise in cyclic AMP levels may not be linked to protein secretion but rather to a stimulation of protein synthesis by pancreozymin[32] and acetylcholine. In view of the observations that cholinergically innervated organs respond to their agonist by elevation of cyclic GMP levels (Dr. P Greengard, personal communication), it could be suggested[31] that the exocrine pancreatic cell might respond to pancreozymin by elevation of levels of cyclic GMP (rather than cyclic AMP), since the end result of stimulation of the pancreas by peptide hormones or acetylcholine is the same.[21] The secretory response to cholinergic agents and pancreozymin has been shown to be calcium-dependent.[8,18,24]

It has become apparent that all attempts to identify and characterize peptide hormone receptors rely upon the preservation or reconstitution of the binding activity for the hormone throughout fractionation and purification procedures. This is frequently impossible and the only case of the reconstitution of peptide hormone binding activity in an apparent receptor protein is that of the human chorionic gonadotropin receptor.[17] The problem remains as to how to identify the hormone-binding protein of the receptor during and after purification if binding activity cannot be maintained. One solution to the problem is to affinity-label the hormone-binding protein of the receptor with radiolabeled hormone under conditions where the biologic response to the hormone can be measured (in tissue or intact cells) and where appropriate controls for specificity of labeling can be performed. Following affinity labeling, biochemical and chemical characterization of the tagged receptor can be accomplished without the necessity of the normally restrictive experimental conditions necessary to maintain binding activity. In addition, peptide hormone receptor sites in tissue or on cells covalently tagged with the hormone, will allow for the morphologic identification of the receptor site, either by autoradiographic or immunochemical techniques, which have not been previously applied to receptor localization. The affinity labeling of pancreozymin receptor sites in the exocrine pancreas will be presented in Results and Discussion.

The Labeling of Biologically Active Sites

Irreversible labeling has been used as a tool to characterize many types of biologically active sites. Two excellent reviews of active-site labeling are those of Baker[1] and Singer.[40] The types of active-site labeling experiments can be divided into two categories depending on the degree of resolution of the active site required. The first type is the location or mapping, by covalent tagging, of an active site within the linear amino acid sequence of a protein. The labeling of the catalytic site of an

enzyme is included in this category. Specific amino
acids that are tagged in such an experiment can be
identified as comprising the boundaries of the active
site or as being essential for the catalytic activity
of the site. The labeling of antibody-combining sites
or regulatory sites on enzymes also serves to locate
these sites within the linear amino acid sequence of
the protein by identifying which amino acids are involved in the binding process.

The second type of active-site labeling is the
identification, by covalent tagging, of a single protein in a complex mixture of proteins. This is the
type of labeling we will employ, since we are not
concerned with the location of the pancreozymin-
binding site within the primary sequence of the binding protein, but are concerned only with identifying
the binding protein. Thus we hope to be able to
label the pancreozymin-binding protein specifically
in the presence of many other membrane proteins in
the pancreatic acinar cell plasma membrane.

There are two widely used methods of labeling
biologically active sites: the labeling of an unusually reactive functional group, such as an enzyme's
catalytic site, and affinity labeling. The labeling
of an unusually reactive functional group is the most
common technique for labeling enzyme-active sites.
The catalytic site of an enzyme usually contains one
or more functional groups (such as the nucleophilic
groups -SH, -OH, -NH$_2$, and -COOH) of exceptionally
high reactivity. Thus, reagents designed to react
with nucleophiles (such as alkylating agents) will
react with the unusually reactive groups present in
enzyme active sites in preference to the same groups
of normal reactivity present in the rest of the protein. This technique applies only to enzymes, where
unusually reactive functional groups can be expected
to be present. In the case of the active sites of
antibodies, regulatory subunits of enzymes, and
hormone receptor sites, there is no reason to expect
the presence of a reactive nucleophile since no known
catalytic activity is directly associated with these
active sites. Affinity-labeling is the method most
frequently used for tagging an active site that is
a binding site (for an antigenic determinant, a
regulatory molecule, or a hormone) but is not a catalytic site. It is this method which we have chosen
to label pancreozymin-binding sites.

Affinity-labeling of hormone receptor sites consists of two parts: that concerned with the binding of hormone to receptor (affinity part) and that involved in covalent bond formation (labeling part). In the case of peptide hormone receptor sites, the hormone itself provides the affinity that holds the labeling moiety in proximity to the binding site, thus insuring specific labeling of the binding site. The labeling moiety must be attached to the hormone in the form of an easily prepared chemical derivative, which does not seriously interfere with biologic activity and which must be capable of reacting with the protein to which the peptide hormone is bound. The high affinity of peptide hormones for their receptor sites (insulin $K_{dissociation} = 10^{-7}$ M,[6] ACTH $K_{dissociation} = 10^{-7}$ M,[10] human chorionic gonadotropin $K_{dissociation} = 10^{-10}$ M[17]) should result in highly specific labeling of these sites, since the enhancement of reaction with the binding site compared to random reaction elsewhere can theoretically be of the order of the binding constant to the site.[40]

In order for an affinity label to tag its binding site, the reactive functional group attached to the hormone must be capable of reacting with whatever functional groups are found at the hormone-binding site. In the case of labeling enzyme catalytic sites, alkylating agents have served as excellent affinity-labels where the alkylating agent is attached to a substrate that is specific for the enzyme. Thus, tosyllysine chloromethyl ketone is a specific active-site label for trypsin. In the case of peptide hormone receptors, however, there is no reason to expect the presence of any particular reactive functional group (such as a nucleophile) at the binding site, since no catalytic activity is known to be associated directly with the binding site. In spite of this, alkylating derivatives of peptide hormones have been used to label their receptor sites. Bromoacetyl oxytocin has been found to act as a specific irreversible inhibitor of the action of neurohypophyseal hormones in toad bladder and rabbit kidney.[42] Chlorambucil bradykinin was without a blocking effect on bradykinin receptors[11] and chlorambucil angiotensin II was found to inhibit the action of angiotensin II in guinea pig ileum irreversibly, but caused no permanent changes in rat blood pressure.[29] In some uterine preparations, however, the latter authors observed that chlorambucil angiotensin elicited a permanent

agonist response. The lack of activity of an alkylating agent in effecting antagonism may be due to lack
of interaction with the hormone receptor site because
of the absence of reactive nucleophiles. The antagonism observed may be a consequence of the fact that
the alkylating agent seeks out and reacts with nucleophiles outside the receptor vicinity if none are
located in the receptor site, thus causing nonspecific disruption of cellular functions. The agonist
response reported by Paiva and associates[29] probably
indicates the labeling of a nucleophile at the angiotensin receptor site in the uterus.

We believe that a less discriminating, more reactive reagent could be more capable of specifically
labeling a hormone-binding site where nucleophiles
may not be present. In our own experiments with an
indiscriminate, highly reactive, photoactivatable
affinity-labeling derivative of pentagastrin, we
consistently observe irreversible agonist activity.

Indiscriminately reactive reagents can be generated
by the photolysis of several chemically stable functional groups. These include alkyl carbenes from
aliphatic diazo compounds, aryl nitrenes from aryl
azides, and reactive triplet states from aryl ketones.
All of these have been used successfully as photoaffinity labels. (See Knowles[26] for a discussion of
carbene and nitrene affinity labels and Galardy and
associates[12,13] for the use of aryl ketone triplet
state affinity labels.) There are two distinct ad-
vantages of photoaffinity-labeling reagents compared
to conventional chemical affinity-labeling reagents.
First, carbenes, nitrenes and aryl ketone triplet
states can react with almost any carbon-hydrogen
bond, and although we cannot be certain if nucleophiles are present in peptide hormone binding sites
on receptors, we can guarantee the presence of carbon-
hydrogen bonds, thus insuring labeling within the
binding site once the hormone is bound to that site.
Second, photogenerated active site reagents are inert
before photolysis in contrast to chemically reactive
affinity-labeling reagents which can begin reacting
with nucleophiles immediately upon their introduction
into the system. With photoaffinity labels, binding
constants, binding specificity, and biologic activity
and specificity can be measured before photolysis,
thus providing evidence for the specificity of the
interaction with the receptor.

The photoaffinity labeling of biologically active
sites has been reviewed by Knowles.[26] More recent
developments in this field include labeling of a
myeloma protein,[33] labeling of cyclic AMP binding
sites,[16] labeling of ouabain-binding sites on Na+ -
K+ ATPase,[36] labeling of pentagastrin-binding sites
on serum albumin,[13] the preparation of a reagent for
the photoaffinity-labeling of insulin receptor sites,[28]
and a critique of the photoaffinity-labeling technique.[35]

We are currently using aryl nitrenes for photoaffinity labeling, although the relative merits of
nitrenes, carbenes, and ketone triplet states do not
dictate the preferential use of any one of these
reagents over the others. The scheme for the photoaffinity labeling of peptide hormone receptor sites
is shown schematically in Figure 1. Our results
demonstrate that we can affinity-label pancreozymin
receptors in the exocrine pancreas, which results in
the irreversible activation of the discharge of
exportable protein.

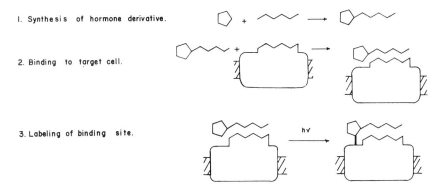

1. Synthesis of hormone derivative.

2. Binding to target cell.

3. Labeling of binding site.

Figure 1. A schematic plan for the photoaffinity labeling of
a peptide hormone–binding site. In 1, a peptide hormone derivative is prepared which can, upon photoactivation, covalently
bond to a protein. In 2, the hormone derivative is allowed to
interact with its receptor site on a protein in a cell plasma
membrane. In 3, photolysis results in the formation of a
covalent bond from the hormone to the protein to which it is
bound.

Photoaffinity Labeling of Pancreozymin Receptor Sites

Although the natural secretagogue for the pancreatic acinar cell is pancreozymin, its secretory activity is retained in C-terminal fragments of the peptide. Caerulein, a decapeptide isolated from frog skin[9] whose sequence is nearly identical to that of pancreozymin's C-terminus, has equal or greater potency compared to pancreozymin. The C-terminal peptapeptide common to pancreozymin, gastrin, and caerulein retains the full secretory activity of pancreozymin but is of much lower potency. The potencies of pancreozymin and caerulein, and of 2-nitro-5-azidobenzoyl pentagastrin,[13] the peptide we have used to photoaffinity-label peptide hormone receptors on pancreatic acinar cells, are shown in Figure 2. In the following sections we will assume that receptor sites for photoactivatable pentagastrin and for pancreozymin are identical. Definitive tests of this assumption will, however, require the use of pancreozymin in competitive binding experiments.

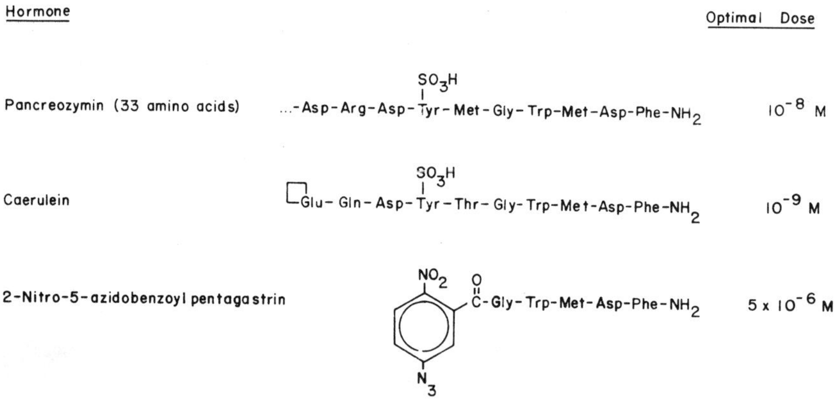

Hormone		Optimal Dose
Pancreozymin (33 amino acids)	...-Asp-Arg-Asp-$\overset{SO_3H}{\underset{\mid}{Tyr}}$-Met-Gly-Trp-Met-Asp-Phe-NH$_2$	10^{-8} M
Caerulein	$\overline{}$Glu-Gln-Asp-$\overset{SO_3H}{\underset{\mid}{Tyr}}$-Thr-Gly-Trp-Met-Asp-Phe-NH$_2$	10^{-9} M
2-Nitro-5-azidobenzoyl pentagastrin	(NO$_2$ azidobenzoyl ring) $\overset{O}{\overset{\parallel}{C}}$-Gly-Trp-Met-Asp-Phe-NH$_2$	5×10^{-6} M

Figure 2. Comparison of primary structure and biologic activity for pancreozymin, caerulein, and a photoactivatable derivative of pentagastrin, 2-nitro-5-azidobenzoylpentagastrin in the stimulation of pancreatic protein secretion. The dose-response optima for secretory protein release from pancreatic lobules is shown (JD Jamieson, RE Galardy, unpublished data).

With this reservation in mind, we have tested photoactivatable nitroazidobenzoyl-pentagastrin as a probe for pancreozymin receptor sites on pancreatic acinar cells. The specific biologic response monitored was the ability of acinar cells to discharge secretory proteins *in vitro*; the morphologic and biochemical features of this process have been summarized recently.[21] For all the experiments described below, the experimental protocol was similar; guinea pig pancreatic lobules (small clusters of acini) were prepared[3] and exposed to nitroazidobenzoyl-pentagastrin in the dark, photolyzed, extensively washed to free the tissue of unphotolyzed peptide, and subsequently monitored for their ability to release secretory proteins pulse-labeled with tritiated leucine in the same manner as that described for pancreatic slices.[19] Photoaffinity labeling by the pentagastrin derivative is irreversible and maximally activates the discharge process in pancreatic acinar cells. Using irreversible photoactivation of secretory protein discharge as an index of receptor occupancy, we have been able to measure the association and dissociation kinetics of nitroazidobenzoyl-pentagastrin with its receptor sites.

Two important photoreactions of aryl azides which probably occur in the photoaffinity labeling of proteins are shown in Figure 3. Figure 3b, the reaction of a photogenerated aryl nitrene with a carbon-hydrogen bond, is the indiscriminate covalent-bond-forming reaction which insures labeling of a hormone-binding site if nucleophiles are not present in the binding site.

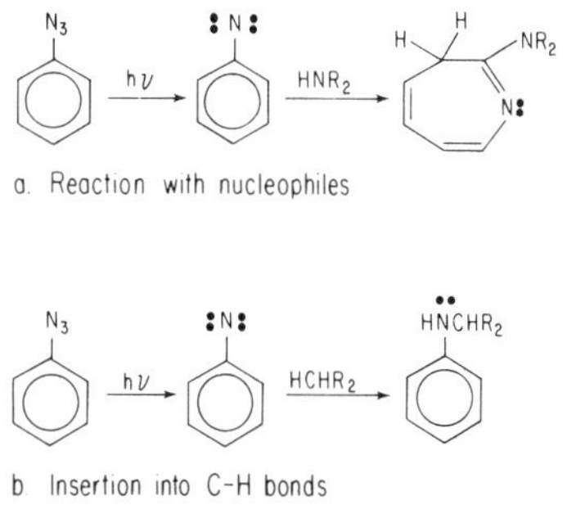

Figure 3. Two photoreactions of aryl azides. In 3a, the photogenerated nitrene has reacted with an amine nucleophile (such as a lysine ε-amino group) to form a substituted azepine ring system. In 3b, the photogenerated nitrene has inserted into a carbon-hydrogen bond to form a substituted aniline.

a. Reaction with nucleophiles

b. Insertion into C–H bonds

R.E. Galardy

RESULTS

Irreversible Activation of the Discharge Process

As shown in Table 1, photolysis of pancreatic lobules in the presence of photoactivatable pentagastrin
results in the irreversible activation of the discharge process. Activity could not be removed by extensive washing after photolysis, was maximum as indicated by lack of enhancement of discharge by optimal
doses of caerulein, and could only be reduced by metabolic inhibition, a characteristic of normally-induced
discharge in pancreatic acinar cells.[20] Incubation of
pancreatic lobules continuously over the assay period
in the dark with unphotolyzed pentagastrin derivative
or with previously photolyzed derivative gave maximal
secretory responses, but the activity was readily
reversible by washing.
Electron microscopic examination of tissues stimulated reversibly and irreversibly, indicated that discharge occurred via exocytosis of zymogen granules and
that the majority of granules were released over the
assay period. These findings are in accord with previous morphologic observations on pancreatic lobules
stimulated to discharge maximally *in vitro* with cholinergic agents or pancreozymin.[20] Photolysis does not
compromise cell structure or function, a conclusion
confirmed by separate biochemical studies on the
ability of photolyzed tissue to incorporate amino
acids into proteins.

Dose-Response for the Photoactivation of Discharge

A comparison was made of the secretory response of
pancreatic lobules to unphotolyzed pentagastrin derivative with that obtained after photolysis with the
derivative. As shown in Figure 4, sigmoidal log-dose-
responses were obtained under both conditions with
similar dose optima which suggests that irreversible
binding due to photolysis did not alter hormone-
receptor interaction. Assuming that binding to the
receptor is the rate-limiting step in the activation
of the discharge process, the dissociation constant
for photoactivatable pentagastrin binding to its
receptor sites is estimated to be $K_d = 5 \times 10^{-7}$ M,
(equal to the concentration of hormone at one-half
maximal stimulation). Dose-responses in this system

Table 1. Irreversible stimulation of protein discharge by affinity labeling[a]

Treatment of tissue after photolysis	% Discharge of Secretory Proteins in three hours		
	Unphotolyzed tissue	Photolyzed tissue	Tissue Photolyzed with 5×10^{-6} M NAB-pentagastrin
None	8	13	53[c]
10^{-9} M caerulein	60	54	51
5×10^{-6} M NAB-pentagastrin (in the dark)[b]	66	63	56

[a] Pancreatic lobules were tested for their secretory response without prior photolysis, without added pentagastrin derivative, and after photolysis for 10 seconds at 4C with the indicated concentration of the derivative. Photolysis with the derivative was followed by extensive washing in derivative-free medium (six changes of 100 ml each, over 90 minutes) prior to assaying for secretory protein release (line 1 of Table). In line 2, the ability of pancreatic lobules to respond to 10^{-9} M caerulein present continuously in the assay medium over the three-hour assay period was measured to determine if photolysis itself hinders release and to see if discharge activation by the photoactivatable derivative was maximum. Similar experiments were performed in which lobules were exposed for the three-hour assay to the photoactivatable derivative in the dark or to prephotolyzed derivative (line 3).

[b] Prephotolyzed NAB-pentagastrin had the same potency as unphotolyzed peptide.

[c] This response is completely blocked by performing the discharge assay at 4C or at 37C under 5% CO_2/95% N_2.

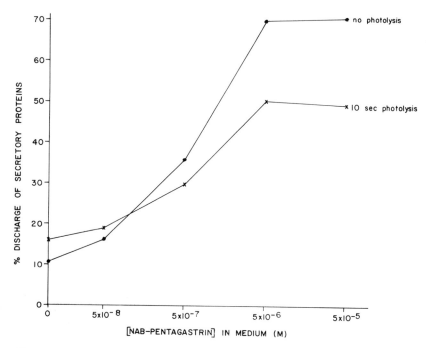

Figure 4. Dose-response curves for discharge of secretory proteins by photoactivatable pentagastrin. Assay as in Table 1.
Photolyzed set: pancreatic lobules photolyzed with increasing
concentrations of the derivative for 10 seconds and washed
extensively prior to assay. Unphotolyzed set: pancreatic
lobules exposed to increasing concentrations of the derivative
in the dark continuously for the assay period. Differences
in net output of secretory proteins are due to animal variations and are not significant.

for caerulein and pancreozymin are also sigmoidal in shape but shifted to the left in comparison to the curves for photoactivatable pentagastrin, with dose optima at 10^{-10} and 10^{-9} M, respectively.

Kinetics of Association and Dissociation of Nitroazidobenzoyl-Pentagastrin from Pancreatic Lobules

Using irreversible photoactivation of secretory protein discharge as an index of receptor occupancy, the association and dissociation kinetics of nitro-azidobenzoyl-pentagastrin at its dose optimum (5×10^{-6} M) with binding sites on pancreatic lobules, was measured (Figs. 5 & 6). The time of exposure to the derivative required to elicit one-half maximal discharge (after photolysis) was about two minutes at 4C (Fig. 5). The half-time for dissociation of activity on the other hand was about 28 minutes at 4C (Fig. 6). The dissociation rate constant, k_d, can be calculated to be 4×10^{-4}/sec based on the data in Figure 6 which show first-order dissociation kinetics (assuming that dissociation of activity is identical to dissociation of the pentagastrin deri-vative from its receptor sites).

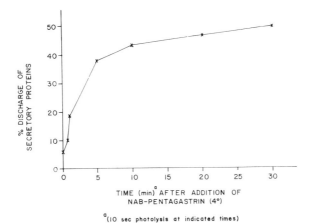

Figure 5. Association time for photoactivatable pentagastrin with pancreatic lobules. Pancreatic lobules were incubated for the indicated times in the dark with 5×10^{-6} M nitroazidobenzoyl-pentagastrin at 4C, photolyzed for 10 seconds, washed, and assayed for secretory protein discharge as in Table 1.

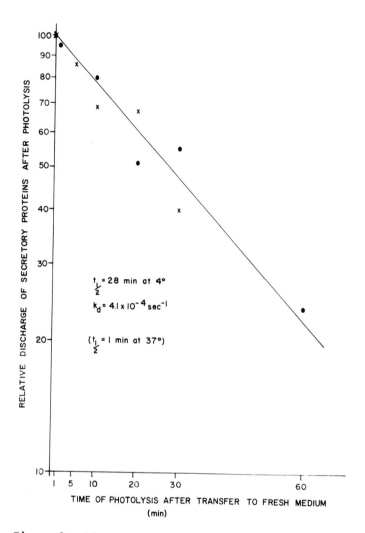

Figure 6. Dissociation time for photoactivatable pentagastrin from pancreatic lobules. Pancreatic lobules were preincubated for 30 minutes at 4C in the dark with 5x10^{-6} M photoactivatable pentagastrin, then transferred to a large volume of hormone-free medium for the indicated times, photolyzed for 10 seconds, washed, and assayed for secretory protein discharge as in Table 1.

Since we have not yet obtained quantitative data on the absolute numbers of photoactivatable penta-gastrin receptors in pancreatic lobules, we cannot directly calculate an association rate constant from Figure 5. We can make the approximation, however, that the fraction of total photoactivatable penta-gastrin bound to its receptor sites at equilibrium is small, and thus derive k_a, the association rate constant, in the same manner as Bockaert and associates[2] for vasopressin receptor sites in renal plasma membranes. This method gives $k_a = 4.4 \times 10^3 /M/$ sec.

The key assumptions underlying these calculations of association and dissociation kinetics are that photolysis quantitatively converts reversibly bound peptide to irreversibly bound peptide and that irreversible activation of the discharge process is a true index of receptor occupancy. The identity of dose-responses for unphotolyzed derivative in the dark and for photoaffinity-labeled tissue after extensive washing, suggests that these assumptions may be valid.

DISCUSSION

The irreversible agonist effect associated with photoaffinity labeling of pancreozymin receptors with 2-nitro-5-azidobenzoyl-pentagastrin clearly indicates that the hormone-binding site on the pancreozymin receptor has been tagged, probably by a covalent bond between the peptide and the binding protein. The identity of the dose-responses to nitroazidobenzoyl-pentagastrin in the dark and after photoaffinity labeling, suggests that the photoaffinity labeling and the normal activation of the secretory process are limited by the same step, presumably the binding of the hormone to its receptor.

The association and dissociation kinetics for the interaction of photoactivatable pentagastrin with its receptor site have been measured, assuming that irreversible activation of the secretory protein discharge is an index of receptor occupancy. The semi-log plot of the dissociation process is linear (Fig. 6) and shows no interference from other, non-specific components, which suggests that the population of receptors examined is homogeneous. The fact that we observe maximal stimulation of secretory protein discharge by photoaffinity labeling implies that this homogeneous receptor population is the only receptor population involved in mediating discharge for pentagastrin, that is, for pancreozymin. The lack of interference from nonspecific binding components is to be expected, since nonspecific binding of the photoactivatable pentagastrin is not detected by the discharge assay. Thus a direct measurement of the binding kinetics of a peptide hormone to its receptor without interference from nonspecific components has been realized. This is not usually found when direct binding measurements are made with radiolabeled peptide hormones where nonspecific components may interfere with the determination of the binding parameters of the true receptor site.[23]

The calculated dissociation constant for the binding of photoactivatable pentagastrin to its receptor site ($k_d = 4 \times 10^{-4}$/sec) is very similar to that found for insulin binding to liver plasma membranes ($k_d = 6.6 \times 10^{-4}$/sec)[23] and to fat cell plasma membranes ($k_d = 7.4 \times 10^{-4}$/sec).[5] However, the calculated association rate constant for the binding of photoactivatable pentagastrin to its receptor site ($k_a = 4.4 \times 10^3$/M/sec), differs from that found for insulin in the other systems ($k_a = 1.3 \times 10^6$/M/sec [23] and $k_a = 1.5 \times 10^7$/M/sec).[5] Our association rate constant of 4.4×10^3/M/sec, estimated from kinetic data, does not agree entirely with that ($k_a = 0.8 \times 10^3$/M/sec) calculated from an equilibrium dissociation constant of 5×10^{-7} M and the dissociation rate constant of 4×10^{-4}/sec. This may be a consequence of an experimental error in the discharge assay (10%-20% in the kinetic experiments) or of our lack of knowledge as to whether irreversible activation of discharge is really a measure of receptor occupancy. Quantitative binding studies with radiolabeled pentagastrin and pancreozymin may clear up this discrepancy.

It is interesting to note that the dissociation rate constant found for photoactivatable pentagastrin is of the same order as that found by other investigators for insulin,[5,23] but that our association rate is slower by several orders of magnitude. If the association and dissociation rates of pancreozymin with its receptor are comparable to those of insulin, then the difference in potency between pentagastrin and pancreozymin (about three orders of magnitude) is probably due entirely to the slow association of pentagastrin to the receptor relative to pancreozymin. This hypothesis requires that full biologic activity resides in the pentapeptide, but that the requirements for association of the hormone to the receptor, which determine the potency, reside further from the C-terminus than the fifth amino acid residue.

In conclusion, we believe that we have affinity labeled the pancreozymin receptor site on pancreatic acinar cells using the photoactivable affinity label, 2-nitro-5-azidobenzoyl-pentagastrin. The affinity labeling irreversibly stimulates the cells to discharge secretory protein. Using irreversible stimulation of the discharge process as an index of receptor occupancy, we have measured the association and dissociation rates for the binding of photoactivatable pentagastrin to its receptor. We hope to provide further quantitation of the properties of the pancreozymin receptor by preparing radiolabeled and photoactivatable derivatives and analogs of pancreozymin equal in potency to the native hormone. Our goal is the morphologic localization and the biochemical characterization of the pancreozymin receptor.

SUMMARY

The affinity label, 2-nitro-5-azidobenzoyl-pentagastrin mimics pancreozymin in stimulating the secretion of exportable protein from acinar cells of the guinea pig pancreas *in vitro*. Photolysis of this photoactivatable derivative of pentagastrin in the presence of pancreatic lobules (small clusters of acini) causes irreversible stimulation of the secretion process. This irreversible agonist activity cannot be removed by extensive washing and is blocked only by metabolic inhibition. We have measured the association and dissociation kinetics of nitroazidobenzoyl-pentagastrin with its binding sites in pancreatic lobules, using irreversible agonist activity as an index of binding-site occupancy. We believe that the pentagastrin binding sites that we have affinity-labeled, are the hormone-binding sites on pancreozymin receptors.

Acknowledgment

This research was supported by USPHS Grant AM-17389 from the National Institutes of Arthritis and Metabolic Diseases.

References

1. Baker BR: *Design of Active Site Directed Irreversible Enzyme Inhibitors*, New York: Wiley, 1967.
2. Bockaert J, Roy C, Rajerison R, Jard S: Specific binding of ^{3}H-lysine vasopressin to pig kidney plasma membranes. *J Biol Chem* 248:5922-5931, 1973.
3. Castle JD, Jamieson JD, Palade GE: Radioautographic analysis of the secretory process in the parotid acinar cell of the rabbit. *J Cell Biol* 53:290-311, 1972.
4. Cuatrecasas P: Interaction of insulin with the cell membrane: The primary action of insulin. *Proc Natl Acad Sci USA* 63:450-457, 1969.
5. Cuatrecasas P: Insulin-receptor interactions in adipose tissue cells: Direct measurement and properties. *Proc Natl Acad Sci USA* 68:1264-1268, 1971.
6. Cuatrecasas P: Isolation of the insulin receptor of liver and fat cell membranes. *Proc Natl Acad Sci USA* 69:318-322, 1972.
7. Cuatrecasas P: Insulin receptor of liver and fat cell membranes. *Fed Proc* 32:1838-1846, 1973.
8. Eimerl S, Savion N, Heichal O, Selinger Z: Induction of enzyme secretion in rat pancreatic slices using the ionophore A-23187 and calcium. *J Biol Chem* 249:3991-3993, 1974.
9. Erspamer V: Biogenic amines and active polypeptide of the amphibian skin, in Elliot WH (ed), *Annu Rev Pharmacol*, California: Annual Reviews, Inc., 11:327-350, 1971.
10. Finn FM, Widnell CC, Hofmann K: Localization of an adrenocorticotropic hormone receptor on bovine adrenal cortical membranes. *J Biol Chem* 247:5695-5702, 1972.
11. Freer RJ, Stewart JM: Alkylating analogs of peptide hormones: 1. Synthesis and properties of p-[N, N-bis (2-chloroethyl) amino] phenylbutyryl derivatives of bradykinin and bradykinin potentiating factor. *J Med Chem* 15:1-5, 1972.
12. Galardy RE, Craig LC, Printz MP: Benzophenone triplet: A new photochemical probe of biological ligand-receptor interactions. *Nature [New Biol]* 242:127-128, 1973.

13. Galardy RE, Craig LC, Jamieson JD, Printz MP: Photoaffinity labeling of peptide hormone binding sites. *J Biol Chem* 249:3510-3518, 1974.
14. Goldfine ID, Roth J, Birnbaumer L: Glucagon receptors in β-cells: Binding of ^{125}I-glucagon and activation of adenylate cyclase. *J Cell Biol* 247:1211-1218, 1971.
15. Grossman MI: Nervous and hormonal regulation of pancreatic secretion, in de Rueck AVS, Cameron MP (eds), *Exocrine Pancreas*, London: Churchill Limited, 1962, pp 208-220.
16. Guthrow CE, Rasmussen H, Brunswick DJ, Cooperman BS: Specific photoaffinity labeling of the adenosine 3': 5'-cyclic monophosphate receptor in intact ghosts from human erythrocytes. *Proc Natl Acad Sci USA* 70:3344-3346, 1973.
17. Haour F, Saxena BB: Characterization and solubilization of gonadotropin receptor of bovine corpus luteum. *J Biol Chem* 249:2195-2205, 1974.
18. Hokin LE: Effects of calcium omission on acetylcholine-stimulated amylase secretion and phospholipid synthesis in pigeon pancreas slices. *Biochim Biophys Acta* 115:219-221, 1966.
19. Jamieson JD, Palade GE: Condensing vacuole conversion and zymogen granule discharge in pancreatic exocrine cells: Metabolic studies. *J Cell Biol* 48:503-522, 1971.
20. Jamieson JD, Palade GE: Synthesis, intracellular transport, and discharge of secretory proteins in stimulated pancreatic exocrine cells. *J Cell Biol* 50:135-158, 1971.
21. Jamieson JD: Transport and discharge of exportable proteins in pancreatic exocrine cells: *In vitro* studies, in *Current Topics in Membranes and Transport*, New York: Academic Press, 3:273, 1973.
22. Johnson H, Sherratt HSA, Case RM, Scratcherd T: The effects of secretin, pancreozymin, and acetylcholine on the concentration of adenosine 3':5' cyclic monophosphate in cat pancreas, abstracted. *Biochem J* 120:8P, 1971.
23. Kahn CR, Freychet P, Roth J, Neville DM: Quantitative aspects of the insulin-receptor interaction in liver plasma membrane. *J Biol Chem* 249:2249-2257, 1974.
24. Kanno T: Calcium dependent amylase release and electrophysiological measurements in cells of the pancreas. *J Physiol* 226:353-371, 1972.
25. Knodell RG, Toskes PP, Reber HA, Brooks FP: Significance of cyclic AMP in the regulation of exocrine pancreas secretion. *Experientia* 26:515-517, 1970.
26. Knowles J: Photogenerated reagents for biological receptor-site labeling. *Accts Chem Res* 5:155, 1972.

27. Kulka RG, Sternlicht E: Enzyme secretion in mouse pancreas mediated by adenoside-3' 5'-cyclic phosphate and inhibited by adenosine-3'-phosphate. *Proc Natl Acad Sci USA* 61:1123-1128, 1968.

28. Levy D: Preparation of photo-affinity probes for the insulin receptor sites in adipose and liver cell membranes. *Biochim Biophys Acta* 322:329-336, 1973.

29. Paiva TB, Paiva ACM, Freer RJ, Stewart JM: Alkylating analogs of peptide hormones   II. Synthesis and properties of p-(N, N-bis (2-chloroethyl) amino) phenylbutyryl derivatives of angiotensin II. *J Med Chem* 15:6-8, 1972.

30. Pohl SL, Birnbaumer L, Rodbell M: The glucagon sensitive adenyl cyclase system in plasma membranes of rat liver. Properties. *J Biol Chem* 246:1849-1856, 1971.

31. Rasmussen H: Cell communication, calcium ion, and cyclic adenosine monophosphate. *Science* 170:404-412, 1970.

32. Reggio H, Cailla-Deckmyn H, Marchis Mouren G: Effect of pancreozymin on rat pancreatic enzyme biosynthesis. *J Cell Biol* 50:333-343, 1971.

33. Richards FF, Lifter J, Hew CL, Yoshioka M, Konigsberg WH: Photoaffinity labeling of the combining region of myeloma protein 460: II. An interpretation of the labeling patterns. *Biochemistry* 13:3572-3575, 1974.

34. Ridderstap AS, Bonting SL: Cyclic AMP and enzyme secretion by the isolated rabbit pancreas. *Pfluegers Arch* 313: 62-70, 1969.

35. Ruoho AE, Kiefer H, Roeder PE, Singer SJ: The mechanism of photoaffinity labeling. *Proc Natl Acad Sci USA* 70:2567-2571, 1973.

36. Ruoho A, Kyte J: Photoaffinity labeling of the ouabain binding site on (Na+ + K+) adenosinetriphosphatase. *Proc Natl Acad Sci USA* 71:2352-2356, 1974.

37. Schatz H, Otto J, Hinz M, Maier V, Nierle C, Pfeiffer EF: Gastrointestinal hormones and function of pancreatic islets: Studies on insulin secretion, ^{3}H-leucine incorporation and intracellular free leucine pool in isolated pancreatic mouse islets. *Endocrinology* 94:248-253, 1974.

38. Schimmer BP, Ueda K, Sato GH: Site of action of adrenocorticotropic hormone (ACTH) in adrenal cell cultures. *Biochem Biophys Res Commun* 32:806-810, 1968.

39. Schwartz IL, Shlatz LJ, Kinne-Saffran E, Kinne R: Target cell polarity and membrane phosphorylation in relations to the mechanism of action of antidiuretic hormone. *Proc Natl Acad Sci USA* 71:2595-2599, 1974.

40. Singer SJ: Covalent labeling of active sites, in Anfinsen CB, Anson ML, Edsall JT, Richards FM (eds), *Advances in Protein Chemistry*, 22:1, 1967, New York: Academic Press.

41. Turkington RW: Stimulation of RNA synthesis in isolated mammary cells by insulin and prolactin bound to Sepharose. *Biochem Biophys Res Commun* 41:1362-1367, 1970.

42. Walter R, Schwartz IL, Hechter O, Dousa T, Hoffman PL: Bromoacetyl-oxytocin, an irreversible inhibitor of neurohypophyseal hormone-stimulated adenylate cyclase, and possible affinity label for hormone receptors. *Endocrinology* 91:39-48, 1972.

43. Wolff J, Jones AB: The purification of bovine thyroid plasma membranes and the properties of membrane bound adenyl cyclase. *J Biol Chem* 246:3939-3947, 1971.

HORMONAL ACTIONS ON GASTROINTESTINAL SMOOTH MUSCLE: INTERACTION OF GASTRIN AND METIAMIDE

Sidney Cohen

Gastrointestinal Section, Department of Medicine
of the University of Pennsylvania, at the Hospital
of the University of Pennsylvania, Philadelphia,
Pennsylvania

Each of the gastrointestinal hormones has been shown to affect the motor function of the various portions of the gastrointestinal tract. The effect of each hormone is either excitatory or inhibitory depending upon the specific luminal structure or sphincter being evaluated. The smooth muscle from each structure, studied *in vitro*, reflects the motor function observed *in vivo*. The purpose of this discussion is to review several aspects of hormonal action on gastrointestinal smooth muscle and to discuss the interaction of gastrin I with the H_2 antagonist, metiamide.

METHODS

Studies In Vitro

All studies *in vitro* were performed on the opossum, *Didelphis virginiana*. The opossum was selected because of the demonstration by Christensen and associates[1] that it had a smooth muscle distal esophagus and a physiologic lower esophageal sphincter (LES). We had shown that the opossum had circulating gastrin and a LES that responded to hormonal stimulation.[4] In each opossum, the LES was located as a high pressure zone of about 1.5 cm in length with a mean pressure of approximately 35 mm Hg. Standard intraluminal pressure measurements made with perfused catheters, were employed to locate the sphincter.

The opossums were then killed and the circular muscle from the LES and the adjacent esophagus and stomach was studied *in vitro*.

Muscle strips, 0.5 cm in width and 1.0 cm in length, were mounted in muscle chambers containing Krebs-Ringer solution at 37C-38C bubbled with 95% O_2 and 5% CO_2. The muscle was mounted to record tension from the circular layer. In all experiments, the muscles were studied at their length of optimal tension development, Lo.[4,5] To determine the Lo for a specific muscle, the muscle was gradually increased in length by a screw micrometer. At each increase in length, the passive tension was recorded. In addition, the active tension in response to 10^{-4} M acetylcholine was recorded. The muscle length (Lo) at which the peak active tension (Po) was obtained, was maintained for the duration of the experiment. The active tensions were corrected for muscle weight. An important aspect of studying the muscles *in vitro* was the performance of full dose-response curves for each hormone. Because of the nature of the hormonal effects on the muscle, single doses might have missed the entire range of response.

Studies In Vivo

The methodology employed *in vivo* has been described previously.[2,4] Studies were performed with polyvinyl catheters used (1.4 mm internal diameter), with side-recording orifices (1.4 mm diameter). Each catheter was perfused with distilled water at 1.2 ml to 2.0 ml/min by an infusion pump. All sphincteric pressure measurements were obtained from the portion of the high pressure zone demonstrating the peak pressure. All pressures were expressed with intra-abdominal pressure used as baseline.

RESULTS

There are several specific aspects of hormone action on gastrointestinal smooth muscle that relate to the observations concerning the interaction of gastrin I and metiamide on LES smooth muscle.

*The Hormone Dose-Response Curves of Gastrointestinal
Smooth Muscle*

The effect of gastrin I on the circular smooth
muscle of the LES, gastric antrum, and the pyloric
sphincter was demonstrated and the response expressed
as a percent of maximum response achieved on the LES
muscle, was plotted against the log dose of gastrin I
(residues 2-17) (Fig. 1). The LES muscle responded
at a lower threshold dose and achieved a greater
tension at a lower dose than muscle from the gastric

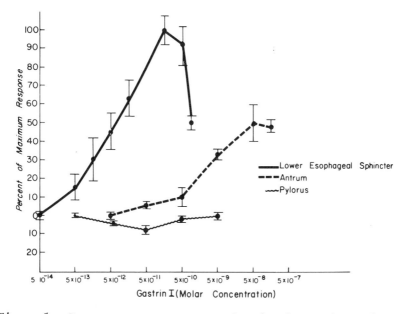

Figure 1. Dose-response curves, at Lo, for increasing molar
concentrations of gastrin I and active tension. (Lo = muscle
length at which peak active tension was obtained.) Active
tension is expressed as a percent of maximum response of lower
esophageal sphincter (LES) muscle. LES muscle responds at a
lower threshold dose and achieves a greater maximum tension.
Pyloric muscle shows no statistically significant change in
active tension. Each point represents the mean ± SE for 20
experiments. (Reproduced, with permission of the *American
Journal of Physiology* 222:775-781, 1972.)

antrum. The pyloric sphincter did not respond at
any dose of gastrin I. These dose-response curves
performed on isolated circular muscle at Lo, illustrated that each portion of the gastrointestinal
tract responded specifically to each gastrointestinal
hormone *in vitro*. Furthermore, it is important to
note that at doses of the hormone greater than that
which gave the maximum response, there was a prominent phase of diminished muscle response. This
phenomenon is best seen with the LES muscle in this
Figure. This diminished response at higher doses
has been called autoinhibition. Autoinhibition has
been observed characteristically with gastrointestinal
hormones acting upon smooth muscle, *in vitro* or upon
motor activity, *in vivo*. It has also been observed
with other hormone responses. The phenomenon of
autoinhibition has been ascribed to the combining of
the hormone with a low-affinity inhibitory receptor.
As will be discussed, there is now direct support
for this supposition.

Hormonal Interaction

    As seen with hormones acting at other areas, the
gastrointestinal hormones interact at each motor
organ. The characteristics of these interactions,
summarized in Table 1, may change with further experiments on other areas of the gut.
    Selectivity of hormonal interaction is illustrated
in Figure 2, in which is shown the antagonistic action of either secretin or gastrin on the agonist
effects of the other hormones acting on the gastric
antrum or on the pyloric sphincter muscles. The
hormone did not nonselectively diminish the effect
of all agonists on a muscle. Secretin reduced the
response of antral circular muscle to gastrin to
approximately 5% of its control value. Secretin
at concentrations of $3x10^{-9}$ M and $3x10^{-7}$ M (not
shown), however, had no significant effect on the
LES response to histamine, dimethylphenylpipera-
zinium (DMPP), or acetylcholine. Similar selectivity
of interaction was seen with the pyloric sphincter
muscle. Here, gastrin selectively reduced the effect
of secretin acting on the pyloric muscle but had no
effect on the other agonists. It was of special
interest that the response to DMPP, a ganglionic

Table 1. Characteristics of hormone interaction on gastro-intestinal smooth muscle

---

1. A hormone which contracts muscle but gives only a small-to-moderate increase in tension may either:
    a. Antagonize the effect of another hormone (cholecystokinin or secretin antagonizes gastrin on LES muscle); or
    b. Give an additive effect with another hormone (secretin and cholecystokinin show an additive effect on the pyloric sphincter muscle).
2. A hormone may have no effect on muscle tension when given alone but may antagonize the effect of another hormone when given in combination. (Gastrin antagonizes secretin or cholecystokinin on the pyloric sphincter.)
3. Hormonal interactions are highly selective; a hormone with an antagonistic effect does not nonspecifically reduce the action of nonhormonal agonists.
4. True potentiation of hormones on gastrointestinal smooth muscle, *in vitro,* has not been demonstrated.

---

stimulant, was not altered. DMPP acted at a site proximal to the action of gastrin on the postganglionic cholinergic nerve. This observation indicated that hormone antagonism at a postganglionic site occurred without altering neural function through other stimuli. This finding of the highly selective interaction of hormones suggested that the specific receptors for gastrin and secretin were closely related, an observation supporting the hormone receptor hypothesis of Grossman.[3]

Interaction of Gastrin and Metiamide

The discussion to this point has focused on the selectivity of hormone interactions and the specificity of hormones acting at each portion of the gastrointestinal tract. These points have suggested unique characteristics of the gastrointestinal hormone receptor on the smooth muscle of the gut. Most recently, studies using metiamide and burimamide have indicated a close relationship between the histamine and the hormone receptors at the parietal cell. The purpose

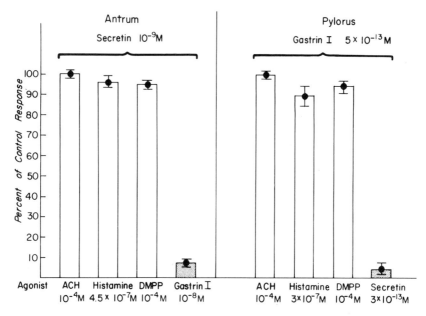

Figure 2. (left) -- Percent of maximum gastrin I and other
agonist control response in presence of 10^{-9} M secretin on
antral muscle. Molar concentration of secretin was selected
as that concentration that provided a near-maximum inhibition
of a maximum gastrin I response. Molar concentration of agonists, shown along the bottom, is that concentration which
produces a maximum response on antral muscle. Each bar represents mean ± SE for 10 separate experiments. Secretin
significantly inhibits a maximum gastrin I response ($p < 0.001$),
but does not affect the response to other agonists ($p > 0.05$).

　　　(right) -- Percent of maximum secretin and other
agonist control responses in presence of 5×10^{-13} M gastrin on
pyloric muscle. Molar concentration of gastrin I was chosen
as that concentration which gave near-maximum inhibition of
a maximum secretin response. Molar concentration of agonist,
shown on bottom, is that concentration which produces a maximum response on pyloric muscle. Each bar represents a mean
± SE for 10 separate experiments. Gastrin I significantly
inhibits a maximum secretin response ($p < 0.001$), but does not
affect response to other agonists. (Reproduced, with permission of the *American Journal of Physiology* 222:775-781,
1972.)

of this portion of the discussion is to provide data
suggesting a similar yet unique relationship between
the gastrin and histamine receptors at the LES. These
studies were performed to determine whether metiamide
had a similar antagonistic effect on gastrin acting
at the LES as seen at the parietal cell.

In Figure 3 is shown the effect of metiamide on
both acid secretion and LES pressure during the

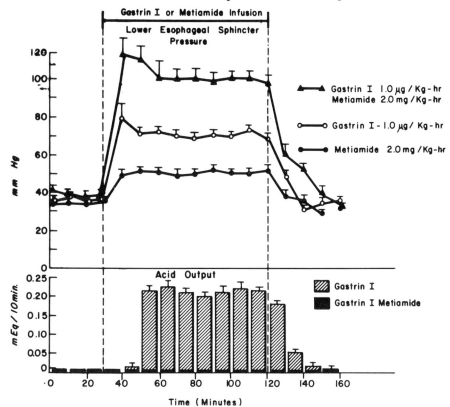

Figure 3. Lower esophageal sphincter (LES) and gastric acid
secretory responses to constant intravenous infusions of (a)
gastrin I; (b) metiamide; and (c) gastrin I plus metiamide.
Each value represents the mean + SE for values obtained in
eight opossums. Gastrin I, alone, and metiamide, alone, gave
sustained increases in LES pressure. The maximum LES response
to gastrin I was increased in the presence of metiamide. Acid
secretion was absent under basal conditions but increased
during gastrin infusion. Metiamide antagonized the acid
secretory response to gastrin I.

constant infusion of gastrin I in the anesthetized
opossum.   There was no basal secretion of acid in
any of the opossums, but a modest secretory response
to gastrin I infusion could be elicited.   Gastrin I
gave a sustained increase in LES pressure with some
fade after the initial 10-15 minute period.   Metiamide, alone, increased LES pressure.   In the presence of a metiamide infusion, acid secretion in response to gastrin I was abolished.   LES pressure
showed a potentiated response to metiamide and
gastrin I.
   The constant intravenous infusion of metiamide gave
a prolonged dose-related increase in LES pressure
(Fig. 4).   The maximum increase in pressure, 18.7 ± 1.5
mm HG, was a moderate yet significant change in LES
tone.   The possible mechanism of this effect was next
investigated.

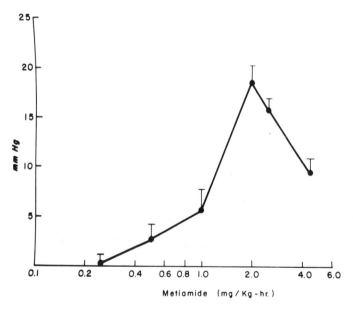

Figure 4.   Lower esophageal sphincter dose-response curve to
continuous intravenous infusions of metiamide.

Studies on the LES circular muscle, *in vitro*, were next performed to evaluate the interaction of metiamide with either gastrin I or histamine. Initially, studies were performed with various concentrations of metiamide alone. No increase in muscle tension was seen with concentrations to 10^{-2} M. This observation suggested that the effect of metiamide *in vivo* was not due to direct smooth muscle stimulation. In Figure 5 is shown the dose-response curve of LES circular muscle to histamine, alone, and in the presence of metiamide or diphenhydramine. As shown, diphenhydramine, an H_1 antagonist, could abolish the LES muscle response to histamine.[6] The histamine response in the presence of metiamide showed augmentation of the maximal response without significant change in the threshold or lower dosage muscle responses. This observation suggested that metiamide antagonized the effect of histamine at an inhibitory H_2 receptor. Thus, histamine acted at both an excitatory H_1 receptor and an inhibitory H_2 receptor.

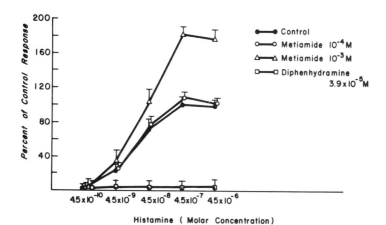

Histamine (Molar Concentration)

Figure 5. Lower esophageal sphincter circular smooth muscle response to histamine in the presence of metiamide or diphenhydramine. Each point represents the mean + SE for a minimum of 10 observations. Diphenhydramine was chosen at a dosage which totally abolished the maximum effect of histamine. Metiamide at 10^{-3} M augmented the maximal response to histamine but did not alter the threshold response. Metiamide (10^{-4} M) had no effect on the histamine dose-response curve.

The presence of an inhibitory H_2 receptor could not
be recognized by examination of the dose response
curve to histamine alone.

The interaction of metiamide and gastrin I on LES
circular muscle is seen in Figure 6. Metiamide had
two effects. At the lower dosage (10^{-4} M), metiamide
abolished the phase of autoinhibition without altering
other portions of the gastrin I dose-response curve.
At the higher dose (10^{-3} M), metiamide not only
abolished the phase of autoinhibition but in addition,
the maximal response was greatly increased. As noted
previously, metiamide alone had no effect on muscle
tension.

The presence of an inhibitory H_2 receptor sensitive
to both histamine and gastrin I could be shown *in
vitro*. With KCl-contracted LES muscles, histamine

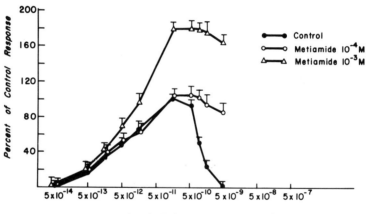

Gastrin I (Molar Concentration)

Figure 6. Lower esophageal sphincter circular muscle response
to gastrin I in the presence of metiamide. Each point represents the mean + SE for a minimum of 10 observations. Metiamide
(10^{-4} M) abolished the phase of autoinhibition or the diminished
response beyond the maximum gastrin I activity. No change in
the maximum active tension was observed with 10^{-4} M metiamide.
Metiamide (10^{-3} M) significantly augmented the maximum gastrin
response and also abolished the phase of autoinhibition. No
change in threshold response was observed with either concentration of metiamide.

or gastrin I gave no additional increase in tension. When diphenhydramine was given together with histamine, an inhibition of the KCl contracture was observed. This inhibition could be antagonized by metiamide. Similarly, gastrin I gave an inhibitory response if atropine was first administered to the KCl-contracted muscle. Again, the inhibitory response could be blocked by metiamide. These studies more directly demonstrate an inhibitory response that occurs with either histamine or gastrin I and that is antagonized by metiamide.

Excitatory H_1 and inhibitory H_2 receptors have been demonstrated in the cardiovascular system of certain animals.[7] The presence of excitatory and inhibitory histamine and hormone receptors is analogous to the alpha- and beta-adrenergic receptors. In the adrenergic system, different effects at these receptors may be observed in different organ systems. The presence of excitatory and inhibitory hormone receptors should also be considered as the possible mechanism of various hormone interactions. Competitive or noncompetitive hormone effects may be better explained by an inhibitory hormonal action seen only during an excitatory hormone response.

The studies with metiamide and its interaction with histamine or gastrin I suggest several points that should be considered in evaluating the responses to the gastrointestinal hormones. First, since the phase of autoinhibition of the gastrin dose-response curve could be selectively blocked, multiple receptors for the same hormone at the same organ must be considered. Second, the true maximal hormone response on muscle *in vitro*, or on motor function *in vivo*, may actually be reduced by hormone interaction with an inhibitory receptor. Third, the shared interaction of histamine and gastrin I with metiamide at the LES suggests a relationship between the receptors for these agents, without one necessarily acting through the other as proposed for gastric acid secretion. Fourth, other structures with excitatory H_1 receptors may have inhibitory H_2 receptors at which gastrointestinal hormones may be shown to act.

SUMMARY

1.   Each gastrointestinal hormone has a specific
      effect on each portion of the gastrointestinal
      tract. These effects are best seen in the dose-
      response relationships of the smooth muscle,
      itself.
2.   Gastrointestinal hormones may antagonize the
      effect of another hormone or may show an addi-
      tive effect with another hormone. No true
      potentiation of hormone responses has been ob-
      served on muscle strips *in vitro*.
3.   The antagonism of one hormone for another is
      selective. Hormones do not alter the response
      to other agonists.
4.   Studies with metiamide suggest the presence of
      both excitatory and inhibitory gastrin receptors
      at the LES. Antagonism of the inhibitory
      receptor augments the maximal excitatory re-
      sponse to gastrin.
5.   A relationship between the histamine and gastrin
      receptor mechanism has now been observed within
      smooth muscle, as well as at the parietal cell.
      This relationship may be independent of gastrin
      acting through histamine.
           The presence of excitatory and inhibitory
      receptors to the same hormone at the same struc-
      ture, as well as the unexplained relationship
      between histamine and gastrin receptors, suggests
      that the hormone receptor mechanism is more
      complex than previously reported.

Acknowledgments

   This work was supported by Research Grant 5 R01 AM 16280-02
and Research Career Development Award 5 K04 AM 70576-02 from
the National Institutes of Health.

References

1.   Christensen J, Lund GF: Esophageal responses to distension
         and electrical stimulation. *J Clin Invest* 48:408-419,
         1969.

2. Cohen S, Lipshutz WH: Hormonal regulation of human lower esophageal sphincter competence: interaction of gastrin and secretin. *J Clin Invest* 50:449-454, 1971.
3. Grossman MI: Hypothesis: Gastrin, cholecystokinin and secretin act on one receptor. *Lancet* 1:1088-1092, 1970.
4. Lipshutz WH, Cohen S: Physiological determinants of lower esophageal sphincter function. *Gastroenterology* 61:16-24, 1971.
5. Lipshutz WH, Cohen S: Interaction of gastrin I and secretin on gastrointestinal circular muscle. *Am J Physiol* 222:775-781, 1972.
6. Lipshutz W, Tuch AF, Cohen S: A comparison of the site of action of gastrin I on lower esophageal sphincter and antral circular smooth muscle. *Gastroenterology* 61: 454-460, 1971.
7. Wood CJ, Simkins MA (eds), *International Symposium on Histamine H_2-receptor Antagonists*, London: Smith Kline & French Laboratories, 1973.

THE EFFECT OF PENTAGASTRIN ON CANINE GASTRIC MYOELECTRIC AND MOTOR ACTIVITY

Keith A. Kelly

Sections of Gastroenterologic and General Surgery
and of Surgical Research, Mayo Clinic, Mayo
Foundation, and Mayo Medical School, Rochester,
Minnesota

The motor effects of pentagastrin on the proximal portion of the stomach differ from those on the distal portion in keeping with the differing physiologic roles of the two regions.

PROXIMAL REGION OF STOMACH

The actions of pentagastrin on the proximal region of the stomach are illustrated in a conscious, fasted dog with a vagally innervated, separated pouch of the gastric fundus and orad corpus. In control studies, the pouch was filled through its watertight cannula with 75 ml of isotonic sodium chloride, and the pressure across its wall was measured. A baseline pressure of about 10 cm of water was present, on which were superimposed two types of phasic changes in pressure, the slower with an amplitude of 15 to 30 cm of water and a duration of 1 to 3 minutes, and the faster with an amplitude of 5 to 15 cm of water and a duration of 12 to 20 seconds (Fig. 1).

Pentagastrin, 0.1 µg/kg/min given intravenously, inhibited the phasic changes of pressure in the pouch within two minutes after the initiation of infusion (Fig. 2). The inhibition lasted throughout the 15 minutes that pentagastrin was given, the phasic pressures gradually returning to the control 30 minutes later.

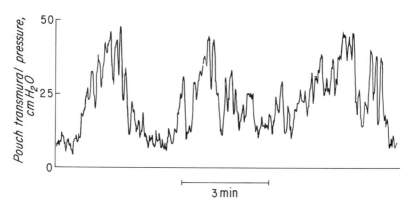

Figure 1. Sustained and phasic changes in pressure occur in a vagally innervated, separated pouch of the canine gastric fundus and orad corpus. (Reproduced, with permission of Mitchell Press.[10])

These effects of pentagastrin on the vagally innervated, fundal pouch are similar to those found when we studied the whole stomach.[15] We measured gastric transmural pressure in conscious dogs whose gastric fundus and corpus were distended to 500 ml by an intragastric bag passed *per os*. A prompt decrease in mean transmural pressure of the intact stomach occurred during pentagastrin infusion, just as in the fundal pouch (Fig. 3).

The inhibition of proximal gastric contractions and the decrease in intragastric pressure brought about by pentagastrin, enhance gastric accommodation to distention and probably account for the pentagastrin-induced slowing of gastric emptying of liquids described earlier by Hunt and Ramsbottom[6] in man, and by us[3] and by Cooke, Chvasta, and Weisbrodt[2] in dogs. Decreases in intragastric pressure slow the rate of gastric emptying by decreasing the driving force behind the emptying. Intraduodenal pressure and resistance to flow across the pylorus also influence the rate of emptying,[12] but others have shown that pentagastrin does not stimulate duodenal or pyloric contractions.[4,8]

The hypothesis that pentagastrin slows gastric emptying of liquids by relaxing the proximal portion of the stomach rather than by inducing antral contractions, is also consistent with our observation that pentagastrin slows emptying of both isotonic

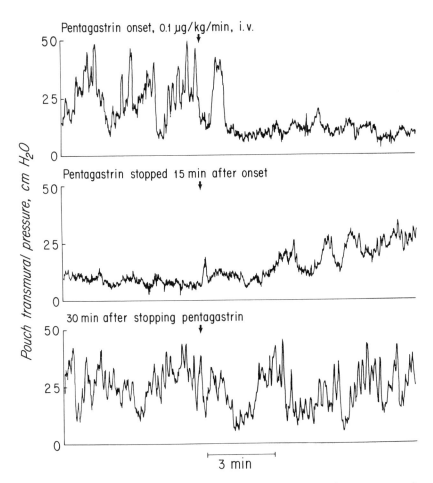

Figure 2. Pentagastrin inhibits phasic changes in pressure in a vagally innervated canine fundal pouch.

sodium chloride and isotonic sodium bicarbonate
(pH >8.0) even after excision of the distal antrum
and pylorus (Figs. 4 & 5).[3] The experiments with
NaHCO$_3$ indicate that the effect is not due to the
release of secretin by passage into the duodenum
of acid secreted in the stomach in response to
pentagastrin.

DISTAL REGION OF STOMACH

Pentagastrin increases the frequency of the cycles
of the pacesetter potential in the distal region,
whether the cycles are being generated by the natural
gastric pacemaker (Fig. 6)[9] or at more slowly os-
cillating sites surgically separated from the pacemaker and so not driven by it.[1] The faster

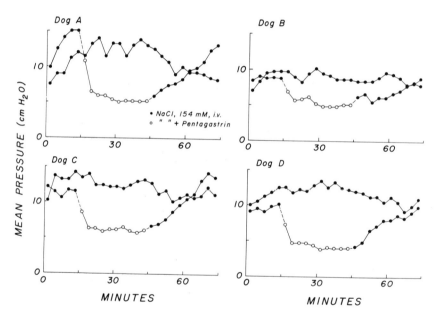

Figure 3. Pentagastrin decreases gastric transmural pressure.
In tests in which sodium chloride alone is infused, each point
is a mean pressure over three minutes. In tests in which
pentagastrin is added to sodium chloride, each point is an
overall mean of three 3-minute mean pressures from three
separate experiments. (Reproduced, with permission of
Gastroenterology.[15])

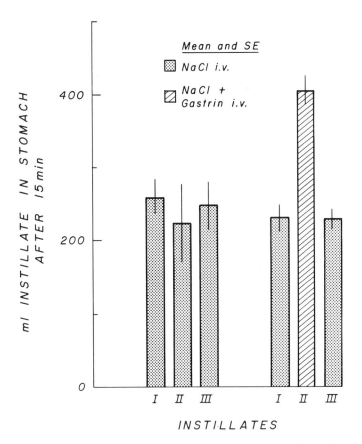

Figure 4. Pentagastrin slows gastric emptying of 500 ml of 154 mM sodium chloride after antrectomy. The overall means in this figure and in Figure 5 are of two tests in each of four dogs.[3]

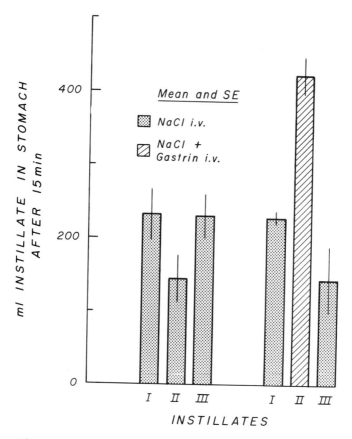

Figure 5. Pentagastrin slows gastric emptying of 500 ml of 165 mM sodium bicarbonate after antrectomy.[3]

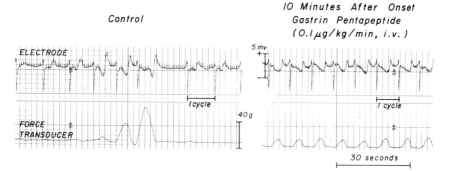

Control

10 Minutes After Onset
Gastrin Pentapeptide
(0.1 μg/kg/min, i.v.)

ELECTRODE

5 mv

1 cycle

1 cycle

40 g

FORCE
TRANSDUCER

30 seconds

Figure 6. Gastrin pentapeptide (pentagastrin) increases the frequency of the canine antral pacesetter potential and causes action potentials to appear with every cycle (upper panel), stimulating a steady series of medium-amplitude contractions (lower panel). Electric recordings are from extracellular, monopolar silver electrodes, and force recordings are from strain gauges implanted adjacent to electrodes. (Reproduced, with permission of Mitchell Press.[10]

frequencies stimulated by pentagastrin at the distal sites, however, are always slower than those stimulated at the pacemaker.

In addition to these effects on frequency, my colleague, Dr. C.F. Code, has observed that pentagastrin converts irregular rhythms of the pacesetter potential to a regular rhythm, in both the intact and the isolated, perfused stomach (CF Code, personal communication). He has proposed that gastrin be used to correct disturbed rhythms of the gastric pacesetter potential.

Pentagastrin also abolishes the interdigestive myoelectric complex (IDMEC),[11] the intense band of action potentials and contractions that begins in the gastroduodenal area every 1½ to 2 hours during fasting and moves slowly aborad from stomach to cecum.[14]

In place of the IDMEC in the stomach, pentagastrin stimulates a regular sequence of pacesetter potentials with action potentials and thus a steady series of peristaltic contractions (Fig. 6).[5,7,8,10,13] The increased frequence of peristalsis and the consequent antral propulsion and retropulsion brought about by pentagastrin serve to mix and grind gastric solids.

SUMMARY

Pentagastrin inhibits the phasic contractions of
the proximal portion of the stomach, thereby en-
hancing gastric accommodation to distention and
slowing gastric emptying of liquids. Concurrently,
pentagastrin increases the frequency of the gastric
pacemaker, abolishes the interdigestive myoelectric
complex, and induces a regular sequence of peristaltic
contractions in the distal part of the stomach, which
enhances gastric mixing and grinding of solids.

Acknowledgments

This investigation was supported in part by Research Grant
AM-2015 from the National Institutes of Health, Public Health
Service.

References

1. Bedi BS, Kelly KA, Holley KE: Pathways of propagation of
       the canine gastric pacesetter potential. *Gastroenter-
       ology* 63:288-296, 1972.
2. Cooke AR, Chvasta TE, Weisbrodt NW: Effect of pentagastrin
       on emptying and electrical and motor activity of the
       dog stomach. *Am J Physiol* 223:934-938, 1972.
3. Dozois RR, Kelly KA: Effect of a gastrin pentapeptide
       on canine gastric emptying of liquids. *Am J Physiol*
       221:113-117, 1971.
4. Fisher RS, Lipshutz W, Cohen S: The hormonal regulation of
       pyloric sphincter function. *J Clin Invest* 52:1289-
       1296, 1973.
5. Gregory RA, Tracy HJ: The constitution and properties of
       two gastrins extracted from hog antral mucosa. *Gut*
       5:103-117, 1964.
6. Hunt JN, Ramsbottom N: Effect of gastrin II on gastric
       emptying and secretion during a test meal. *Br Med J*
       4:386-387, 1967.
7. Isenberg JI, Grossman MI: Effect of gastrin and SC 15396
       on gastric motility in dogs. *Gastroenterology* 56:450-
       455, 1969.
8. Jacoby HI, Marshall CH: Gastric motor-stimulating activity
       of gastrin tetrapeptide in dogs. *Gastroenterology*
       56:80-87, 1969.

9. Kelly KA: Effect of gastrin on gastric myo-electric activity. *Am J Dig Dis* 15:399–405, 1970.

10. Kelly KA: Canine gastric motility and emptying: Electric, neural, and hormonal controls, in *Proceedings of the Fourth International Symposium on Gastrointestinal Motility*, Vancouver: Mitchell Press, 1974, pp 463–470.

11. Marik F, Code CF: Neural and humoral control of the inter-digestive myoelectric complex, abstracted. *Rendi R Gastroenterol* 5:152–153, 1973.

12. Nelsen TS, Kohatsu S: The stomach as a pump. *Rendi R Gastroenterol* 3:65–71, 1971.

13. Sugawara K, Isaza J, Woodward ER: Effect of gastrin on gastric motor activity. *Gastroenterology* 57:649–658, 1969.

14. Szurszewski JH: A migrating electric complex of the canine small intestine. *Am J Physiol* 217:1757–1763, 1969.

15. Wilbur BG, Kelly KA: Gastrin pentapeptide decreases canine gastric transmural pressure. *Gastroenterology* 67:1139–1142, 1974.

GASTROINTESTINAL HORMONES AND BLOOD FLOW

John C. Bowen, Wan-Fen Fang,
Wieslaw Pawlik, Eugene D. Jacobson

Programs in Surgery and Physiology,
The University of Texas Medical School
at Houston, Houston, Texas

When a conscious dog with implanted vascular trans-
ducers is exposed to the sight and smell of food,
his cardiac output rises abruptly, and blood flow
to his gastrointestinal tract is increased. The
presence of food in the upper gut may or may not
evoke an increase in splanchnic blood flow.[1] These
two facts suggest that the major extrinsic regulator
of gastrointestinal blood flow is the rapidly acting
autonomic nervous system which drives the heart to
increase its minute-volume of blood and which simultaneously relaxes the splanchnic arterioles to accept
the higher flow.

When the secretory organs of the gastrointestinal
tract are stimulated to elaborate their juices, the
metabolism of their tissues also increases. The
altered metabolic environment around the smooth
muscle of the splanchnic arterioles induces vasodilation and increased blood flow.[4] This suggests
that the major intrinsic regulator of gastrointestinal blood flow is the need of parenchymal cells for
nutrients, expressed through changes in the chemical
environment of the minute blood vessels, which leads
to an increased flow of blood through the tissues.
The local chemical messengers that signal relaxation
of vascular smooth muscle and an augmented perfusion
of gastrointestinal tissues with blood, are altered
concentrations of oxygen, carbon dioxide, electro-
lytes (such as potassium and magnesium), and several
putative vasodilator tissue substances (for example,
histamine, bradykinin, ATP, cyclic AMP, E and A type
prostaglandins).

391

If the rapid general increase in gastrointestinal blood flow at meal time is regulated by the autonomic nervous system, and the moment-by-moment changes in blood flow through areas of metabolizing gastrointestinal tissue are controlled by local tissue substances, what role is left for the gastrointestinal hormones-- gastrin, secretin and cholecystokinin (CCK)--as normal circulatory regulators? The answer is "not much." It is true that activation of secretion by a hormone will evoke an increase in blood flow through the stimulated organ,[5] but the effect is secondary to the metabolic sequelae of increasing secretion. Thus, for example, blood flow in the gastric mucosa is increased when the stomach is stimulated to secrete its juices by gastrin; it is increased much more, however, when the stomach is stimulated to secrete at the same rate by histamine.[6] The difference in mucosal blood flow evoked by these two agents that stimulated the same rate of gastric secretion, is attributable to the difference in vaso- dilator potencies between the secretagogues: histamine is a more effective dilator than is gastrin.

Furthermore, at the concentrations in the plasma achieved by gastrin, secretin, and CCK, when these hor- mones are driving the stomach, pancreas, and gallblad- der to respond maximally, there is little effect upon the general circulation other than that of the acti- vated target organ. Thus, for example, infusion of 0.1 µg/kg/min pentagastrin intravenously will drive the dog stomach to secrete nearly maximally, but will not alter superior mesenteric artery blood flow nor systemic arterial blood pressure.

Despite the above opinions that current evidence indicates little role for the gastrointestinal hor- mones as direct physiologic regulators of the circu- lation, two points remain to be considered on the topic. First, the entire circulation is continually exposed to varying plasma concentrations of these hormones. At least three times daily in adults, cir- culating levels of gastrin, secretin, and CCK reach peak values. One inference from this is that these hormones are either rapidly metabolized or are well tolerated agents in the circulation and in tissues and are not likely to evoke untoward side effects or allergic reactions, especially if their use as possible circulatory drugs were to be fairly brief.

The second point is this: these hormones do possess vasoactive properties; all three polypeptides are

vasodilator substances. Although intravenous infusion
of these hormones does little in the general circulation, intra-arterial infusion of the same dose of hormone is attended by prompt dilator responses in that
regional circulation. The amplification of dosage
provided by alteration of the route of administration
should be obvious; even in as large an artery as the
superior mesenteric, intra-arterial infusion increases
the intestinal plasma concentration of a hormone ten-
fold over intravenous administration of the same dose
of drug.

Thus, we are no longer in the realm of physiology.
We are no longer concerned with the normal regulation
of gastrointestinal blood flow by gastrointestinal
hormones. The focus of the remainder of this paper
is upon the potential use of gastrointestinal hormones
as vasodilator drugs in the circulation of the gut.
The following is a pharmacologic report.

The intestinal circulation is the locus of much
human vascular disease. When severe vasospasm grips
this circulation in an elderly person with congestive
cardiac failure, the outlook is hopeless for survival,
at least with current therapies.[7] Since radiologists
are able to insert catheters into the intestinal circulation to make the angiographic diagnosis of this
dread disorder, there is no sound reason why they
cannot leave the catheter in the superior mesenteric
artery for continuous infusion of a dilator drug to
overcome the intestinal ischemia. Several agents
come to mind as candidates for that dilator drug in
this circumstance--isoproterenol, glucagon, and
prostaglandin E_1, among others.

The object of our study was to explore pharmacologic
effectiveness of gastrin, secretin, and CCK as selective vasodilator agents in the intestinal circulation.

Subjects of our study were 30 mongrel dogs, weighing 15-20 kg each and of either sex. The dogs were
anesthetized intravenously with pentobarbital sodium
(30 mg/kg). After performing a midline laparotomy
in each dog, we exposed a segment of mid-small intestine of about 10 cm length, ligated its ends and
isolated its arterial and venous supplies.

The instrumentation implanted in or connected to
the dog included: 1) electromagnetic blood flow transducer (Micron) applied around the mesenteric artery
branch to the gut segment; the transducer was connected via cables to amplifiers and a polygraphic

recorder (Hewlett-Packard) to allow continual measurement of blood flow;   2) arteriovenous oxygen analyzer
(Oxford) connected via cannulas to the venous blood
draining the intestinal segment and to the systemic
arterial blood; this apparatus was also connected to
the recorder to allow continual measurement of the
arteriovenous oxygen content difference in the blood
flowing across the gut;   3) pressure transducer (Sanborn) interposed between the femoral artery and the
recorder to allow continual measurement of systemic
arterial pressure;   4) a constant-flow infusion pump
(Harvard) connected to a twig of the artery under
study to allow intra-arterial administration of agents
at fixed rates.   From the aforementioned measurements
we were able to calculate mesenteric vascular resistance (arterial pressure/mesenteric blood flow) and
intestinal oxygen consumption (mesenteric blood flow
times arteriovenous oxygen content difference).

   The agents employed in our studies were: 1) pentagastrin (Peptavlon, kindly   supplied by Mr. B Mollov,
Ayerst);   2) synthetic secretin (Schwartz/Mann);
3) the synthetic octapeptide of CCK, to be referred
to as CCK-OP (kindly supplied by Dr. Miguel Ondetti,
Squibb);   4) glucagon (Lilly);   5) acetylcholine
chloride (Sigma); and   6) atropine sulfate (Burroughs
Wellcome).

   The design of these experiments was as follows: an
infusion of saline (0.2 ml/min) was begun into the
mesenteric artery branch and continued for 30 min
(control); then, CCK-OP, pentagastrin, glucagon or
acetylcholine was infused in the same volume into the
vessel for 10 minutes.   In the 24 dogs receiving
either CCK-OP, pentagastrin, glucagon, or acetylcholine,
we injected atropine (0.5 mg) intravenously, and the
hormone or acetylcholine infusion was repeated after
waiting 10 minutes.   In the six experiments with
secretin infusion (0.03 µg/kg/min), a hiatus of 10
minutes was followed by infusion of a higher dose
(0.3 µg/kg/min).   The doses of other agents infused
were 0.1 µg/kg/min for CCK-OP, 0.15 µg/kg/min for
acetylcholine and 0.5 µg/kg/min for pentagastrin and
glucagon, which produced an approximate increase of
50% in blood flow.

   Results from one experiment appear in Figure 1.   In
this dog CCK-OP was infused directly into the superior
mesenteric artery branch to the gut segment.   The
hormone caused an approximate increase of 50% in blood

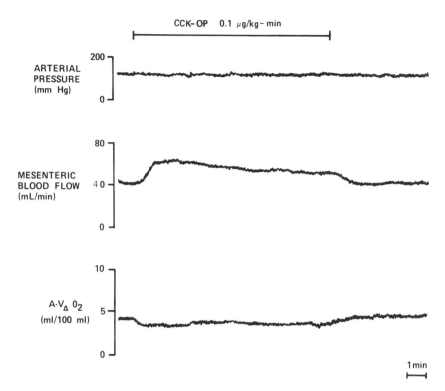

Figure 1. Results from one experiment showing the effects of direct intra-arterial infusion of CCK-OP on systemic arterial blood pressure, blood flow through a branch of the superior mesenteric artery, and the arteriovenous oxygen content difference.

flow, a lesser decline in the arteriovenous oxygen content difference and no change in systemic arterial pressure.

There are five important inferences not immediately apparent from a glance at this polygraphic record:

1. Although the dose of CCK-OP infused was approximately that which would stimulate pancreatic exocrine secretion of enzymes maximally (and, therefore, is an amount which may be equivalent to the endogenous CCK released during the feeding cycle), the concentration of hormone in the mesenteric arterial blood is far beyond anything normally experienced by that circulation. Since the branch of the

mesenteric circulation siphons off about 1% of the
cardiac output, the hormone concentration in that
blood is at least 100 times anything occurring normally. This is a pharmacologic dose of the hormone
because of the route of administration.
        2. The route of administration also guarantees
restriction of the circulatory effects of CCK-OP to
the intestinal vasculature. Infusing the agent into
the mesenteric artery means that the hormone must be
cleared by the intestine, the liver, and the lung as
well as diluted by the entire circulating blood volume before it reaches any other peripheral circulation. Therefore, the hormone has little effect on
blood flow to any organ other than the gut by merit
of the route of administration. This is evident by
the lack of change of systemic arterial pressure
during CCK-OP infusion; had the hormone vasodilated
the circulations of brain, kidney, and skeletal muscle the way it dilated the intestinal circulation,
there would have been a severe hypotensive response
to CCK-OP. Furthermore, intravenous infusion of
CCK-OP in the same dose results in no increase in
intestinal blood flow.
        3. There was a reciprocal change in blood flow
and arteriovenous oxygen content difference with
CCK-OP; blood flow increased as the oxygen difference
decreased. This indicates that some of the augmented
blood flow to the gut did not perfuse capillaries at
a rate which permitted normal extraction of oxygen
by adjacent cells. In effect this is a "physiologic
shunt" with some of the blood either perfusing vessels
in regions of low cell density or perfusing capillaries
at a velocity too high for normal extraction rates.
Therefore, some arterialized blood reached the venous
side, and the arteriovenous oxygen content difference
decreased. It should also be noted that some of the
augmented blood flow does enter capillaries from
which oxygen can be extracted at normal or increased
rates, and thus, the fall in oxygen difference is not
of as great a magnitude as the increase in blood flow.
        4. Intestinal vascular resistance, which is the
quotient of systemic arterial pressure divided by
blood flow can be calculated from the data in the
figure. During CCK-OP infusion, systemic arterial
pressure did not change. Hence, the change in resistance with CCK-OP is the reciprocal of the change in
blood flow. Since blood flow increased by about 50%,

intestinal vascular resistance decreased to the same
degree. This tells us that CCK-OP is a vasodilator
drug as employed in this experiment. This also tells
us the anatomic locus of action of the drug in the
intestinal microcirculation: CCK-OP relaxed the
smooth muscle of the arteriolar wall, since most of
the resistance to flow is generated by the arterioles.
    5. Another important calculation is that of oxy-
gen consumption by the gut. This is the product of
blood flow times the arteriovenous oxygen content
difference. Since the blood flow increased propor- ·
tionately more than the oxygen differenced during
infusion of the drug, oxygen consumption was increased
by CCK-OP,   although not as much as the increase in
blood flow. This means that the hormone increased
the density of perfused capillaries, so intestinal
cellular extraction of oxygen increased. It is obviously desirable to employ a drug in intestinal
ischemic disease which increases both total blood
flow to the gut and the nutrient component of that
circulation, thereby allowing correction of tissue
hypoxia.
Results from 30 animal experiments are summarized
in Table 1. In each paired set of experiments (1
and 2, 3 and 4, 5 and 6, 7 and 8, 9 and 10) a different series of six dogs was used. The major findings
are:
    1. CCK-OP and pentagastrin increased intestinal
blood flow about 50% and increased oxygen consumption
about 25% during intra-arterial infusion. These and
other increases noted in the table were highly significant ($p < 0.01$ or less).
    2. Atropine blocked the vasodilator and oxygen
uptake responses to both hormones.
    3. These antagonistic effects of atropine ap-
pear specific insofar as atropine also abolished the
vasodilator and oxygen uptake responses to acetylcholine but not to glucagon.
    4. Synthetic secretin in doses of 0.03 and 0.3
μg/kg/min infused into the intestinal vessel altered
neither blood flow nor oxygen consumption. These
doses would create a plasma concentration of the
hormone 100 to 1000 times endogenous levels at peak
pancreatic secretory rates.
Our findings indicate that CCK-OP and pentagastrin
are potent vasodilators of the mesenteric circulation,
capable of increasing both total blood flow to the gut

Table 1. Effect of gastrointestinal hormones and acetylcholine on intestinal blood flow and oxygen consumption

	Agent	Blood Flow	Oxygen Consumption
1.	CCK-OP	↑↑	↑
2.	CCK-OP after atropine	--	--
3.	Pentagastrin	↑↑	↑
4.	Pentagastrin after atropine	--	--
5.	Acetylcholine	↑↑	↑
6.	Acetylcholine after atropine	--	--
7.	Glucagon	↑↑	↑
8.	Glucagon after atropine	↑↑	↑
9.	Secretin lower dose	--	--
10.	Secretin higher dose	--	--

and tissue uptake of oxygen. The vasodilator effects appear to be mediated through cholinergic receptors, as evidenced by similar responses to acetylcholine, antagonism by atropine, and lack of effect of atropine against glucagon. Furthermore, other gastrointestinal smooth muscle responses to CCK and gastrin are considered to be mediated through cholinergic receptors.[9]

Our finding that synthetic secretin was such a weak dilator in this circulation is at variance with other reports of vasodilator responses to the hormone in this vasculature.[2,3,8] Previous investigators used GIH secretin, however, which is contaminated with CCK and VIP, both of which are vasodilator agents in the intestinal vessels.

In summary, we used two synthetic gastrointestinal hormone moieties -- CCK-OP and pentagastrin -- as pharmacologic dilators of the intestinal circulation. These agents appear to have some promise as selective vasodilators of the ischemic bowel.

SUMMARY

We explored the pharmacologic effects of cholecysto-kinin-octapeptide (CCK-OP), pentagastrin, and synthetic secretin on the mesenteric circulation. Direct infusion of these hormones was performed into a branch of the superior mesenteric artery in anesthetized dogs. We measured blood flow through the vessel, systemic arterial pressure, and the arteriovenous oxygen content difference, and we calculated oxygen consumption across the gut segment. CCK-OP and pentagastrin increased blood flow and oxygen consumption without altering systemic arterial blood pressure. Atropine blocked these effects of the hormones. Acetylcholine reproduced the same effects as the hormones which were also antagonized by atropine. Glucagon infusion increased blood flow and oxygen consumption in the gut segment; these responses to glucagon were not altered by atropine. Synthetic secretin had little effect on blood flow and oxygen consumption. CCK-OP and pentagastrin appear to have promise as intestinal vasodilator drugs.

Acknowledgments

These investigations were supported by USPHS grant AM 15977-03.

References

1. Bynum TE, Jacobson ED: Blood flow and gastrointestinal function. *Gastroenterology* 60:325-335, 1971.
2. Fara JW, Rubinstein EH, Sonnenschein RR: Intestinal hormones in mesenteric vasodilation after intraduodenal agents. *Am J Physiol* 223:1058-1067, 1972.
3. Fasth S, Filipsson S, Hultén, Martinson J: The effect of the gastrointestinal hormones on small intestinal motility and blood flow. *Experientia* 29:982-984, 1973.
4. Jacobson ED, Swan KG, Grossman MI: Blood flow and secretion in the stomach. *Gastroenterology* 52:414-420, 1967.
5. Jacobson ED: Secretion and blood flow in the gastrointestinal tract, in *Handbook of Physiology,* sec 6, vol 2. Washington DC: The American Physiological Society, 1967, pp 1043-1062.
6. Jacobson ED, Chang ACL: Comparison of gastrin and histamine on gastric mucosal blood flow. *Proc Soc Exp Biol Med* 130:484-486, 1969.
7. Price WE, Rohrer GV, Jacobson ED: Mesenteric vascular diseases. *Gastroenterology* 57:599-604, 1969.
8. Ross G: Cardiovascular effects of secretin. *Am J Physiol* 218:1166-1170, 1970.

9. Vizi SE, Bertaccini G, Impicciatore M, Knoll J: Evidence
    that acetylcholine released by gastrin and related
    polypeptides contributes to their effect on gastro-
    intestinal motility. *Gastroenterology* 64:268-277,
    1973.

RELEASE OF GI HORMONES

GASTRIN TURNOVER IN GASTRINOMA TISSUE: *IN VITRO* INCUBATION, SUBCELLULAR FRACTION AND MONOLAYER CULTURE STUDIES

N.S. Track, C. Creutzfeldt,
U. Junge, W. Creutzfeldt

Division of Gastroenterology and Metabolism,
Department of Medicine, University of Göttingen,
Göttingen, Germany

The classical studies of mammalian protein turnover were performed with pancreatic exocrine cells. The predominance of these cells in the pancreas, the characteristic appearance of their zymogen granules and the availability of routine enzyme determination techniques, made these cells very attractive to work with. From these studies, a comprehensive scheme of protein (enzyme) turnover in the pancreatic exocrine cells was proposed.[6,7] Whether this scheme is applicable to other enzyme and hormone-producing cells remains to be established.

Study of gastrointestinal and pancreatic polypeptide hormone turnover has been hindered by the sparse distribution of hormone-producing cells in their tissue sources. Hormone-producing cells stained with specific antibodies stand as small islands in the sea of other cells. The development of techniques to isolate the conveniently clustered pancreatic B-cells in the islets of Langerhans[8,9] made it possible to study their proinsulin/insulin turnover.

The ability to measure minute hormone quantities by radioimmunoassay provided the opportunity to assess the effects of certain conditions upon tissue hormone contents. This laboratory has been involved in extensive biochemical and morphologic studies of proinsulin/insulin turnover in insulin-producing cells (normal rat pancreatic islets, tolbutamide degranulated islets and human insulinoma tissue).[3,12] The results

403

of these studies were the basis of a proposal that
human insulinomas have a more rapid turnover of proinsulin and insulin than normal pancreatic islet
tissue, apparently as a consequence of defective insulin storage and release mechanisms. The question
arises if all polypeptide hormone-producing cells in
the gut have the same turnover characteristics as
the insulin-producing cells. The limited information
about gastrin turnover in antral and duodenal G-cells
and gastrinoma tissue prompted the initiation of
these present studies. Concurrent studies in our
laboratory[4] have shown that gastrin synthesis starts
immediately with stimulation of the G-cells, which
leads to an increase of the antral gastrin concentration during the release phase. This suggests that
the gastrin-producing G-cell has a much faster hormone turnover than the insulin-producing B-cell.

   This report describes results from incubations of
gastrinoma tissue *in vitro* and from gastrinoma cells
maintained in monolayer cultures. Tissue was incubated in pulse/chase experiments in an attempt to
incorporate ^{3}H-glutamic acid into gastrin components,
follow its turnover, and measure the endogenous
gastrin release.

   Cultured gastrinoma cells were used to study the
effect of the incubation time and the addition of
amino acids and secretin upon gastrin release.

MATERIALS AND METHODS

   L- [3-^{3}H] -glutamic acid (27 ci/mM) was obtained
from New England Nuclear, Boston, Mass.; human serum
albumin from Behringwerke AG, Marburg/Lahn; trypsin
from Serva Feinbiochemica, Heidelberg; collagenase
(150 U/mg) from Worthington, Free Hall, NJ; minimal
essential medium (Eagle) (MEM), Leibovitz (L15) and
fetal calf serum from Flow Laboratory, Bonn; Instagel
liquid scintillator from Packard Instruments Co., Inc.,
Downers Grove, Ill.; sucrose and all other reagents
from E. Merck, Darmstadt. Natural human big gastrin
(G-34) and little gastrin (G-17) were gifts from
Professor R.A. Gregory, Liverpool. Synthetic secretin was a gift from Dr. R. Rapun, Schwarz/Mann,
Orangeburg, NY.

   Gastrinoma tissue was excised from three patients
during operations in the Department of Surgery,

University of Göttingen. The tissue was placed in Krebs-Ringer bicarbonate buffer (pH 7.4) and transferred to the laboratory where it was cut into 5 - 10 mg pieces. Human antral tissue was obtained from two patients with carcinoma of the gastric corpus.

Pieces of gastrinoma tissue were incubated in pulse/chase experiments as outlined in detail for insulinoma tissue[3] with the following modifications: During the 15-minute pulse periods ^{3}H-glutamic acid (100 μci/ml) replaced the ^{3}H-leucine. Human serum albumin was used instead of bovine serum albumin, and L-leucine (20 μg/ml) was added to all incubation media. Tissue pieces from all three tumors were incubated also for a 60-minute pulse period with ^{3}H-glutamic acid.

Homogenates of tumor tissue and human antral tissue were separated into subcellular fractions by differential centrifugation as described previously.[3]

Cell debris, mitochondrial, secretory granule, and microsomal pellets were resuspended in 0.3 M sucrose and then together with the 100,000 G supernatant (S-100) placed in a water bath at 100C for 10 minutes. These boiled extracts of all subcellular fractions and the media samples were assayed for total IRG content by radioimmunoassay[11] with synthetic human gastrin I used as reference standard.

The total IRG content for each fraction was divided by the total content of the five fractions from one homogenate to determine the percentage distribution for each individual fraction.

All samples were chromatographed upon Sephadex G10 (2.5x20.0 cm) in 0.05 M NH$_4$HCO$_3$ to remove any free ^{3}H-glutamic acid that might be present in the extract. The lyophilized G10 void volume fractions were chromatographed upon Sephadex G50 (1x200 cm) in 100 mM phosphate buffer (pH 7.4). IRG and radioactivity were determined in successive 1.0-ml fractions from the beginning of the void volume (fraction 53) to the excluded volume (fraction 170). The column was calibrated with natural human big gastrin (G-34) and little gastrin (G-17). Their elution positions are marked above the G50 patterns.

The void volume of the 15-minute pulse medium sample from Case 2 contained a peak of both IRG and radioactivity. These fractions were pooled, lyophilized and reconstituted in M acetic acid. A portion of the sample was chromatographed upon Sephadex G50 (1x100 cm) in M acetic acid, and another portion upon Sephadex G100 (1x100 cm) in M acetic acid.

Tumor tissue, subcellular fractions, and cultured cells were fixed and processed for ultrastructural studies as described in detail elsewhere.[3]

A 5x5 mm piece of each tumor was washed twice in cold Hank's solution, finely minced, and washed three more times with ice-cold Hepes buffer.[5] To this mince 10 ml of a trypsin/collagenase buffer (trypsin 0.5%, collagenase 0.2%, glucose 0.05%) in 0.1 M phosphate buffered saline (pH 7.4) were added, and the material was stirred for 20 minutes at 37C. The supernatant was decanted onto 10-ml ice-cold L15 plus 20% FCS. This procedure was repeated twice. The cells were then centrifuged for five minutes at 150 G and the pellet was washed four times in L15. Seventy-one percent of the cells were viable after this isolation procedure when tested by trypan blue staining.

Cells were cultured in petri dishes (diameter 60 mm) at a cell concentration of $7x10^5$ cells/ml in a 95% air/5% CO_2 atmosphere at 35C. Both of the culture media employed (MEM, L15) were supplemented with glutamine 2 mM, Gentamycin 50 µg/ml and Amphotericin-B 5 µg/ml. The media were changed after 24 hours, after five days, and at the time of the experiments.

RESULTS

Immunoreactive (IRG) release and gastrinoma tissue contents are outlined for the three tumors in Tables 1 and 2. Two tumors had initially high IRG contents (Cases 1 and 2, Table 1), whereas the third (Case 3)

Table 1. IRG release and net synthesis during 60-minute incubations of gastrinoma tissue *in vitro*

Case	Tissue IRG Content		IRG Released into 60-min medium (ng/mg)	IRG Net (ng/mg)	Synthesis (% of initial content)
	Initial (ng/mg)	Incubated (ng/mg)			
1. Bau.	108.0	102.0	173.5	167.5	155
2. Braun.	75.2	58.6	70.8	54.2	72
3. Schd.	2.05	1.96	1.02	0.93	45

was low. An extremely high IRG release from all three
tumors was detected in the 60-minute incubation media.
These values together with those of the incubated
tissue content, revealed that in all three tumors a
net synthesis of IRG had occurred. In the pulse/
chase experiments, a remarkable net synthesis was
found during the 15-minute pulse period amounting to
50% and 32% of the initial tissue content (Table 2).
During the subsequent chase period (80 minutes) lower
values were found.

The subcellular IRG distribution for the incubated
gastrinoma tissue samples were compared with those
found for two normal nonincubated human antral
samples (Table 3). In cases 1 and 3, the secretory
granules contained the highest percentages of IRG.
The three gastrointestinal S-100 fractions contained
a higher percentage of the total IRG than the two
human antral ones. Ultrastructural examination of
the secretory granule fraction from Case 2 revealed
that it contained granules of different electron
densities and intact membranous sacs (Fig. 1). This
granule population was comparable to that found in
the intact gastrinoma cells (Fig. 2). This ultrastructural similarity of granules was found also in
Case 1 (secretory granule fraction, Fig. 3; intact
gastrinoma cells, Fig. 4).

Table 2. IRG release and net synthesis during 15-minute and
subsequent 80-minute incubations of gastrinoma
tissue *in vitro*

Case	Incubation time (min)	Tissue IRG Content		IRG Released into Medium (ng/mg)	IRG Net Synthesis	
		Initial (ng/mg)	Incubated (ng/mg)		(ng/mg)	% of initial content
2. Braun.	15 pulse	75.2	44.4	68.6	37.8	50
	+80 chase	44.4	31.8	17.1	4.5	10
3. Schd.	15	2.05	1.39	1.33	0.67	32
	+80	1.39	1.03	0.53	0.17	12

Microsomal, secretory granule, S-100 fractions and media samples from the three tumor incubations were analyzed by Sephadex G50 column chromatography. G50 IRG and radioactivity patterns from Case 2 (15-minute pulse samples) are depicted in Figure 5. G-34 was the prominent component in the microsomal, secretory granule, and S-100 fractions. The microsomes, in addition, contained G-17, a small peak between G-17 and G-34, and one peak larger than G-34. G-17 was detected in the secretory granules. No radioactivity was found in the microsomal, secretory granule or S-100 G50 fractions. Also, none was found in the chase samples. In the 15-minute pulse medium, IRG activity was associated with other areas besides those of G-34 and G-17. Both IRG and radioactivity eluted in the void volume. Radioactivity was detected also in the G-17 peaks. The pooled void volume fractions were chromatographed upon Sephadex G50 and G100 in molar acetic acid. Although some of the IRG and radioactivity still eluted in the void volume of both columns, major G-17 peaks now appeared (Fig. 6). No other peaks of IRG or radioactivity were found.

Table 3. Percentage IRG distribution in gastrinoma and human antral subcellular fractions

Case	Incubation time (min)	Percentage of Total IRG in				
		Cell debris	Mitochondria	Secretory granules	Microsomes	S-100
1. Bau.	60	11.9	28.2	40.4	6.8	12.7
2. Braun.	60	5.4	19.7	23.3	3.7	47.9
	15	9.6	16.9	23.4	4.5	45.6
	+20	10.8	17.3	21.7	3.6	46.6
	+80	8.9	14.8	23.6	5.7	47.0
		8.6	17.2	23.0	4.4	46.8
3. Schd.	60	13.2	19.5	53.3	6.2	7.8
	15	12.3	21.5	51.4	7.2	7.6
	+20	13.2	20.2	53.5	6.1	7.0
	+80	15.2	15.4	52.8	6.9	9.7
		13.4	19.2	52.8	6.6	8.0
Human antrum						
4. Fan.	-	12.5	33.5	50.6	2.4	1.0
5. Hol.	-	15.9	26.4	51.6	4.2	1.7

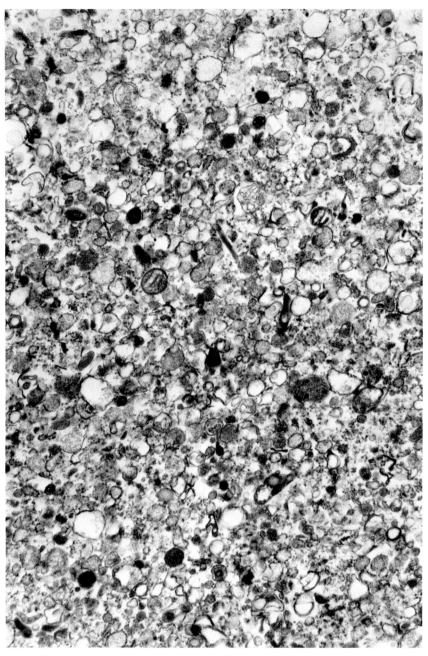

Figure 1. Secretory granule fraction of gastrinoma
tissue showing secretory granules of different electron
density, intact membranous sacs and few mitochondria.
(×20,200) (Case 2, Table 1).

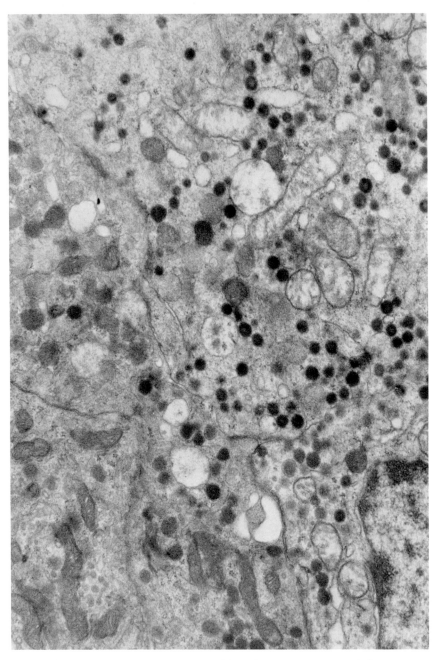

Figure 2. Four adjacent cells of a gastrinoma with different types of secretory granules: small electron dense granules and large membranous sacs containing filamentous material (Type II gastrinoma). (×20,200) (Case 2, Table 1).

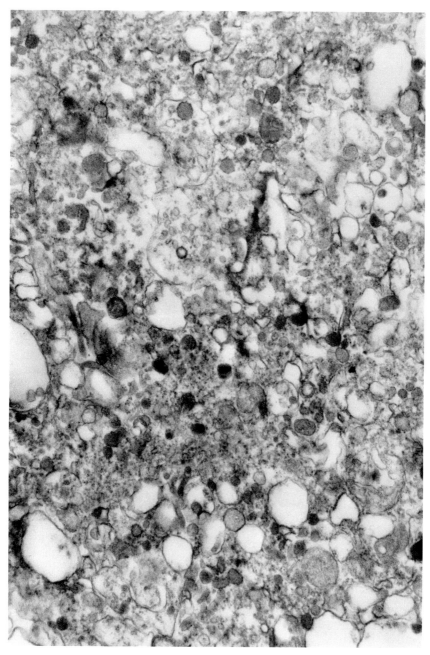

Figure 3. Secretory granule fraction of gastrinoma
tissue showing secretory granules, membranous sacs.
(×20,200) (Case 1, Table 1).

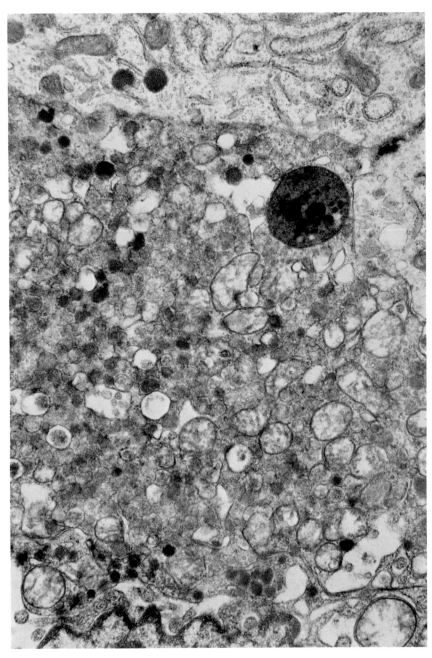

Figure 4. Three adjacent cells of a gastrinoma. The secretory
granules of the cell in the center show the characteristic
granule population of an antral G-cell: few electron dense
granules and membranous sacs filled partially or completely
with gray filamentous material. Since other tumor cells (not
shown) contain only electron-dense granules, this is a Type II
gastrinoma. (×20,200) (Case 1, Table 1).

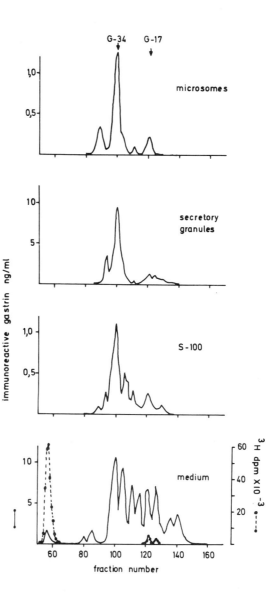

Figure 5. Sephadex G50 IRG (——) and radioactivity (o---o) patterns from 15-minute pulse incubation tissue subcellular fractions and medium (Case 2). All samples were chromatographed first upon Sephadex G10 to remove free ³H-glutamic acid. The G50 column (1x200 cm) was eluted with 100 mM phosphate buffer (pH 7.4). The elution positions of natural human big gastrin (G-34) and little gastrin (G-17) are denoted above the G50 patterns. The void volume of the column commenced at fraction 53.

413

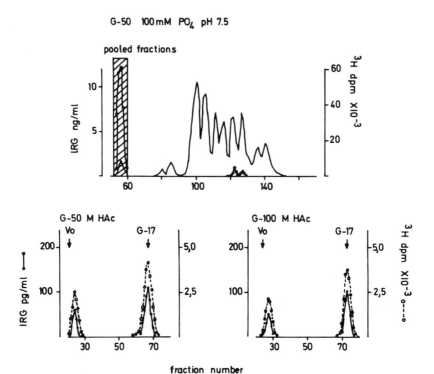

Figure 6. Sephadex G50 and G100 IRG (●——●) and radioactivity (o---o) patterns of the pooled void volume peak from the 15-minute pulse medium of Case 1 (Fig. 5). The G50 void volume fractions (top, hatched column) were pooled, lyophilized and reconstituted in molar acetic acid (HAc). Part of the sample was chromatographed upon G50 (1x100 cm) and eluted with molar acetic acid (bottom, left), whereas another part was chromatographed upon G100 (1x100 cm) eluted with molar HAc (bottom, right). The void volume (Vo) and elution position of natural human little gastrin (G-17) are denoted above the column patterns.

G50 IRG patterns of the subcellular fractions and medium from the 15-minute pulse incubations from Case 1 are shown in Figure 7. The microsomal, secretory granule fractions and medium contained only G-17. The S100 pattern revealed the presence of G-34 and a component between it and the major G-17 peak. No radioactivity was detected in any of the tissue or media samples of this tumor. G50 patterns of sub-cellular fractions and media from the pulse and chase samples of Case 3, revealed the presence of only G-17. No radioactivity was detected in any of the tissue or media samples of this tumor. Monolayer cultures were derived from two tumors (Cases 1 and 2). After three days in culture, the clumped, round, floating cells started to attach to the bottom of the dish and form a monolayer of polygonal, epithelial cells with a rather clear cytoplasm. After five days, the bottom of the dish was covered to 70% with the mono-layer which did not grow further and remained un-changed for 15 days. Ultrastructural analysis of both cultures of gastrinoma cells (Case 1, Fig. 8; Case 2, Fig. 9) demonstrated that they contained granules of varying electron density and intact mem-branous sacs comparable to those seen in the original tumor tissue (Case 1, Fig. 4; Case 2, Fig. 2). No mitoses or other signs of cell multiplication were seen. No fibroblasts or other cells were observed.

The monolayer cultures of the two tumors released large amounts of IRG. Three cultures from the gastrinoma of Case 2 released 220, 260 and 400 ng/ culture in four days. Unfortunately, these cultures were lost because of contamination. The cultures from the other tumor (Case 1) were maintained for 15 days and then fixed for ultrastructural studies. In these cultures, the initial release amounted to 100, 140, 340 and 380 ng/culture in 14 days. Starting on the fifth day of culture, an experiment was begun to evaluate the effect of amino acids upon IRG re-lease during different incubation times, varying from 30 minutes to 24 hours. Cultures 1 and 3 were incubated with MEM, cultures 2 and 4 with L15, an amino-acid-rich medium. Within 30 minutes after the medium was changed, the IRG content reached levels of 44 to 62 ng/culture (Fig. 10). Significant IRG levels were observed when the cells were incubated for longer periods up to 24 hours (Fig. 10); however, these levels were generally lower than those in the

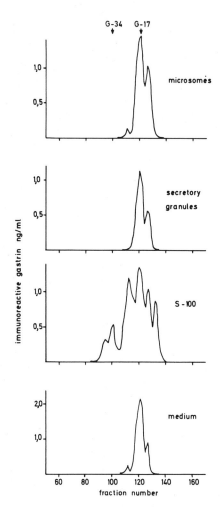

Figure 7. Sephadex G50 IRG
patterns from 15-minute pulse
incubation tissue subcellular
fractions and medium (Case 1).
The G50 column (1x200 cm) was
eluted with 100 mM phosphate
buffer (pH 7.4). The elution
positions of natural human
big gastrin (G-34) and little
gastrin (G-17) are denoted
above the G50 patterns. The
void volume of the column
commenced at fraction 53.

416

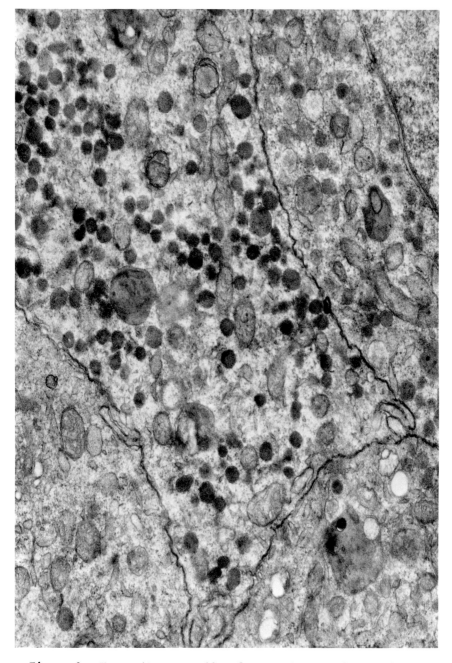

Figure 8. Four adjacent cells of a monolayer culture of a gastrinoma; well-granulated cells, one containing mainly electron dense granules, the other mainly membranous sacs with filamentous material. Monolayer culture, maintained for 15 days, of the same tumor as seen in Fig. 4. (×20,200) (Case 1, Table 1).

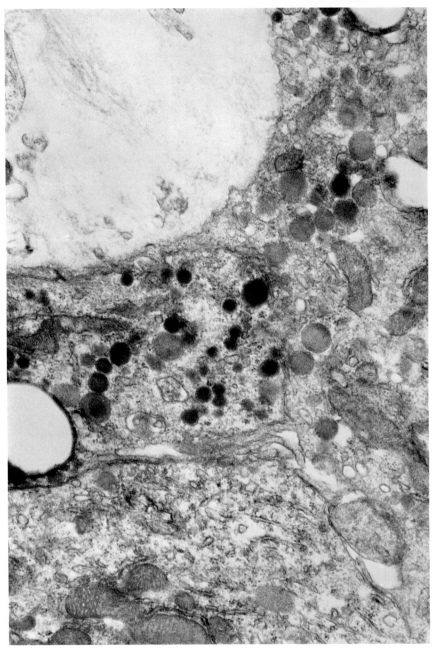

Figure 9. Three adjacent cells of a monolayer culture of a gastrinoma. The two well-granulated cells show different granule populations. The one, electron-dense granule, the other, pale granules and some membranous sacs containing only little filamentous material. Monolayer culture, maintained for four days, of the same tumor as seen in Figure 2. (Case 2, Table 1).

first 30 minutes. Cells cultured in L15 (amino-acid-rich medium) did not release more IRG than cells in MEM. In a separate experiment, the addition of glycine alone (3 mM) was also without any effect. The time-corrected IRG release values (ng IRG/h/culture) showed a decrease with longer incubation periods (Fig. 11).

Sephadex G50 column chromatography of the supernatant from a six-day-old culture after a 24-hour incubation separated the total IRG into big gastrin (G-34) and little gastrin (G-17) (Fig. 12). G-34 represented 85% of the total IRG released.

The effect of secretin upon IRG release in an 11-day-old culture is shown in Figure 13. The addition of secretin (15 ng/ml) caused an increase of 56% and 70% in cultures 3 and 4, respectively, over the previous six-hour IRG release.

DISCUSSION

The term human gastrinoma covers a wide spectrum of tumor tissue.[2] Gastrinomas vary in their ultrastructural appearance, their IRG content, and distribution of tissue IRG components. Because of these differences it is not possible to compare absolute IRG content or release values from one tumor to

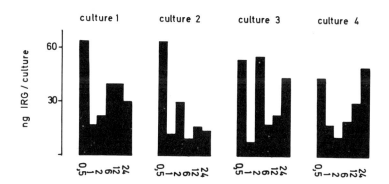

Figure 10. Total IRG release during different incubation periods from gastrinoma cells maintained in monolayer cultures for five days. MEM (+20% FCS) was used in cultures 1 and 3. L15 (+20% FCS) was used in cultures 2 and 4.

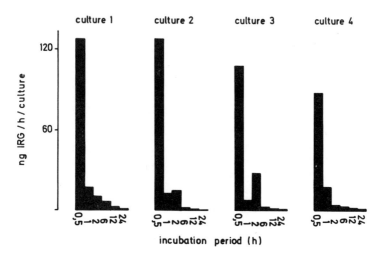

Figure 11. IRG release/hour during different incubation periods from gastrinoma cells maintained in monolayer culture for five days. MEM (+20% FCS) was used in cultures 1 and 3. L15 (+20% FCS) was used in cultures 2 and 4.

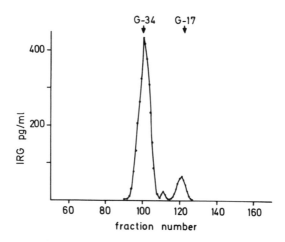

Figure 12. Sephadex G50 gel filtration pattern of IRG released during 24 hours from gastrinoma cells maintained in monolayer culture for six days. The elution positions of natural human big gastrin (G-34) and little gastrin (G-17) are noted above the IRG pattern.

420

another. Therefore, it is only meaningful to consider *relative* changes in one tumor compared to another.

Gastrinoma cells have a very rapid IRG turnover as demonstrated by the net synthesis results (Tables 1 & 2). The speed at which the cells work can be seen by comparing the 15- and 60-minute values. It is clear that a major net synthesis occurs in the first 15 minutes. Following the release for an additional 80 minutes shows that the cells do not maintain this high initial rate. Incubations of human insulinoma tissue never demonstrated a net hormone synthesis.[3]

Subcellular fractionation of gastrinoma tissues reveals that a higher proportion of the total IRG is found in the cytoplasm (S-100) when compared to normal human antrum. The proportion of the total IRG in the secretory granule fractions of two tumors were in the same range as those of the antral tissue; in the third tumor it was lower. In this case, almost half of its total IRG was found in the S-100. Granules resembling those in the original tumor tissue were identified in the secretory granule fractions.

Incorporation results from the pulse/chase experiments were disappointing. Only in the 15-minute pulse medium from one tumor (Case 2) was any radioactivity recovered with IRG components. The presence of both IRG and radioactivity in the G50 elution position of little gastrin (G-17) suggests that this material has been synthesized in the cells and released within 15 minutes. The major peak of radioactivity in the void volume lost a major portion of its IRG and radioactivity when chromatographed in molar acetic acid.

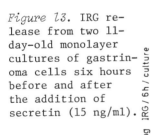

Figure 13. IRG release from two 11-day-old monolayer cultures of gastrinoma cells six hours before and after the addition of secretin (15 ng/ml).

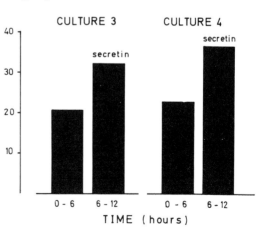

This IRG and radioactivity had the elution position
of G-17, which indicates that in the incubation medium the radioactive G-17 must be bound to a larger
protein, perhaps albumin, which results in its elution in the void volume.

From the considerable net synthesis during the incubations, one would expect that radioactivity should be
recovered in the tissue fractions, at least in the
initial 15-minute pulse period. A possible explanation
for the lack of incorporation may be the metabolism
of L- [3-^{3}H] -glutamic acid in the tumor tissue. First,
only a small proportion of the radioactivity added is
going to diffuse into the cells. Second, these gastrinoma cells have active transaminases which can cause a
rapid detritiation, by hydrogen exchange, leaving nonradioactive glutamic acid. If this nonradioactive glutamic acid is then incorporated into IRG components,
no radioactivity would be measurable! Such a hydrogen
exchange mechanism has been described for alanine[1] and
aspartic acid (Walter, personal communication).

Gastrinoma cells were maintained in monolayer culture over a period of 15 days. The lack of cell multiplication *in vitro* is in contrast to that of other
gastrinoma cultures reported.[10] There is no obvious
explanation why the gastrin release is higher in the
first 30 minutes of incubation than during 24 hours,
and why, accordingly, the time-corrected IRG release
decreases with incubation time. A rapid increase of
IRG release 30 minutes after medium change was found
also in other cultures.[10] Changes in the medium or IRG
degradation with time may be the cause of this effect.

It has been supposed that the immediate increase
in IRG in serum of patients with Zollinger-Ellison
syndrome during a secretin test, is due to direct
effect of secretin upon gastrinoma cells. This has
now been confirmed *in vitro*. Secretin concentrations
comparable to serum levels obtained during a secretin
test cause a pronounced increase of IRG release.
Amino acids or glycine alone have no effect.

Feeding studies in rats indicate that their antral
G-cells have a rapid IRG turnover rate in response
to the stimulation.[4] The biphasic serum response is
comparable to other hormones but the increase in
antral IRG content is unique. These present studies
of three human gastrinomas indicate that these tumor
cells have an *extremely* rapid IRG turnover. This

enhanced turnover may be a characteristic of gastrin-producing cells or may be a common characteristic of all gastrointestinal hormone cells. Further turnover studies with other gastrointestinal hormones are necessary to answer this question.

SUMMARY

Gastrinoma tissue from three tumors was incubated in pulse/chase experiments. A net synthesis of immunoreactive gastrin (IRG) was detected in the 15-minute incubation samples. Only in the 15-minute pulse medium from one tumor was radioactivity found with an IRG component, little gastrin (G-17). Subcellular fractions from one tumor contained mainly big gastrin (G-34) whereas the other two contained mainly G-17.

A higher proportion of the total cellular IRG was detected in the 100,000-G supernatants (S-100) of the gastrinoma tissue, compared to normal human antrum. Ultrastructural control of the secretory granule fractions revealed that their granules resembled those of the intact gastrinoma cells.

Cells of two gastrinomas were maintained in monolayer culture for up to 15 days. The cells did not multiply in the culture and their ultrastructural appearance was similar to the original tumor cells. Large amounts of IRG, mainly big gastrin (G-34), were released into the medium. Gastrin release was stimulated by secretin but remained unchanged after the addition of amino acids or glycine alone.

References

1. Babu UM, Johnston RB: D_2O-alanine exchange reactions catalyzed by alanine racemase and glutamic pyruvic transaminase. *Biochem Biophys Res Commun* 58:460-466, 1974.

2. Creutzfeldt W, Arnold R, Creutzfeldt C, Track NS: Pathomorphological, biochemical and diagnostic aspects of gastrinomas (Zollinger-Ellison syndrome). *Human Pathology*, in press.

3. Creutzfeldt C, Track NS, Creutzfeldt W: In vitro studies of the rate of proinsulin and insulin turnover in seven human insulinomas. *Eur J Clin Invest* 3:371-384, 1973.

4. Creutzfeldt W, Track NS, Creutzfeldt C, Arnold R: The
    secretory cycle of the G-cell: Ultrastructural and
    biochemical investigations of the effect of feeding
    in rats, in Thompson JC (ed), *Gastrointestinal
    Hormones*, Austin: University of Texas Press, 1975,
    pp 197-211.

5. Good NE, Winget GP, Winter W, Connolly TN, Izawa S, Singh
    RM: Hydrogen ion buffers for biological research.
    Biochemistry 5:467-477, 1966.

6. Jamieson JD, Palade GE: Condensing vacuole conversion
    and zymogen granule discharge in pancreatic exocrine
    cells: Metabolic studies. *J Cell Biol* 48:503-522,
    1971.

7. Jamieson JD, Palade GE: Synthesis, intracellular transport,
    and discharge of secretory proteins in stimulated pan-
    creatic exocrine cells. *J Cell Biol* 50:135-158,
    1971.

8. Keen H, Sells RA, Jarrett RJ: A method for the study of
    the metabolism of isolated mammalian islets of
    Langerhans and some preliminary results. *Diabetologia*
    1:28-32, 1965.

9. Lacy PE, Kostianovsky M: Method for the isolation of
    intact islets of Langerhans from the rat pancreas.
    Diabetes 16:35-39, 1967.

10. Lichtenberger LM, Lechago J, Dockray GJ, Passaro E Jr:
    Gastrin release from Zollinger-Ellison tumor cells in
    tissue culture, abstracted. *Gastroenterology* 66:
    851, 1974.

11. Mayer G, Arnold R, Feurle G, Fuchs K, Ketterer H, Track
    NS, Creutzfeldt W: Influence of feeding and sham
    feeding upon serum gastrin and gastric acid secretion
    in control subjects and duodenal ulcer patients.
    Scand J Gastroenterol 9:703-710, 1974.

12. Track NS, Frerichs H, Creutzfeldt W: Release of newly
    synthesised proinsulin and insulin from granulated
    and degranulated isolated rat islet. The effect of
    high glucose concentration. *Horm Metab Res*, in
    press.

MECHANISMS OF RELEASE OF ANTRAL GASTRIN

H.T. Debas, J.H. Walsh,
M.I. Grossman

VA Wadsworth Hospital Center
and UCLA School of Medicine,
Los Angeles, California

Under physiologic conditions, release of gastrin
depends mainly on vagal activity, gastric distension,
and on the action of food on the gastrin cell (G-cell).
The unifying concept that all three of these stimuli
act by a cholinergic mechanism is no longer tenable.
In this review, we will discuss what is known of the
mechanisms by which vagal stimulation, distension of
the stomach and local contact with food, act to
release gastrin.

VAGAL RELEASE OF GASTRIN

The cephalic phase of gastrin release is probably
a purely vagal phenomenon. Thus, vagal denervation
of the antrum abolishes gastrin response to sham
feeding.[14] Hypoglycemic release of gastrin, however,
may involve more than the vagal pathways because it
is not abolished by vagotomy.[2,12] Several studies
implicate an adrenergic mechanism to explain this
persistence of gastrin response after vagotomy in
man. Brandsborg and associates[1] have shown that if
the concentrations of adrenalin in the blood that
occur after insulin-induced hypoglycemia are simu-
lated by infusion of exogenous adrenalin, an amount
of gastrin is released that is comparable to the
amount released after infusion of insulin. Release
of gastrin by catecholamines has been demonstrated
in both dog[11] and man.[13]

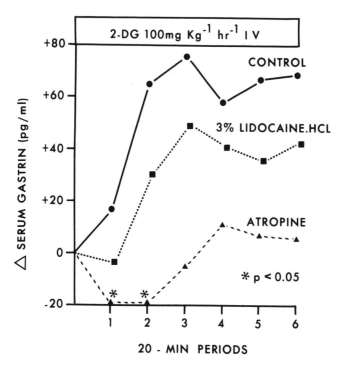

Figure 1. Mean serum gastrin elevation over basal (pg/ml) during intravenous infusion of 2DG alone (control), and following treatment with atropine SO4 (0.2 mg/kg intravenously), or with topical 3% lidocaine HCl in the AP. Each point is the mean of four experiments on four dogs.

We studied release of gastrin in dogs by continuous administration of 2DG (100 mg/kg/hr). Serum gastrin increased within 20 minutes of the start of the infusion (Fig. 1) in dogs with innervated antral pouches (AP), and reached a plateau at 40 minutes. The increase in serum gastrin concentration in these dogs (mean 70 pg/ml) was 30% of their mean response to distension with acetylcholine. Pretreatment with intravenous atropine sulphate (0.02 mg/kg) abolished the gastrin response to 2DG during the first hour. A small gastrin response (11 pg/ml) was seen after the first hour. This small response could represent the noncholinergic response to hypoglycemia, since atropine in this dose has a duration of action of over two hours. We attempted to block the response to 2DG by instillation of 3% solution of lidocaine HCl at pH 7.3 into the AP before and during 2DG

426

infusion. Distension of the AP was prevented by
using a barostat adjusted to 0 pressure position.
Under these circumstances, we were unable to abolish
the gastrin response to 2DG, although some reduction
in response did occur. The results of our experiments can be interpreted as showing either that lumi-
nally applied lidocaine (3% solution) failed to gain
access to the deeply located nerve endings, or that
lidocaine is incapable of blocking release of acetylcholine from these nerve endings.

The amount of gastrin released by any mode of
vagal stimulation is substantially smaller than can
be released by food or topical acetylcholine in the
antrum. This could mean either that vagal stimulation is incapable of maximal release of gastrin, or
that the release we measure is the net result of the
activation of inhibitory and stimulatory mechanisms.
Evidence is rapidly accumulating to suggest that
vagal pathways can inhibit as well as stimulate
release of gastrin. In man, atropine enhances gastrin release that is produced by insulin hypoglycemia.[9] Cairns, Deveney, and Way[3] have recently
shown that they could preferentially block these
inhibitory fibers by cooling the cervical vagi and
thereby augment the increase in gastrin that follows
insulin hypoglycemia.

In summary, vagal release of gastrin appears to be
cholinergic. Hypoglycemic release of gastrin is not
entirely vagal in either man or dogs, and the nonvagal mechanism is probably adrenergic. The amount
of gastrin released by vagal stimulation is substantially lower than the amount released by food. This
may be due in part to activation of inhibitory as
well as secretory fibers during vagal stimulation.

RELEASE BY DISTENSION

Distension of the pyloric gland area of the stomach
initiates both long (vagovagal) and local reflexes.[8,10]
These reflexes have both their effectors and receptors in the pyloric gland area and may be designated
as pyloropyloric reflexes. Evidence for these reflexes is presented in Figure 2 which shows gastrin
response to distension of an AP with 0.1 M NaHCO$_3$
before and after vagal denervation. Vagal denervation of the AP greatly reduces its ability to respond
to distension. There is, however, a small but significant response which persists and which is probably

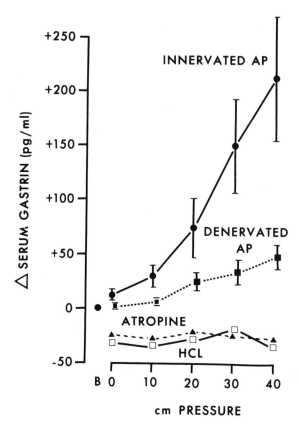

Figure 2. Pyloro-pyloric reflexes. Mean (± SE) rise in serum gastrin over basal in response to antral distension with 0.1 M NaHCO$_3$ before and after vagal denervation of the AP. Each point represents the mean of at least two experiments on each of three dogs.

due to activation of short reflexes. The pyloropyloric reflexes are cholinergic and are completely abolished by systemic atropine. When the AP is distended with 0.1 M HCl instead of 0.1 M NaHCO$_3$, the response to distension is completely abolished. We presume that acid blocks release of gastrin by acting at the efferent side of these reflexes.

We have recently shown[6] that distension of a vagally innervated pouch of the oxyntic gland area releases gastrin from a vagally innervated pouch of the pyloric gland area (Fig. 3). We have called this the oxyntopyloric reflex. Acidification of the AP completely abolishes the gastrin response, and here we are certain that the site of action of acid is on the efferent side of the reflex. In one dog, we have distended the lesser curve Pavlov pouch (PP) with saline which becomes rapidly

428

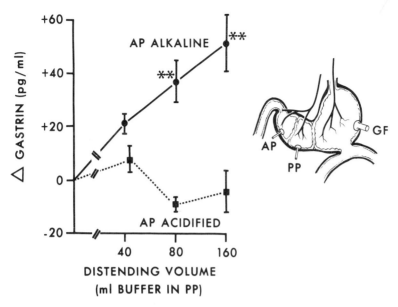

Figure 3. Oxynto-pyloric reflex for gastric release. Mean (± SE) rise in serum gastrin over basal in response to distension of PP with different volumes of tris buffer with the AP either alkalinized or acidified. Each point is the mean of seven experiments on three dogs when the AP is alkaline and three experiments on three dogs when the AP is acid. Asterisks indicate significance of difference between the two curves (two asterisks p <0.01).

acidified by H⁺ secretion from the PP (pH 2.0), and the gastrin response was unaffected (Fig. 4). Acid therefore has no effect on the afferent side of the reflex. Similarly, the afferent side of the pyloro-oxyntic reflex for acid secretion[8] is unaffected by acid, and was in fact demonstrated by distending an AP with acid, thus eliminating the gastrin mechanism.

In summary, gastrin is released not only by distension of the pyloric gland area (pyloropyloric reflexes) but also by distension of the oxyntic gland area (oxyntopyloric reflexes). These reflexes are cholinergic. Acid blocks gastrin response to these reflexes by acting at their efferent and not their afferent side.

RELEASE BY FOOD

Release of gastrin by the presence of food in the
stomach is due to the cooperative effects of distension and the effect of specific chemical components
of the food. Although these chemicals are capable
of releasing gastrin under conditions when no pressure is operating, they require background pressure
for maximal effectiveness.[7] We are reasonably certain that the distension component has a cholinergic
mechanism. We do not know the mechanism involved in
the chemical action of food on the G-cell. Theoretically, these specific chemical substances in food

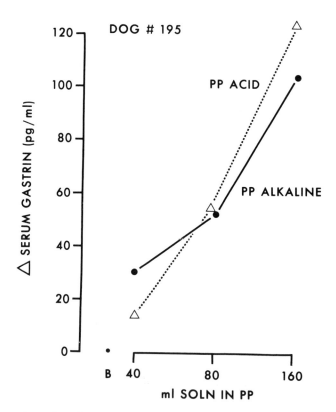

Figure 4. Rise in serum gastrin over basal in response to
distension of PP with different volumes of either alkaline
or acid fluid while the AP is alkaline.

(polypeptides, amino acid, alcohol, etc) can act on
the G-cell either by a direct action on the micro-
villi that project into the lumen, or by activating
chemoreceptors that initiate a local reflex, or by
both of these mechanisms. The local reflex mechanism, if it exists, could have a cholinergic or noncholinergic mediation.

In the intact dog atropine abolishes the acid response to a protein meal but causes only a small decrease in the release of gastrin.[4] In dogs with
isolated AP, we sought to determine whether gastrin
release by chemical stimulation was blocked by atropine. In one study the AP was distended by 0.4 M
glycine at 30-cm distension (Fig. 5). Gastrin response was studied while the animals received either
saline or different doses of atropine sulfate by
intravenous injection every half hour. The gastrin
response to glycine was blocked by even the smallest
dose of atropine used (0.007 mg/kg given intravenously). In a different group of dogs, also with
isolated AP, we irrigated the AP with 6% Bovril meat
extract solution at pH 7.0 (Fig. 6), but avoided
distension by adjusting the fluid level in the barostat to the level of the pouch. Atropine (0.2 mg
kg[-1] given intravenously), completely abolished
gastrin response to Bovril.

The findings of these studies with isolated AP are
clearly different from those in the intact dog where
atropine fails to suppress food-stimulated gastrin
response. There are at least two theoretical possibilities to explain this discrepancy: 1) in the
intact dog intestinal gastrin is released and its
release is not atropine-sensitive; or 2) food causes
release from the intestine of a substance that acts
on the antrum to release gastrin via a noncholinergic
mechanism. The first explanation can be discarded
since no increase in serum gastrin occurs when antrectomized dogs are fed.[5] The second possibility
is under active investigation.

We also found that gastrin response to Bovril could
not be abolished by pretreating the AP with 3% solution of lidocaine and by using a Bovril solution containing 3% lidocaine (Fig. 6). There was, however,
partial inhibition which suggested that some local
neural mechanism might be involved.

The major blow to the concept that all gastrin release is cholinergic came from work on humans by

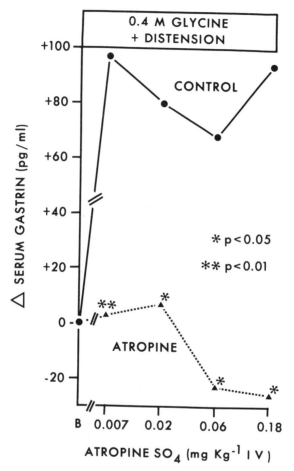

Figure 5. Mean rise in serum gastrin over
basal in response to distension (30 cm) of
the AP with 0.4 M glycine at pH 7.0, while
injections of either saline (control) or
different doses of atropine SO4 were given
intravenously every 30 minutes. Each point
is the mean of two experiments on each of
three dogs. Asterisks indicate statistical
significance of the difference between control and atropine experiments. One asterisk
signifies *p* <0.05; two asterisks *p* <0.01.

Walsh and associates.[15] They showed that in man atropine enhanced rather than inhibited the increase in serum gastrin response to a meal. These findings indicate either that food releases gastrin by a noncholinergic mechanism, or if a cholinergic mechanism is involved, that it is atropine-resistant. Experimental models are needed to test these two hypotheses. The increase in serum gastrin response to food after atropine has been ascribed to a rise in gastric pH. An equally plausible explanation, however, is that atropine is blocking a cholinergic inhibitory mechanism. The enhancement by atropine of gastrin release by insulin hypoglycemia is not due to differences in pH brought about by atropine.[12]

In unpublished studies still in progress, we have shown that vagotomy in the intact dog greatly enhances the release of gastrin by food, and that this enhancement could be blocked by systemic atropine. These findings suggest that a local cholinergic mechanism is involved in the response to food. The clear implication of these findings is that in the nonvagotomized dog, the vagus exerts an inhibitory influence on this local cholinergic mechanism.

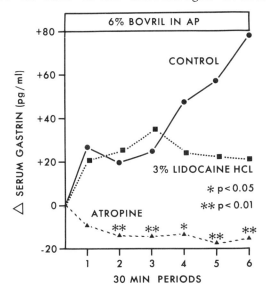

Figure 6. Mean rise in serum gastrin over basal in response to perfusion of AP with 6% Bovril at pH 7.0; and following pretreatment with atropine SO4 (0.2 mg/kg intravenously) and topical anesthesia with 3% lidocaine HCl in the AP. Asterisks have the same significance as in Figure 5.

SUMMARY

   The mechanism of gastrin release by food is, at
least in part, either not cholinergic or is cholinergic but atropine-resistant. Assuming that the
mechanism is noncholinergic, we do not know as yet
whether the chemicals in food act directly on the
G-cell or via short noncholinergic nervous paths
(e.g., purinergic). In dogs with isolated antral
pouches, we were unable to find an atropine-resistant mechanism for gastrin release by glycine or
Bovril meat extract. Since an atropine-resistant
mechanism exists in the intact dog, the possibility
exists that food releases an intestinal stimulant of
antral gastrin whose action is atropine-resistant.

References

1. Brandsborg O, Brandsborg M, Christensen NJ: Plasma adrena-
       line and serum gastrin: Studies in insulin induced
       hypoglycemia and after adrenaline infusions. *Gastroent-
       erology*, in press.
2. Byrnes D, Scratcherd T: Vagotomy and gastrin secretion.
       Gut 13:848, 1972.
3. Cairns D, Deveney CW, Way LW: Mechanism of release of
       gastrin by insulin hypoglycemia. *Surg Forum* 25:325-
       327, 1974.
4. Csendes A, Walsh JH, Grossman MI: Effects of atropine and
       of antral acidification on gastrin release and acid
       secretion in response to insulin and feeding in dogs.
       Gastroenterology 63:257-263, 1972.
5. Debas HT, Slaff GF, Grossman MI: Intestinal phase of gas-
       tric acid secretion: Augmentation of maximal response
       of Heidenhain pouch to gastrin. *Gastroenterology*,
       in press.
6. Debas HT, Walsh JH, Grossman MI: Evidence for an oxynto-
       pyloric reflex for release of gastrin. *Gastroenterology*,
       in press.
7. Debas HT, Csendes A, Walsh JH, Grossman MI: Release of
       antral gastrin, in Chey WY, Brooks FP (eds), *Endocrin-
       ology of the Gut*, Thorofare NJ: Charles B. Slack, Inc.,
       1974, pp 222-232.
8. Debas HT, Konturek SJ, Walsh JH, Grossman MI: Proof of a
       pyloro-oxyntic reflex for stimulation of acid secretion.
       Gastroenterology 66:526-532, 1974.

9. Farooq O, Walsh JH: Atropine enhances gastrin release produced by insulin hypoglycemia in man, abstracted. *Gastroenterology* 66:872, 1974.

10. Grossman MI, Robertson CR, Ivy AC: Proof of a humoral mechanism for gastric secretion: The hormonal transmission of the distension stimulus. *Am J Physiol* 153:1-9, 1948.

11. Hayes JR, Ardill J, Kennedy TL, Shanks RG, Buchanan KD: Stimulation of gastrin release by catecholamines. *Lancet* 1:819-821, 1972.

12. Stadil F: Effect of vagotomy on gastrin release during insulin hypoglycaemia in ulcer patients. *Scand J Gastroenterol* 7:225-231, 1972.

13. Stadil F, Rehfeld JF: Release of gastrin by epinephrine in man. *Gastroenterology* 65:210-215, 1973.

14. Tepperman BL, Walsh JH, Preshaw RM: Effect of antral denervation on gastrin release by sham feeding and insulin hypoglycemia in dogs. *Gastroenterology* 63:973-980, 1972.

15. Walsh JH, Yalow RS, Berson SA: The effect of atropine on plasma gastrin response to feeding. *Gastroenterology* 60:16-21, 1971.

VAGAL CONTROL OF GASTRIN RELEASE

Horst D. Becker, David D. Reeder,
James C. Thompson

Department of Surgery, The University of Texas Medical
Branch, Galveston, Texas and the Kliniken der Universität
Göttingen, Klinik und Poliklinik fur Allgemeinchirurgie,
Göttingen, Germany

A continuous interplay between the vagus nerve and
the antral hormone, gastrin, seems to be essential
for the optimal activation of the parietal cell mass
during the acid secretory response to a meal. It
has been shown previously that the vagus nerve acts
on the release of gastrin and on the parietal cell.
In the following we report studies on the effect of
direct electrical vagal stimulation on gastrin release,
the importance of vagal innervation for the release
of gastrin from the antrum by different stimuli, and
the effect of different forms of vagotomy on the basal
and postprandial levels of serum gastrin.

VAGAL RELEASE OF GASTRIN

In two sets of experiments we studied the characteristics of gastrin release from the gastric antrum by
direct electrical stimulation of the antral branches
of the vagus. Gastrin concentrations were measured
(by radioimmunoassay) directly in the venous outflow
of the antrum as previously described.[4,8]
In five dogs we tested the effect of vagal stimulation and antral acidification on the release of gastrin
(Fig. 1). The mean basal serum gastrin concentration
increased immediately after the electrical stimulation
(5 V, 5 msec, 10 impulses/sec) was begun. Near peak
gastrin levels of 463 ± 178 pg/ml were observed two minutes after the initiation of the vagal stimulation.
Antral acidification caused a stepwise decrease in
gastrin levels.

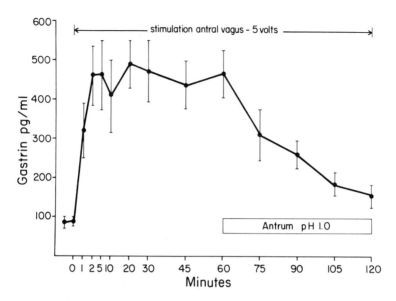

Figure 1. Serum gastrin concentrations in the antral vein during electrical stimulation of the antral vagus (five dogs). (Reproduced, with permission of *Surgery*.[4])

In a second group of six dogs we tested the effect of prior and subsequent antral acidification on the gastrin release from the antrum (Fig. 2). The stimulus was 10 V this time, since stimulation with 5 V caused only a very small increase in gastrin release. Acidification of the antrum did not abolish the gastrin release during electrical stimulation of the vagal branches. Neutralization of the antrum caused a further increase of gastrin concentration in the venous outflow of the antrum.

Our results in dogs show by direct measurement in the venous blood draining the gastric antrum that electrical stimulation of the antral vagus branches results in a gastrin release from the antrum. Acidification of the antrum diminishes but does not totally abolish the vagal release of gastrin.

These studies confirm the results of other groups who found an increase in serum gastrin levels after electrical vagal stimulation.[5] They showed that the magnitude of gastrin release depends on the frequency of the applied stimuli.

Sham feeding, the most physiologic manner of vagal stimulation, has been shown to increase peripheral

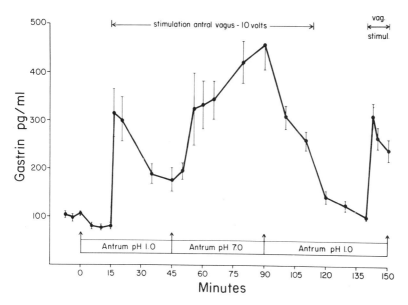

Figure 2. Effect of antral acidification on vagal release of gastrin (six dogs). (Reproduced, with permission of *Surgery.*[4])

serum gastrin levels in dogs[12,15] and in patients with duodenal ulcer disease.[7,9] An increase of serum gastrin concentration could be achieved only if gastric acid were kept away from the antrum by diverting the gastric juice. In normal man, however, an increase of serum gastrin during sham feeding was not observed.[7]

VAGAL INFLUENCE ON LOCAL GASTRIN RELEASE

The local release of gastrin from the mucosa of the antrum by various stimuli is under cholinergic control. It has been shown that denervation of an innervated antral pouch in dogs causes a pronounced diminution of gastrin release from the antrum during stimulation with acetylcholine (Ach) or by distension.[6]

In six dogs with innervated antral pouches (AP) and denervated main stomachs, equipped with a gastric fistula (GF), we tested the effect of atropine on the release of gastrin from the antrum, induced by

439

continuous perfusion of the AP with acetylcholine (Ach)
0.1% pH 7.0.   Basal serum gastrin levels of 67±6 pg/ml
increased during Ach-perfusion to a maximum of 230±51
pg/ml at time 60 minutes (Fig. 3).   Fifteen minutes
after the intravenous injection of 0.05 mg/kg atropine,
gastrin had decreased to 115±24 pg/ml (p <0.01) and
remained decreased during the next 90 minutes.   GF-
acid secretion increased during antral perfusion from
a basal of 0.11 mEq/15 min to 1.69±0.45 mEq/15 min.
The decrease of acid secretion after administration
of atropine was greatly delayed, compared to the decrease in serum gastrin levels.

We next studied the effect of vagal denervation on
the calcium-induced gastric secretion and hypergastrinemia in cats, since we found that hypercalcemia causes
an increase in serum gastrin levels and gastric secretion in cats, as it does in man.   In four cats with
gastric fistula we infused calcium gluconate at a
rate of 10 mg/kg/hr for 180 minutes; after truncal

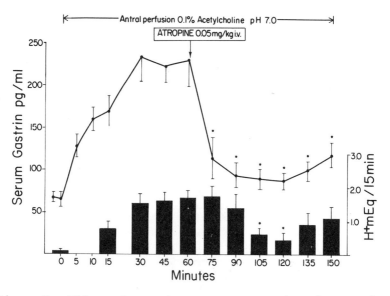

Figure 3.   Effect of atropine on serum gastrin release and
gastric secretion induced by antral perfusion with Ach (six
dogs).

vagotomy we repeated the studies in triplicate
(Fig. 4). Truncal vagotomy caused a small but significant rise in basal serum gastrin levels, whereas
the calcium-induced hypergastrinemia was strongly
inhibited. These results show that vagal innervation plays a permissive role in gastrin release,
even after parenteral administered stimuli.[1]

EFFECT OF DIFFERENT TYPES OF VAGOTOMY ON GASTRIN RELEASE

Previous studies by several groups have shown that
all types of vagotomy result in an increase of basal
serum gastrin levels in man,[3,11,13,14] and dogs.[10,16]
The present studies were undertaken to determine the
effect of selective proximal vagotomy (SPV), selective gastric vagotomy (SGV) and truncal vagotomy (TV)
on the release of serum gastrin and on Heidenhain
pouch (HP) secretion in response to food.

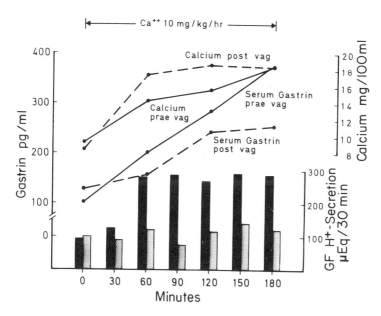

Figure 4. Effect of vagotomy on calcium-induced hypergastrinemia in four cats. Acid secretion from gastric fistulae
shown in bar graphs: solid bars = prevagotomy; stippled
bars = postvagotomy.

Six dogs were prepared with a gastric fistula, HP
and pyloroplasty. After the food studies were done
in duplicate, SPV was performed. After the dogs
recovered from the operation, the food studies were
repeated, followed by SGV. After another set of
food studies intrathoracic truncal vagotomy was
done.

The mean basal serum gastrin concentration increased
after SPV from 98±4 pg/ml to 110±10 pg/ml (Fig. 5).
Dissecting the antral vagus branches resulted in a
further significant increase of basal serum gastrin
concentration, which was not altered by truncal
vagotomy. The serum gastrin response to food was
increased by all three types of vagotomy; the highest
postprandial serum gastrin levels were found after
truncal vagotomy.

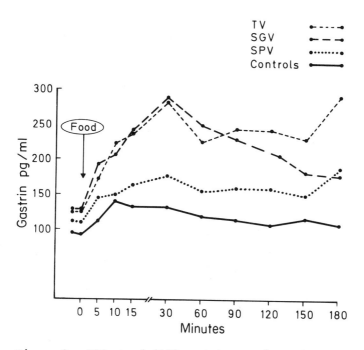

Figure 5. Effect of different types of vagotomy on serum
gastrin concentration in dogs (six Heidenhain pouch dogs).

In order to quantitate the postprandial release of
gastrin, we calculated the integrated serum gastrin
output after a standard meal for the two 90-minute
periods and the total 180-minute period of the studies.
As shown in Figure 6, serum gastrin output after
truncal vagotomy was much higher than after the other
two forms of vagotomy, especially during the second
90-minute period.

In a similar way we calculated the HP-acid output
after food. As shown in Figure 7, the amount of acid
secreted by the HP roughly paralleled the increase in
serum gastrin levels after the first two operations.
However, after dissection of the extragastric fibers
to perform the truncal vagotomy, we found a significant decrease in HP-acid secretion (Fig. 7), whereas
the gastrin output showed a further increase, compared to SGV.

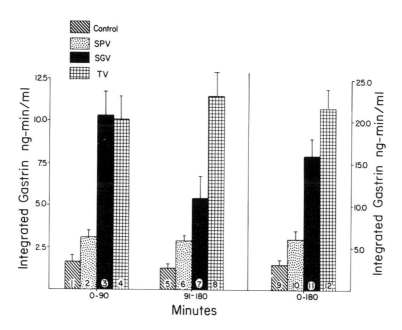

Figure 6. Integrated postprandial serum gastrin output after different types of vagotomy in dogs (six
Heidenhain pouch dogs).

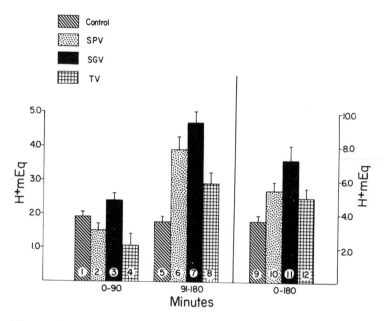

Figure 7. Postprandial HP-acid output after different types of vagotomy in dogs (six Heidenhain pouch dogs).

The conclusion drawn from this series of experiments was that all types of vagotomy cause an increase of basal and postprandial serum gastrin levels, which may be due to a decreased acid inhibition of the antrum, a stasis in the antrum, or an increase in gastrin content in the antral mucosa after vagotomy.[2]

SUMMARY

1) Electrical stimulation of the antral vagal branches causes a strong release of gastrin from the antrum, which is inhibited, but not abolished by antral acidification.
2) Vagotomy decreases gastrin release in cats induced by hypercalcemia.

3) HSV and SGV cause an increase in basal and postprandial serum gastrin values in dogs. Dissection of the extragastric vagal fibers (TV) results in a further increase in post-prandial serum gastrin, but a diminished HP-acid output.

Acknowledgments

This work is supported in part by the Deutsche Forschungs-gemeinschaft, a grant from the National Institutes of Health (AM 15241) and by a grant from the John A. Hartford Foundation, Inc.

References

1. Becker HD, Konturek SJ, Reeder DD, Thompson JC: Effect of calcium and calcitonin on gastrin and gastric secretion in cats. *Am J Physiol* 225:277-280, 1973.
2. Becker HD, Reeder DD, Thompson JC: Effect of vagotomy on gastrin content of gastric fundus and antrum and pancreas in rats. *Surg Forum* 24:359-360, 1973.
3. Becker HD, Reeder DD, Thompson JC: Effect of truncal vagotomy with pyloroplasty or with antrectomy on food stimulated gastrin values in patients with duodenal ulcer. *Surgery* 74:580-586, 1973.
4. Becker HD, Reeder DD, Thompson JC: Direct measurement of vagal release of gastrin. *Surgery* 75:101-106, 1974.
5. Brooks FP, Lanciault G: The role of the vagus nerve in gastrin release, in Chey WY, Brooks FP (eds), *Endocrinology of the Gut,* Thorofare NJ: Charles B. Slack, Inc, 1974, pp 233-240.
6. Debas HT, Csendes A, Walsh JH, Grossman MI: Release of antral gastrin, in Chey WY, Brooks FP (eds), *Endocrinology of the Gut,* Thorofare NJ: Charles B. Slack, Inc., 1974, pp 222-232.
7. Fuchs K, Arnold R, Becker HD, Meier G, Creutzfeldt W: Untersuchungen zur vagalen Gastrinfreisetzung bei Patienten mit Ulcus duodeni und Normalpersonen. *Langenbecks Arch Chir (Suppl Chir Forum)* 91:67, 1974.
8. Jackson BM, Reeder DD, Thompson JC: Dynamic characteristics of gastrin release. *Am J Surg* 123:137-142, 1972.

9. Knutson U, Olbe L, Ganguli PC: Gastric acid and plasma
    gastrin responses to sham feeding in duodenal ulcer
    patients before and after resection of the antrum and
    duodenal bulb. *Scand J Gastroenterol* 9:351-356, 1974.

10. Konturek SJ, Becker HD, Thompson JC: Effect of vagotomy
    on hormones stimulating pancreatic secretion. *Arch
    Surg* 108:704-708, 1974.

11. Korman MG, Hansky J, Coupland GAE, Cumberland NH: Serum
    gastrin response to insulin hypoglycemia: Studies
    after parietal cell vagotomy and after selective
    gastric vagotomy. *Scand J Gastroenterol* 8:235-239,
    1973.

12. Nilsson G, Simon J, Yalow RS, Berson SA: Plasma gastrin
    and gastric acid response to sham feeding and feeding
    in dogs. *Gastroenterology* 63:51, 1972.

13. Stadil F, Rehfeld JF: Gastrin response to insulin after
    selective, highly selective, and truncal vagotomy.
    Gastroenterology 66:7, 1974.

14. Stern DH, Walsh JH: Gastrin release in postoperative ulcer
    patients: Evidence for release of duodenal gastrin.
    Gastroenterology 64:363-369, 1973.

15. Teppermann BL, Walsh JH, Preshaw RM: Effect of antral
    denervation on gastrin release by sham feeding and
    insulin hypoglycemia in dogs. *Gastroenterology* 63:
    973-980, 1972.

16. Walsh JH, Csendes A, Grossman MI: Effect of truncal vagot-
    omy on gastrin release and Heidenhain-pouch acid
    secretion in response to feeding in dogs. *Gastroenter-
    ology* 63:593-600, 1972.

ANTRAL ACIDIFICATION AND GASTRIN RELEASE IN MAN

J.A. Chayvialle, R. Lambert,
C. Touillon, F. Moussa

Unité de Recherches de Physio-Pathologie
Digestive, I.N.S.E.R.M. U. 45, Hôpital
Edouard-Herriot, Pavillon H, Lyon, France

Previous studies of the metabolism of gastrin in man have shown an inverse relationship between the acid secretion rate and the fasting serum gastrin level.[27] The exception is in duodenal ulcer (DU) patients who show unstimulated and stimulated acid secretion rates that are higher than those in normal subjects. The mean fasting serum gastrin concentration is the same, however, and the gastrin responses to insulin and a protein meal are greater than the corresponding values in control groups.[9,13,20,24] Berson and Yalow[3] raised the hypothesis that acidification of the antrum might fail to inhibit the release of gastrin in DU patients as it does in normal subjects.

Inhibition of gastrin release by antral acidification is well documented in animals, mainly in dogs. In early studies, acid secretion collected from an innervated (Pavlov) or denervated (Heidenhain) oxyntic pouch was used to monitor the release of gastrin from an isolated (innervated) antral pouch to various stimuli. Woodward and associates[30] observed in Heidenhain pouch dogs a significant acid response to antral irrigation with pH 6.3 liver homogenate, but no response when the same homogenate was brought to pH 5.0. As reported by Andersson and Elwin,[2] antral irrigation with a pH 7.0 solution of 2% choline in Pavlov pouch dogs, evoked an acid response of about 60% of the maximal response to histamine. The acid response was suppressed, however, when a pH 1.0 solution of choline was infused into the antrum. Most of the results obtained in acid secretion studies were later confirmed

447

Table 1. Stimulants of gastrin release in dogs

	Gastrin Estimation	
	Oxyntic Pouch	Radioimmunoassay
Topical	Ethanol-choline-glycine[2,7] Protein[30]	Acetylcholine[16]
Distension	[12,31]	[6]
Vagal	Insulin[23] Sham feeding[1]	Electrical[19] Insulin[5] Sham feeding[21]

by direct (radioimmunologic) estimation of the serum gastrin concentration. Csendes and associates[5] showed that the significant gastrin response to intravenous injection of 0.5 U/kg insulin in Pavlov and antral pouch dogs (94 to 216 pg/ml) was suppressed when the antral pouch was irrigated with 0.1 N HCl. The same inhibitory effect of antral acidification was demonstrated for most stimulants of gastrin release in dogs, as listed in Table 1.

Whether gastrin release in man is dependent to a similar extent on antral pH has not been thoroughly investigated. The present paper will briefly review the information presently available on this relation in man. In addition, some observations on the feedback between antral pH and gastrin release in normal subjects and duodenal ulcer patients will be discussed.

ANTRAL ACIDIFICATION AND GASTRIN RELEASE IN FASTING MAN

This was initially studied in patients with achlorhydria and hypergastrinemia.[32] Ingestion or intragastric infusion of HCl resulted in a decrease of the fasting serum gastrin concentration, which indicated decreased gastrin release or increased catabolism. There was some evidence, however, that in these patients a significant part of the serum gastrin reactivity was not acid-suppressible. In Yalow and Berson's study,[32] the fasting serum gastrin level in a subject with achlorhydria was about 2 ng/ml two hours after infusion of 300 ml HCl (0.1 N) into the stomach, even though a second 150-ml drink of HCl was administered one hour after the test started.

448

Similar studies were made by Ganguli and Hunter[11] in three healthy subjects. Ingestion of 250 ml of 0.05 M HCl resulted 30 minutes later in a moderate and transient decrease of the fasting serum gastrin concentration. Whether this effect was due to direct influence of the acid solution on antral G-cells or to mechanisms involving other gastrointestinal hormones could not be ascertained. In more recent studies, directed at investigating a possible relationship between gastrin and the lower esophageal sphincter pressure, antral acidification of short duration (20 or 30 minutes) was reported to evoke a slight decrease or no change of the basal gastrin level in healthy subjects.[15,17] It remains possible, however, that antral acidification for longer periods could result in a significant decrease in the serum gastrin immunoreactivity, since the predominant molecular forms of circulating gastrin in fasting subjects, namely big and big-big gastrin,[22,33,34] have longer half-lives than the heptadecapeptide.[26,28]

ANTRAL ACIDIFICATION AND STIMULATED GASTRIN RELEASE

Results from previous studies are presently few and conflicting. The gastrin response to insulin-mediated hypoglycemia is greater with than without antral irrigation with bicarbonate. This difference was possibly due to further distension of the antrum, since the volume of the instillate was 200 ml.[13] In other studies, continuous aspiration of the gastric contents was done in an attempt to prevent antral acidification. Feurle and associates[8] reported that this procedure was necessary to observe a significant gastrin response in normal subjects after insulin stimulation. In a study by Stadil and Rehfeld,[24] however, gastric aspiration did not result in a significant increase of the moderate gastrin response observed after the same stimulus. Moreover, the response to insulin was found to be significant even though the pH of the antral content was lower than 1.5. The authors thus suggested that the feedback between antral pH and gastrin release might be less stringent in man than in other species. The same hypothesis was raised by Fordtran and Walsh,[9] since antral alkalinization of the gastric content two or three hours after a protein meal, the time when the

antral mucosa was bathed by ·the meal-induced acid
secretion, did not result in an increased gastrin
response. Thus, the effects of antral acidification
on the gastrin responses to various physiologic
stimuli in man deserve further investigation.

LOW ANTRAL pH AND GASTRIN RELEASE IN NORMAL SUBJECTS
AND DUODENAL ULCER PATIENTS

The gastrin responses to insulin and to a protein
meal were studied in 14 normal volunteers (mean age:
29.9, range: 24-43 years) and in 15 patients with uncomplicated duodenal ulcer (mean age: 41.9, range:
25-55 years) in whom the gastric contents were kept
at pH 1.5.

After an overnight fast, a 16 Fr Levin gastric tube
was positioned in the antrum under fluoroscopy. The
subjects were then allowed to rest for at least 15
minutes before the test was started. They were sitting
throughout the test, and saliva was continuously aspirated. After a 20-minute basal period (I), 0.032 N HCl
was instilled into the stomach at a rate of 5 ml/min.
for 20 minutes (period II). The stomach was then
emptied, and the subjects were given insulin or the
protein meal.

In the group receiving insulin, eight controls and
seven DU patients were injected intravenously with
0.2 U/kg insulin. Instillation of HCl was then continued at a rate of 1.5 ml/min for the remaining 90
minutes (period III).

Nine controls and nine DU patients composed the
group given an acidified protein meal, prepared by
mincing 100 g boiled beef in 0.1 N HCl. The pH of
the mixture was then adjusted to pH 1.5 with 1.0 N
HCl. The meal (final volume : 200-250 ml) was infused through the gastric tube in less than five
minutes. The tube was then flushed with HCl and
with air. No acid solution was instilled during
period III in this meal group.

The intragastric pH was monitored before every
blood sampling by aspirating and reinjecting about
5 ml of the gastric content three times before a 2-ml
sample was kept for pH reading on a Beckman SS-3
pH-meter. Blood was taken through an indwelling
catheter 30, 20, 10 minutes and immediately before,
and 5, 15, 30, 45, 60 and 90 minutes after stimulation. Sera were kept at -40C.

Gastrin was assayed with the radioimmunoassay of
Ganguli and Hunter,[11] with a rabbit antigastrin serum
used (generously given by Dr. PC Ganguli, Manchester)
and natural porcine gastrin (a gift of Prof. RA Gregory)
used as standard and for iodination. Serum samples
were assayed at two or more dilutions. The sensitivity
of the assay was 15 pg/ml of serum and the precision at
the sensitivity limit was 4.8% (coefficient of variation of eight replicates). The within-assay and be-
tween-assay variations, estimated by assaying 17 samples twice in the same assay or in two different
assays, were 8.2% and 6.9% (C.V.). Insulin did not
interfere with the binding of the iodinated gastrin
by the antiserum. Blood glucose level was measured
10 minutes before, and 30 and 60 minutes after insulin.
Student's "t" test for paired or unpaired values was
used for statistical analysis.

The pH of the gastric content during period I (basal)
ranged from 1.4 to 6.4 (median: 2.4) in the controls
and from 1.3 to 6.6 in the DU patients (median: 1.7).
The median pH in both groups during infusion of
0.032 N HCl (period II) was 1.5 (range: 1.4-1.8).
The mean serum gastrin levels for period I (basal)
and for period II (acidification) were not different
in both the control (59.4±5.7 and 55.6±4.7 pg/ml) and
the DU patients (70.2±4.1 and 67.1±5.0 pg/ml) (Fig. 1).
During these two periods, the mean values in normals
and in DU patients were not significantly different.

The gastric pH during period III in all subjects
ranged from 1.4 to 1.8 (median: 1.5).

Following *insulin*, the mean serum gastrin level
rose from 55.6±4.7 to a peak value of 64.3±8.1 pg/ml
in the controls and from 67.1±5.0 to a peak value of
78.0±5.3 pg/ml in the DU patients (Fig. 2). Both
variations were significant (respectively $p < 0.05$
and < 0.01). The individual gastrin responses varied
widely in both groups (Fig. 3). Calculated according
to Stern and Walsh,[25] the mean integrated gastrin
response for period III was not different from zero
in the controls, and reached 550±290 pg/90 minutes
in the DU patients (Fig. 4, NS). After the *protein
meal*, the mean serum gastrin level rose to a peak
value of 66.8±7.7 pg/ml in the controls and to
106.6±20.1 pg/ml in the DU patients (Fig. 5). Both
variations, observed 30 minutes after the meal, were
significant ($p < 0.01$). The mean serum gastrin level
in DU patients 45 and 60 minutes after the meal, was

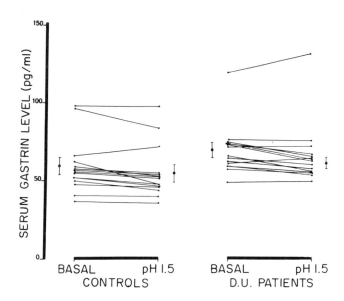

Figure 1. Effect of antral acidification to pH 1.5 on fasting serum gastrin concentration in normal subjects and in duodenal ulcer (DU) patients. ⚕ : mean (± SEM) serum gastrin level for Period I (basal) and Period II (antral instillation of 0.032 N HCl, 5 ml/min for 20 minutes).

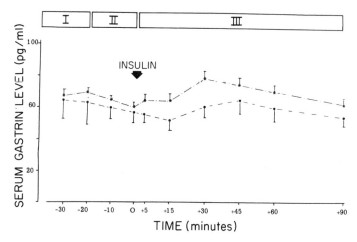

Figure 2. Effect of insulin (0.2 μ/kg) on serum gastrin level in 8 normal subjects (●) and 7 DU patients (*). ⚕ : mean (± SEM). Period I (basal), Period II (instillation of 0.032 N HCl at a rate of 5 ml/min), Period III (instillation of HCl at a rate of 1.5 ml/min).

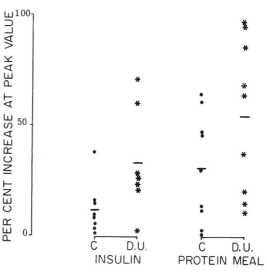

Figure 3. Peak gastrin concentration expressed as percent increase above basal value (mean serum gastrin level for Period II) in normal subjects (•) and DU patients (*) after insulin or a protein meal. Each point represents the value for one subject. The mean variation is given for each group (—). The difference between control and DU patients is significant ($p < 0.05$) after insulin but not after a protein meal.

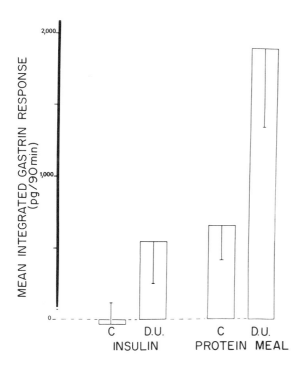

Figure 4. Mean (± SE) integrated gastrin responses to insulin and to a protein meal in controls and DU patients, at a 1.5 pH. Integrated gastrin response calculated according to Stern and Walsh.[25] The difference between duodenal ulcer patient (DU) and control patient (C) observed in the insulin test and in the protein meal test is not significant ($p > 0.05$).

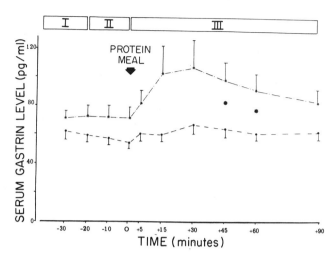

Figure 5. Effect of an acidified protein meal (pH 1.5) on serum gastrin level in 9 normal subjects (•) and 9 DU patients (*). ⟟ : mean (± SEM). Period I (basal), Period II (instillation of 0.032 N HCl at a rate of 5 ml/min), Period III (no intragastric infusion). * = *p* <0.05 for the difference between the values in normals and in DU patients.

significantly higher than the mean value in controls. The individual gastrin responses were again far from uniform in both groups (Fig. 3). The mean integrated gastrin response for period III was 660±240 in the controls and 1910±550 pg/90 min in the DU patients (NS, Fig. 4).

Recently, it was demonstrated that the gastrin response to an amino acid or peptone meal was inhibited in normal subjects and in duodenal ulcer patients when the antral pH was serially lowered from 5.5 to 2.5[29] or 1.0.[18] Since the resting intragastric pH in most DU patients is less than 2.0, the present study was directed to assess whether antral acidification to pH 1.5 would suppress the gastrin responses to insulin and to a protein meal in normals but not in DU patients.

Although insulin-mediated hypoglycemia resulted in a significant rise of the mean serum gastrin concentration in normals, the mean integrated gastrin response to this stimulus was negligible. In contrast, a definite response was observed in the same subjects

when they were given a pH 1.5 protein meal. A similar intragastric pH is likely to occur after a non-
modified meal, since Fordtran and associates[10] observed a mean intragastric pH of about 2.0 in seven DU
patients one hour after a test meal. The present
results, thus, suggest that a significant gastrin
response to protein ingestion may be observed in
normal subjects in spite of antral acidification by
the meal-induced acid secretion.

In agreement with several other studies,[13,20,24]
the gastrin responses to insulin and a protein meal
in the present group of DU patients were higher than
those in normals. Whether this particular reactivity
of DU patients is due to failure of the feedback
between antral pH and gastrin release may be ques-
tioned. Walsh and associates[29] reported that lowering
the pH of an amino-acid meal from 5.5 to 2.5 suppressed
the gastrin response in normal subjects but not in
DU patients. Complete inhibition of the gastrin response to a peptone meal, however, was observed by
Konturek and associates[18] in six DU patients in whom
the antrum was irrigated with the peptone solution
at pH 1.0, which suggests that antral pH did control
the release of gastrin in fed DU patients. In the
present study, the gastrin responses in DU patients
were greater than those in normals, but the patterns
of individual responses in both groups were not essentially different. It thus seems unlikely that specific
alteration of the feedback between antral pH and gastrin release accounts for the exaggerated gastrin
response observed in stimulated DU patients.

LIMITATIONS OF ANTRAL ACIDIFICATION STUDIES IN MAN

In animals, the relationship of antral pH and
gastrin release can be studied quite selectively
allowing for: 1) specific stimulation or acidification of the antral mucosa; 2) evaluation of the
relative importance of combined stimuli, i.e. topical, vagal, distension; 3) absence of interference
from acid secretion or other gastrointestinal hormones on the effects of the gastrin releasing
factors.

In contrast, investigation in intact man meets
several limitations:
1) The specific stimulation of the antrum is
not possible. Significant quantities of gastrin,

mainly big gastrin, can be extracted from the human
duodenal mucosa.[4] The reactivity of these extra-
antral sites has been demonstrated in antrectomized
(Billroth I) patients after ingestion of a protein
meal.[25] In addition, the metabolism and biologic
activity of duodenal gastrin during stimulation or
acidification of the antrum remains to be investigated. To be sure, it is possible that some molecular
forms are less sensitive than the others to intraluminal pH changes.[14]

    2) The existing radioimmunoassays for gastrin
possess immunoreactivity to the various molecular
forms of the hormone. These forms may differ by
their preferential reaction sites, their degradation
rates, and their relative distribution in healthy
and diseased patients.[26,28,34]

    3) The topical stimulation of gastrin release
in man has been performed, with a great variety of
stimuli. Walsh and associates[29] observed no significant gastrin response in nine normal subjects after
ingestion of a pH 2.5 amino acid mixture. In the
present study the mean integrated gastrin response
to a pH 1.5 protein meal was about 660 pg/90 minutes.
Thus, it is likely that a given antral pH may, or
may not, suppress the gastrin response to a given
stimulus, depending on the potency of the stimulus
used.

    4) Since the metabolism of gastrin has been
studied in various clinical groups of patients with
different acid secretory rates, they probably possess
different resting antral pHs. Differing results
suggest the possibility that the rate and degree of
antral acidification from the resting initial pH may
be more important factors influencing gastrin inhibition than the final resulting pH.

Further progress in understanding the physiologic
relation between antral pH and gastrin release in
man will require the following studies: discrimina-
tive analyses of the gastrin producing sites; specific measurement of the molecular forms of gastrin
achieving standardized stimulation of gastrin release;
well controlled manipulation of the antral pH.

SUMMARY

In animals, antral acidification is known to inhibit or suppress the gastrin responses to various stimuli: vagal (electrical, insulin, sham feeding), topical (acetylcholine, proteins), and distension.

In normal human subjects, the fasting serum gastrin level is little or not affected by acidification of the antrum for short periods. The individual gastrin responses to insulin and to a protein meal observed under antral acidification to pH 1.5, are not uniform. Insulin results in a moderate although insignificant response. An acidified protein meal is followed by a definite rise of the serum gastrin level, which suggests that the release of gastrin is only partially inhibited by meal-induced acid secretion in healthy man.

With the intragastric pH kept at 1.5, the gastrin responses to insulin and to a protein meal in duodenal ulcer patients are higher than those in normals. The patterns of individual responses in the two groups are not essentially different, however, which indicates that a specific alteration of the feedback between antral pH and gastrin release is probably not the cause of the exaggerated gastrin responses observed in stimulated duodenal ulcer patients.

References

1. Andersson S, Olbe L: Inhibition of gastric acid response to sham feeding in Pavlov pouch dogs by acidification of antrum. *Acta Physiol Scand* 61:55–64, 1964.
2. Andersson S, Elwin CE: Relationship between antral acidity and gastrin releasing potency of chemical stimulants. *Acta Physiol Scand* 83:437–445, 1971.
3. Berson SA, Yalow RS: Gastrin in duodenal ulcer. *N Engl J Med* 284:445–446, 1971.
4. Berson SA, Yalow RS: Nature of immunoreactive gastrin extracted from tissues of gastrointestinal tract. *Gastroenterology* 60:215–222, 1971.
5. Csendes A, Walsh JH, Grossman MI: Effects of atropine and of antral acidification on gastrin release and acid secretion in response to insulin and feeding in dogs. *Gastroenterology* 63:257–263, 1972.

6. Debas HT, Konturek SJ, Walsh JH, Grossman MI: Proof of a
   pyloro-oxyntic reflex for stimulation of acid secretion.
   Gastroenterology 66:526–532, 1974.
7. Elwin CE, Uvnäs B: Distribution and local release of
   gastrin, in Grossman MI (ed), *Gastrin,* Los Angeles:
   University of California Press, 1966, pp 69–82.
8. Feurle G, Arnold R, Eydt M, Fuchs K, Ketterer H, Creutzfeldt
   W: Unterschiedlicher Anstieg des Serum-Gastrins während
   Insulinhypoglykämie mit und ohne gleichzeitige Aspiration
   des Magensaftes. *Dtsch Med Wochenschr* 98:1879–1880,
   1973.
9. Fordtran JS, Walsh JH: Gastric acid secretion rate and
   buffer content of the stomach after eating. Results
   in normal subjects and in patients with duodenal ulcer.
   J Clin Invest 52:645–657, 1973.
10. Fordtran JS, Morawski SG, Richardson CT: In vivo and in
    vitro evaluation of liquid antacids. *N Engl J Med*
    288:923–928, 1973.
11. Ganguli PC, Hunter WM: Radio-immunoassay of gastrin in
    human plasma. *J Physiol* 220:499–510, 1972.
12. Gregory RA, Tracy HJ: Secretory responses of denervated
    gastric pouches. *Am J Dig Dis* 5:308–323, 1960.
13. Hansky J, Korman MG, Cowley DJ, Baron JH: Serum gastrin
    in duodenal ulcer: II. Effect of insulin hypoglycaemia.
    Gut 12:959–962, 1971.
14. Hansky J, Soveny C, Korman MG: Studies with two gastrin
    antisera of different specificity for gastrins I and
    II. *Digestion* 10:97–107, 1974.
15. Higgs RH, Smyth RD, Castell DO: Lower esophageal sphincter
    response to gastric alkalinization: Does endogenous
    gastrin play a role? abstracted. *Gastroenterology*
    66:710, 1974.
16. Jackson BM, Reeder DD, Thompson JC: Dynamic characteristics
    of gastrin release. *Am J Surg* 123:137–142, 1972.
17. Kline M, Curry N, Sturdevant RAL, McCallum RW: Effect of
    gastric alkalinization on lower esophageal sphincter
    pressure and serum gastrin, abstracted. *Gastroenterology*
    66:724, 1974.
18. Konturek SJ, Biernat J, Olesky J: Serum gastrin and
    gastric acid responses to meals at various pH levels
    in man. *Gut* 15:526–530, 1974.
19. Lanciault G, Bonoma C, Brooks FP: Vagal stimulation,
    gastrin release, and acid secretion in anesthetized
    dogs. *Am J Physiol* 225:546–552, 1973.
20. McGuigan JE, Trudeau WL: Differences in rates of gastrin
    release in normal persons and patients with duodenal
    ulcer disease. *N Engl J Med* 288:64–66, 1973.

21. Nilsson G, Simon J, Yalow RS, Berson SA: Plasma gastrin and gastric acid responses to sham feeding and feeding in dogs. *Gastroenterology* 63:51–59, 1972.

22. Rehfeld JF: Three components of gastrin in human serum: Gel filtration studies on the molecular size of immunoreactive serum gastrin. *Biochim Biophys Acta* 285:364–372, 1972.

23. Shimizu HJ, Morrison RT, Harrison RC: Inhibition of vagally stimulated gastric acid by the pyloric antrum. *Am J Physiol* 194:531–534, 1958.

24. Stadil F, Rehfeld JF: Effect of insulin injection on serum gastrin concentrations in duodenal ulcer patients and normal subjects. *Scand J Gastroenterol* 9:143–147, 1974.

25. Stern DH, Walsh JH: Gastrin release in postoperative ulcer patients: Evidence for release of duodenal gastrin. *Gastroenterology* 64:363–369, 1973.

26. Straus E, Yalow RS: Studies on the distribution and degradation of heptadecapeptide, big, and big big gastrin. *Gastroenterology* 66:936–943, 1974.

27. Trudeau WL, McGuigan JE: Relations between serum gastrin levels and rates of gastric hydrochloric acid secretion. *N Engl J Med* 284:408–412, 1971.

28. Walsh JH, Debas HT, Grossman MI: Pure natural human big gastrin: Biological activity and half life in dog, abstracted. *Gastroenterology* 64:873, 1973.

29. Walsh JH, Richardson CT, Fordtran JS: Diminished inhibition of acid secretion by low pH in duodenal ulcer (DU) patients, abstracted. *Clin Res* 22:371, 1974.

30. Woodward ER, Lyon ES, Landor J, Dragstedt LR: The physiology of the gastric antrum: Experimental studies on isolated antrum pouches in dogs. *Gastroenterology* 27:766–785, 1954.

31. Woodward ER, Robertson C, Fried W, Schapiro H: Further studies on the isolated gastric antrum. *Gastroenterology* 32:868–877, 1957.

32. Yalow RS, Berson SA: Radioimmunoassay of gastrin. *Gastroenterology* 58:1–14, 1970.

33. Yalow RS, Berson SA: Size and charge distinctions between endogenous human plasma gastrin in peripheral blood and heptadecapeptide gastrins. *Gastroenterology* 58:609–615, 1970.

34. Yalow RS, Wu N: Additional studies on the nature of big big gastrin. *Gastroenterology* 65:19–27, 1973.

GASTRIN RELEASE IN MAN AS DETERMINED BY BIOASSAY AND IMMUNOASSAY

Lars Olbe

Surgical Clinic II, Sahlgrenska
Hospital, Göteborg, Sweden

The changes in serum gastrin concentration and the gastric acid responses following *vagal stimulation* have been studied rather extensively both in dogs and in man. Our studies were done to explore the question: in what respect may data obtained from radioimmunoassay of gastrin modify our concepts about gastric acid secretory mechanisms in man?
Studies in dogs during vagal activation by physiologic means (sham feeding) as well as pharmacologic means (insulin hypoglycemia) have shown that:
1) vagal activation by sham feeding or insulin hypoglycemia increases the serum gastrin concentration,
2) the gastrin response is eliminated by denervation of the antrum, antral acidification or atropine treatment,
3) vagally released gastrin has a poor acid secretory effect on denervated fundic mucosa, possibly because of simultaneous vagal release of an inhibitory humoral factor (duodenal?),[10],[15] and
4) gastrin greatly augments the acid response to vagal stimulation in antrum-denervated or antrectomized Pavlov pouch dogs. These results seem to suggest that in dogs, gastrin is released essentially from the antrum via a cholinergic and pH-dependent mechanism, and that the released gastrin facilitates the direct vagal activation of the parietal cell region in producing an acid response.
Similar experiments in man have revealed a more complex picture. Although insulin hypoglycemia produces an increase of serum gastrin concentration

461

in both healthy subjects and ulcer patients, the
increase is significantly higher in the ulcer
patients.[14] The Hansky group[5] has reported that the
insulin-induced gastrin response remained after
proximal gastric vagotomy (gastric vagotomy with
intact antral innervation) but was abolished after
selective gastric vagotomy (vagotomy of the whole
stomach), which is in agreement with the results
obtained in dogs. Stadil and Rehfeld,[13] however,
reported that any type of vagotomy (truncal, selective, or proximal gastric) only moderately interfered
with the insulin-induced gastrin response. They
attributed this nonvagal release of gastrin to an
epinephrine effect. Insulin hypoglycemia liberates
epinephrine that can cause gastrin release in man;
this gastrin release is eliminated by adrenergic
blocking agents. It is unknown whether this nonvagal release of gastrin can produce any acid secretion in the vagotomized patient, but it is interesting that adrenergic blocking agents have been reported
to reduce the gastric acid response to insulin after
vagotomy.[11] Consequently, this mechanism has to be
considered in evaluating "the completeness of vagotomy by the insulin test (cf. data in ref 12).

Stadil and Rehfeld[13] have doubts whether vagal release of gastrin is of any importance for the acid
response to insulin in man since insulin produced
similar increases of serum gastrin concentration
after vagotomy irrespective of antrum innervation.
Such a concept is in agreement with the fact that
antral acidification (acid perfusion of the stomach)
in duodenal ulcer patients did not significantly
reduce (15% reduction) the gastric acid response to
insulin hypoglycemia (Stenquist, Knutson, Olbe, unpublished data). However, antral acidification significantly reduced the gastric acid response to
insulin (by 50%) in healthy subjects. The gastrin
and gastric acid responses to insulin hypoglycemia
in man are not easily interpreted. It seems reasonable to conclude that insulin hypoglycemia produces
both vagal and nonvagal release of gastrin in man
and that the acid response to insulin hypoglycemia
is more dependent on antral gastrin in the healthy
subject than in the duodenal ulcer patient. This
conclusion raises the question whether the small
intestine (duodenum?) of the duodenal ulcer patient
in some way facilitates the release or action of
gastrin: increased or changed intestinal release

of gastrin, reduced or changed metabolism of gastrin, reduced activity of an inhibitory factor with secretin serving as a model.[3]

There are less data available concerning release of gastrin by physiologic vagal activation in man. Sham feeding produced a significant gastrin response in duodenal ulcer patients.[8] After antrectomy, only a statistically insignificant gastrin response remained, which favors the theory that vagal release of gastrin occurs predominantly in the antrum. Sham feeding (by chew and spit technique), however, did not produce any gastrin response in healthy subjects.[2],[9] The vagally released gastrin contributes to the acid sham-feeding response in the duodenal ulcer patient, but only with an additive secretory effect.[6] The facilitating effect of subthreshold - threshold doses of exogenous gastrin on the acid sham-feeding response observed in the antrectomized dog, was not obtained in the antrectomized duodenal ulcer patient. The acid sham-feeding response during optimal conditions for vagal release of gastrin is equivalent to the maximal acid response to pentagastrin in dogs, but in the duodenal ulcer patient the acid sham-feeding response reaches just above half of the maximal acid response to pentagastrin.[7] There is no direct evidence for increased release of intestinal gastrin or reduced metabolism of gastrin in the duodenal ulcer patient compared to the healthy subject. The most conceivable hypothesis covering gastrin and acid secretory data following vagal stimulation in man and dog seems to involve an inhibitory factor (vagally dependent?) blocking both release and action of gastrin and being least effective in the dog, moderately effective in the duodenal ulcer patient, and most effective in healthy man.

It cannot be excluded, however, that vagal activation may change the relative amounts of different gastrins in the serum. Different gastrins (G-13, G-17, and G-34) are reported to have different endogenous potencies.[17] Furthermore, the relative amounts of gastrins in the serum varied with time during continuous stimulation of the canine antrum by acetylcholine. Thus, the total gastrin concentration in serum without specifying relative amounts of different gastrins, does not necessarily reflect the acid secretory effect by the actual serum gastrin population.

Data concerning gastrin release by mechanical and chemical stimulation of the human antrum and intestine are fragmentary. Distension of a neutralized antrum had no acid secretory effect in healthy subjects and a rather poor acid secretory effect in duodenal ulcer patients,[1] with no discernible gastrin response. Similar antrum distension in the dog produced a significant gastrin response and a substantial acid response. A meal results in a pronounced serum gastrin response in man. This gastrin response can be suppressed by secretin, which is similar to results obtained in the dog.[16] The serum gastrin response to a meal in the duodenal ulcer patient is reported higher after truncal vagotomy than after selective vagotomy.[4] These data are still compatible with the hypothetical mechanisms previously discussed in vagal activation of gastric acid secretion.

SUMMARY

The serum gastrin increments and gastric acid responses following vagal activation or antral distension in man and in dogs have been briefly reviewed.

Antral distension has produced increased serum gastrin concentration and acid secretion in dogs, increased acid secretion without changed serum gastrin concentration in duodenal ulcer patients, and no acid response in healthy subjects. Sham feeding has caused a serum gastrin response and a gastric acid response in dogs as well as in duodenal ulcer patients (with gastrin as an augmentative acid secretory factor in the dogs and as an additive acid secretory factor in the duodenal ulcer patients) and a gastric acid response without changed serum gastrin concentration in healthy subjects. Insulin hypoglycemia has produced increased serum gastrin concentration and increased acid secretion in dogs as well as in man, with the finding that the serum gastrin increment is higher and the acid response more resistant to the inhibitory effect of antral acidification in duodenal ulcer patients than in healthy subjects. A conceivable hypothesis covering gastrin and acid secretory data might involve an inhibitory factor (vagally dependent?) that blocks both release and action of gastrin and is least effective in dogs, moderately effective in duodenal ulcer patients, and most effective in healthy man.

References

1. Bergegårdh S, Olbe L: Gastric acid response to antrum distension in man. *Scand J Gastroenterol*, in press.
2. Fuchs K, Arnold R, Becker H, Meier G, Creutzfeldt W: Untersuchungen zur vagalen Gastrinfreisetzung bei Patienten mit Ulcus duodeni and Normalpersonen. *Langenbecks Arch Chir (Suppl Chir Forum)* 91:67-69, 1974.
3. Hansky J, Soveny C, Korman MG: Effect of secretin on serum gastrin as measured by immunoassay. *Gastroenterology* 61:62-68, 1971.
4. Korman MG, Hansky J, Coupland GAE, Cumberland VH: Serum gastrin in duodenal ulcer: IV. Effect of selective gastric vagotomy. *Gut* 13:163-165, 1972.
5. Korman MG, Hansky J, Coupland GAE, Cumberland VH: Serum gastrin response to insulin hypoglycaemia: Studies after parietal cell vagotomy and after selective gastric vagotomy. *Scand J Gastroenterol* 8:235-239, 1973.
6. Knutson U, Olbe L: The effect of exogenous gastrin on the acid sham feeding response in antrum - bulb resected duodenal ulcer patients. *Scand J Gastroenterol* 9:231-238, 1974.
7. Knutson U, Bergegårdh S, Olbe L: The effect of intragastric pH variations on the gastric acid response to sham feeding in duodenal ulcer patients. *Scand J Gastroenterol* 9:357-365, 1974.
8. Knutson U, Olbe L, Ganguli PC: Gastric acid and plasma gastrin responses to sham feeding in duodenal ulcer patients before and after resection of antrum and duodenal bulb. *Scand J Gastroenterol* 9:351-365, 1974.
9. Mignon M, Galmiche JP, Accary JP, Bonfils S: Serum gastrin, gastric acid and pepsin responses to sham feeding in man, abstracted. *Gastroenterology* 66:856, 1974.
10. Preshaw RM: Inhibition of pentagastrin stimulated gastric acid output by sham feeding, abstracted. *Fed Proc* 32:410, 1973.

11. Read RC, Thompson BW, Hall WH: Conversion of Hollander
    tests in man from positive to negative. *Arch Surg*
    104:573-578, 1972.
12. Russell RCG, Faber RG, Bloom SR, Hobsley M: The effect
    of vagotomy on gastrin release in response to insulin
    hypoglycaemia, abstracted. *Br J Surg* 61:328, 1974.
13. Stadil F, Rehfeld JF: Gastrin response to insulin after
    selective, highly selective, and truncal vagotomy.
    Gastroenterology 66:7-15, 1974.
14. Stadil F, Rehfeld JF: Effect of insulin injection on
    serum gastrin concentrations in duodenal ulcer patients
    and normal subjects. *Scand J Gastroenterol* 9:143-
    147, 1974.
15. Stening GF, Grossman MI: Gastric acid response to penta-
    gastrin and histamine after extragastric vagotomy in
    dogs. *Gastroenterology* 59:364-371, 1970.
16. Thompson JC, Reeder DD, Bunchman HH, Becker HD, Brandt
    EN Jr: Effect of secretin on circulating gastrin.
    Ann Surg 176:384-393, 1972.
17. Walsh JH: Biological activity and disappearance rates
    of big, little, and mini-gastrins in dog and man,
    in Thompson JC (ed), *Gastrointestinal Hormones*, Austin:
    University of Texas Press, 1975, pp 75-83.

INHIBITION OF GASTRIN RELEASE AND GASTRIC SECRETION BY GIP AND VIP

Hugo V. Villar, H. Roberts Fender,
Phillip L. Rayford, N. Ian Ramus,
James C. Thompson

Department of Surgery, The University of Texas
Medical Branch, Galveston, Texas

Secretin[10,11] and glucagon[9,14] have been shown to suppress gastric secretion. We have previously shown that infusions of secretin[8,20] and glucagon[1] both act to inhibit the food-stimulated release of gastrin.

Gastric inhibitory polypeptide (GIP)[4-6,15] and vaso-active intestinal polypeptide (VIP)[13,17-19] are members of the secretin-glucagon family of hormones, which resemble the parent hormones both in physiologic actions and amino acid sequences.[11] The purpose of the present study is to determine the effect of GIP and VIP on basal and food-stimulated gastrin levels and to correlate gastrin levels with gastric secretory output.

MATERIALS AND METHODS

Four healthy mongrel dogs weighing between 17 and 25 kg were prepared with standard Heidenhain pouches (HP) and were allowed to recover for three weeks. The dogs were studied in random fashion on three different days of a seven-day period. At random times during the seven-day test period, basal blood specimens for gastrin determinations were drawn and normal saline, GIP (2 µg/kg/hr) or VIP (1 µg/kg/hr) was infused for one hour before each dog was given a standard high-protein high-carbohydrate meal. The infusion was then continued for an additional hour after food. Blood specimens were drawn at regular intervals before

and after feeding for measurement of gastrin. Gastric
secretions from the Heidenhain pouches were collected
at 30-minute intervals for measurement of gastric acid
output.

Gastrin concentrations in serum were measured using
a double-antibody technique which has been described.[12]
The antigastrin-antibody used in the method was developed in white New Zealand rabbits to synthetic human
gastrin I (amino acid residues 2-17) conjugated to
bovine serum albumin. The antibody was used in a
final dilution of 1:80,000 and is immunologically
reactive with all known molecular forms of gastrin
(J Walsh, personal communication). The results of
these measurements are expressed as the concentration
of gastrin (pg/ml) at any given time. Gastric acid
secretions were titrated with 0.1 N NaOH to an end
point of 7.0, with phenol red used as indicator.

Results are expressed as the mean ± one standard
error. Student's "t" test was used to analyze the
data for statistical significance of differences
between means. Differences with a *p* value of less
than 0.05 were considered significant.

RESULTS

The mean basal levels of serum gastrin before infusions of saline, GIP or VIP, were 61±5.4 pg/ml,
54±25 pg/ml and 41±8 pg/ml, respectively. These
levels did not change significantly throughout the
one-hour time interval during the infusion of saline,
GIP, or VIP (Fig. 1).

Mean serum gastrin levels rose to 573±101 pg/ml
15 minutes after feeding in the control group (normal saline infusions) and remained on a plateau
above 500 pg/ml for the next two hours (Fig. 1).
During the GIP infusion, mean serum gastrin levels
also rose immediately after food to values of 484±
179 pg/ml at 15 minutes and declined progressively
for the next two hours, except for a second peak at
90 minutes. Serum gastrin concentration two hours
after feeding was 285±133 pg/ml. This was significantly lower (*p* <0.05) than that of control dogs
that received food and infusion of saline. During
VIP infusion, serum gastrin levels rose to 351±215
pg/ml 30 minutes after feeding and declined rapidly.
Sixty minutes after feeding, mean serum gastrin

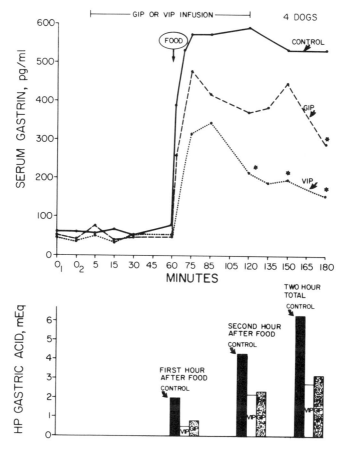

Figure 1. Effect of infusion of GIP (2 μg/kg/hr for 2 hr) and VIP (1 μg/kg/hr for 2 hr) on food-stimulated gastrin response and Heidenhain pouch acid output in four dogs. Asterisks denote points that are significantly different from control values.

levels were 221±113 pg/ml. Two hours after feeding, the serum gastrin level was 154±78 pg/ml. Serum gastrin values during VIP infusion were significantly lower at 60, 90, and 120 minutes after feeding than those dogs in the control group that received food plus saline.

The total HP acid output during the first hour of infusion of saline, GIP and VIP was 2.0, 0.8, and 0.5 mEq, respectively. The total amount of acid during the second hour of infusion was 4.3, 2.3, and 2.2 mEq, respectively. The total two-hour gastric acid output during the infusion of saline, GIP and VIP was 6.3 mEq, 3.1 mEq, and 2.7 mEq, respectively (Table 1).

DISCUSSION

Secretin, glucagon, enteroglucagon, gastric inhibitory polypeptide, and vasoactive intestinal polypeptide are closely related. These hormones have remarkably similar amino acid sequences. Secretin has a molecular weight of 3055 and 27 amino acid residues.[7] Glucagon has a molecular weight of 3485 and 14 of the 29 amino acids are in identical positions with secretin.[3,11] VIP has a molecular weight of 3381 and 28 amino acid residues, nine of which are in positions identical with secretin.[11] GIP is a larger peptide with a molecular weight of 5105 and 43 amino acids of which nine are in common with secretin.[5] Our present studies show that neither GIP nor VIP infusions, at the concentrations used in these experiments, affect basal gastrin levels. When the

Table 1. Food-stimulated Heidenhain pouch acid output (mEq) during control infusion and during test infusions with GIP and VIP

	Saline	GIP	VIP
1st Hour	2.0	0.8	0.5
2nd Hour	4.3	2.3	2.2
Total	6.3	3.1	2.7

dogs were fed and the infusions continued, serum
gastrin concentrations increased rapidly above baseline levels as expected. Within 30 minutes after
food, serum gastrin levels had attained peak values
in each group of dogs (Fig. 1, upper panel). Serum
gastrin concentrations of dogs that received GIP
were significantly lower than that of dogs that received saline at only one time period 120 minutes
after food (one hour after the completion of the
GIP infusion). The serum gastrin response to food
was significantly lower in dogs that received VIP
infusions at 60 (p <0.02), 90 (p <0.02) and 120
(p <0.01) minutes after feeding than the control
group. The difference in gastrin suppression between the VIP and GIP groups was not statistically
significant.

The gastric acid output follows a similar pattern
(Fig. 1, lower panel). Acid output in the control
studies was approximately 50% more than in test
studies in which dogs received either GIP or VIP.
VIP produced a greater suppression of gastric acid
output in response to food than GIP. This suppression, however, was not statistically different.
Pederson and Brown[15] have shown inhibition of hista-
mine- and pentagastrin-induced gastric secretion
with GIP doses ranging from 0.5 to 4 µg/kg/hr,
which are in the same range as the doses used in
this experiment.

VIP has an important vasodilatory activity and a
profound stimulating effect in the small bowel
secretion.[18,19] Increased levels of VIP have been
measured in some patients with watery diarrhea,
hypokalemia and achlorhydria (WDHA syndrome).[2]
GIP is not associated as yet with any disease. GIP
concentrations measured by radioimmunoassay showed
a considerable rise after ordinary meals in man.[5]
Brown and colleagues[5] showed that both glucose and
fat stimulated the release of GIP; they tentatively
identified the GIP-containing cell as the D_1 cell
in the mucosa of the duodenum and jejunum of dog
and man.

The pattern of suppression of food-stimulated
gastric secretion and gastrin release is similar
for all members of the secretin family of hormones
(secretin,[8,20] glucagon,[1] GIP and VIP [this study]).

SUMMARY

GIP and VIP infusions have no effect on basal
levels of gastrin. GIP and VIP suppress food-
stimulated gastrin and gastrin-stimulated acid
secretion. The pattern of suppression of gastric
secretion and gastrin release is similar for all
members of the secretin family of hormones (secretin,
glucagon, GIP, and VIP).

Acknowledgments

This work is supported by a grant from the National
Institutes of Health (AM 15241) and by a grant from the
John A. Hartford Foundation, Inc. N.I. Ramus is the
recipient of a Wellcome Research Travel Grant.

References

1. Becker HD, Reeder DD, Thompson JC: Effect of glucagon
        on circulating gastrin. *Gastroenterology* 65:28-35,
        1973.
2. Bloom SR, Polak JM, Pearse AGE: Vasoactive intestinal
        peptide and watery-diarrhoea syndrome. *Lancet* 2:14-
        16, 1973.
3. Bromer WW, Sinn LG, Behrens OK: The amino acid sequence
        of glucagon: V. Location of amide groups, acid
        degradation studies and summary of sequential evi-
        dence. *J Am Chem Soc* 79:2807-2810, 1957.
4. Brown JC, Dryburgh JR: A gastric inhibitory polypeptide:
        II. The complete amino-acid sequence. *Canad J
        Biochem* 49:867-872, 1971.
5. Brown JC, Dryburgh JR, Pederson RA: Gastric inhibitory
        peptide, in Chey WY, Brooks FP (eds), *Endocrinology
        of the Gut,* Thorofare NJ: Charles B. Slack, Inc., 1974,
        pp 76-82.
6. Brown JC, Pederson RA: A multiparameter study on the
        action of preparations containing cholecystokinin-
        pancreozymin. *Scand J Gastroenterol* 5:537-541,
        1970.
7. Bodansky M, Klausner YS, Said SI: Biological activities of
        synthetic peptides corresponding to fragments of and to
        the entire sequence of the vasoactive intestinal pep-
        tide. *Proc Natl Acad Sci USA* 70:382-384, 1973.

8. Bunchman HH, Reeder DD, Thompson JC: Effect of secretin on the serum gastrin response to a meal in man and in dog. *Surg Forum* 22:303-305, 1971.
9. Dreiling DA, Janowitz HD: The effect of glucagon on gastric secretion in man. *Gastroenterology* 36:580-581, 1959.
10. Greenlee HB, Longhi EH, Guerrero JD, Nelsen TS, El-Bedri AL, Dragstedt LR: Inhibitory effect of pancreatic secretin on gastric secretion. *Am J Physiol* 190:396-402, 1957.
11. Grossman MI: Gastrointestinal hormones: Spectrum of actions and structure-activity relations, in Chey WY, Brooks FP (eds), *Endocrinology of the Gut*, Thorofare NJ: Charles B. Slack, Inc, 1974, pp 65-75.
12. Jackson BM, Reeder DD, Thompson JC: Dynamic characteristics of gastrin release. *Am J Surg* 123:137-142, 1972.
13. Kerins C, Said SI: Hyperglycemic and glycogenolytic effects of vasoactive intestinal polypeptide. *Proc Soc Exp Biol Med* 142:1014-1017, 1973.
14. Melrose AG: Effect of glucagon on gastric secretion in man. *Gut* 1:142-145, 1960.
15. Pederson RA, Brown JC: Inhibition of histamine-, penta-gastrin- and insulin-stimulated canine gastric secretion by pure "gastric inhibitory polypeptide." *Gastroenterology* 62:393-400, 1972.
16. Robinson RM, Harris K, Head CJ, Eiseman B: Effect of glucagon on gastric secretion. *Proc Soc Exp Biol Med* 96:518-520, 1957.
17. Said SI, Makhlouf GM: Vasoactive intestinal polypeptide: Spectrum of biological activity, in Chey WY, Brooks FP (eds), *Endocrinology of the Gut*, Thorofare NJ: Charles B. Slack, Inc., 1974, pp 83-87.
18. Said SI, Mutt V: Potent peripheral and splanchnic vaso-dilator peptide from normal gut. *Nature* 225:863-864, 1970.
19. Said SI, Mutt V: Polypeptide with broad biological activity: Isolation from small intestine. *Science* 169:1217-1218, 1970.
20. Thompson JC, Reeder DD, Bunchman HH, Becker HD, Brandt EN Jr: Effect of secretin on circulating gastrin. *Ann Surg* 176:384-392, 1972.

RELEASE OF SECRETIN AND CHOLECYSTOKININ

J.H. Meyer

Veterans Administration Hospital and
University of California, San Francisco,
California

In the 1960s, it seemed an almost foregone conclusion that bioassayists could ultimately grasp the details of exactly how luminal stimulants release the gut hormones, secretin and cholecystokinin. Seemingly reliable animal models for bioassay had been invented, and relatively pure preparations of secretin and cholecystokinin were available as assay standards. All that had to be done was to find which luminal stimulants mimicked the actions of either hormone. Appropriately, reviews of this subject have become increasingly circumspect in recent years.[18,19] We have since learned that most luminal stimulants produce assay responses characteristic of neither exogenous hormone. We have recognized that the two hormones themselves strongly interact with each other on their target organs and produce mixed responses that are difficult to analyze. We have discovered other gut hormones that could play a role in generating responses to luminal stimuli, and we have not learned how to define precisely the amount of response to a luminal stimulus that is neurally mediated.

Clearly, then, bioassay information cannot tell us with certainty which hormones or how much hormone accounts for an observed response, and independent means are needed to make this assessment. Immuno-assay seems the answer to this problem but still has not been perfected to the level of precision required. And so, bioassay has produced a legacy of descriptive information which still awaits more refined analysis by more precise techniques.

ACID IN THE GUT

When acid is infused into the proximal small bowel, it produces a pancreatic response most similar to that evoked by intravenous exogenous secretin: a copious output of pancreatic bicarbonate is observed with a high ratio of bicarbonate to protein in the juice. The ratio of bicarbonate to protein output is depicted in Figure 1 by plotting pancreatic bicarbonate output against the corresponding pancreatic protein output as the dose of stimulant is increased. Over a range of doses perfused into the gut, acid evokes the secretion of a pancreatic juice with a ratio of bicarbonate to protein output nearer to that of juice stimulated by intravenous secretin than that stimulated by intravenous CCK. However, acid in the gut slightly, but consistently, stimulates more protein secretion relative to bicarbonate output than does intravenous secretin. To explain this observation, many have

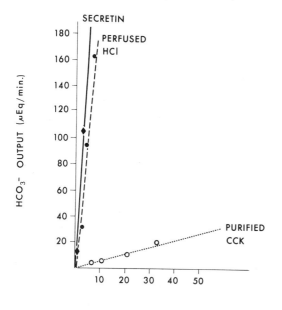

Figure 1. Pancreatic bicarbonate (vertical axis) and protein (horizontal axis) responses to increasing doses of intravenous secretin, of intestinally perfused HCl, or of intravenous purified CCK. Data modified from Debas and Grossman.[9]

postulated that acid releases large amounts of secretin relative to small amounts of CCK. Three lines of evidence support this contention: first, oral ingestion of acid (in man)[4] or perfusion of acid into the proximal bowel (in dog or man)[5-7] produces detectable rises in immunoassayable serum secretin; second, perfusion of acid into the duodenum contracts the canine gallbladder, which indicates that acid also releases CCK[14] and third, the plot of bicarbonate output versus protein output shown in Figure 1 in response to intestinally perfused acid can be almost exactly mimicked by an intravenous mixture of secretin plus CCK with a high constant ratio of secretin to CCK.[2]

Bioassay has yielded much quantitative information about how acid in the gut stimulates pancreatic bicarbonate secretion. Because small increments of intestinally perfused acid produce steep rises in pancreatic bicarbonate outputs, quantitation has been relatively easy, and there is essential agreement among the findings of various investigators.

Whether acid is infused at the pylorus or beyond the ligament of Treitz, pancreatic bicarbonate secretion is strongly stimulated.[16,22,27] This finding indicates that releasable endogenous secretin is rather widely distributed along the proximal gut, a finding which has recently been corroborated by immunoassays for secretin in extracts from segments of small intestine.[3] Secretin is not released at any pH above 4.5.[13,21,25]

When acid is instilled at a pH below 4.5, bicarbonate output from the pancreas varies up to a maximum response with the load (mM/minute) of acid infused. This relationship holds whether weak or strong acid is infused, if the acid is measured as acid titratable to pH 4.5 (Fig. 2).

The dose-response relationship between rate of acid instillation and rate of pancreatic bicarbonate output (Fig. 3) appears to depend on how much acid infused at the pylorus can escape neutralization by the gut mucosa and acidify longer and longer lengths of bowel. Thus bigger loads acidify longer lengths of gut and release more secretin. The bicarbonate response to infused acid in Figure 3 has been translated to doses of intravenous exogenous secretin that give the same rate of bicarbonate secretion. When high, but not lower, doses of acid were diverted from the gut 45 cm beyond the pylorus, pancreatic bicarbonate response was truncated as compared to responses obtained when acid was not diverted. This finding indicates that responses to high loads of undiverted acid are mediated by lengths of gut longer than 45 cm. The findings also indicate that the gut has but a limited capacity to release secretin; as shown, the response generated by acid confined to a proximal 45 cm segment was about equal to 1 U/kg/hr or about 22 mU/kg/hr per cm of gut acidified. Likewise, even when large doses of perfused acid are allowed access to the whole gut, maximum observed or calculated pancreatic bicarbonate responses fall slightly below maximal pancreatic bicarbonate response to exogenous secretin,[9],[16],[22] which indicates that the whole gut, as well, has a limited capacity to release secretin.

Acid normally enters the gut only from the stomach and usually only at appreciable rates as a result of gastric secretion in response to feeding. It is known that during feeding, acid entering the gut from the stomach is brought to pH 4.5 by biliary, pancreatic, and mucosal bicarbonate within 10 cm of the

Figure 2. Pancreatic bicarbonate responses to increasing loads of intestinally perfused HCl or H_3PO_4. Loads were calculated on the basis of titratable acidity (end point pH 4.5) and in each case were varied by infusing acid at a fixed concentration but varying rates of volume flow, or at a fixed rate of volume flow and varying concentration.

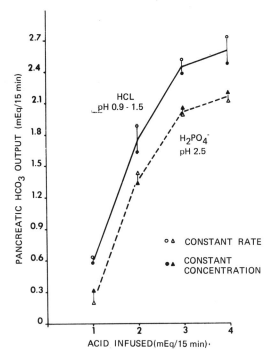

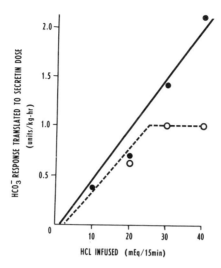

Figure 3. Pancreatic bicarbonate responses
to increasing loads of perfused HCl allowed
access to the entire small gut (solid line)
or diverted from the gut at a point 45 cm
from the pylorus (dotted line). Bicarbonate
response (vertical axis) has been translated
into doses of exogenous secretin that give
the same bicarbonate response in these dogs.

pylorus.[8] Thus, it would be predicted that this 10-
cm length of gut could release no more than 0.3 U/kg/hr
of secretin.[22] Indeed, feeding experiments in dogs
have more directly corroborated the concept that
pancreatic bicarbonate response to feeding is mediated
by 0.4 U/kg/hr of secretin or less.[13]

PRODUCTS OF PROTEIN DIGESTION

Infusion of some individual l-amino acids into the
duodenum stimulates pancreatic enzyme secretion[12] and
gallbladder contraction[17] in man. Similarly in dogs,
individual luminal l-amino acids stimulate a pancreatic
juice low in bicarbonate and volume but rich in protein, a response most characteristic of the actions
of CCK. Since some of the same amino acids most potent in stimulating pancreatic protein secretion in
dogs also contract the canine gallbladder, it is
assumed that amino acids act by releasing CCK.[11]

Quantitation of this pancreatic response to luminal amino acids is difficult because the slope of the dose-response line is shallow and the canine pancreas exhibits spontaneous fluctuations in protein output. Correspondingly, there is some disagreement among investigators as to which amino acids are the most potent stimuli. All agree that phenylalanine and tryptophan are potent. Beyond this there is little agreement except that most investigators have found potency only among the neutral amino acids.[18]

There are many parallels between pancreatic bicarbonate response to intestinally perfused acid, and pancreatic protein response to intestinally perfused amino acids. As with bicarbonate response to acid, protein response to amino acid can be equally well generated when amino acid is instilled at the pylorus or when it is instilled more distally in the jejunum.[10,23] Indeed, immunoassays of gut extracts have confirmed a distribution of CCK along the gut as far caudally as the ileum.[3] As with the bicarbonate response to acid, it appears that the gut has a limited capacity to mediate the protein response to amino acid; even when amino acids are allowed access to the entire gut, the maximum response evoked is less than that which can be stimulated with exogenous CCK.[9,20,23]

As with acid in the gut, the capacity of a finite segment of gut to mediate protein response to amino acid is limited. For example, diverting a high but not a low dose of phenylalanine from the gut diminished the pancreatic protein response (Fig. 4). Phenylalanine was given as a low dose (0.8 mM/15 min) or as a high dose (3.2 mM/15 min) at either a low flow rate and high concentration or a low concentration with a high rate of flow. In either case, the high dose produced more protein output when allowed access to the whole gut than when diverted.

The bulk of protein proteolytic products found in the bowel after a protein meal are not amino acids but peptides.[1]

Peptides in the bowel lumen have long been recognized as pancreatic stimulants,[26] yet little is known about what kind of peptides stimulate. In experiments in which various synthetic oligopeptides were perfused into the gut of dogs receiving an intravenous infusion of secretin, not all peptides stimulated (Fig. 5). Those containing the amino acids phenylalanine or tryptophan, were the most active, whereas those containing only glycine had no apparent effect.

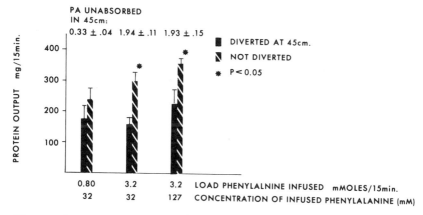

Figure 4. Pancreatic protein output in response to two loads of 1-phenylalanine perfused at the pylorus and allowed access to the whole bowel or diverted from the bowel at a point 45 cm from the pylorus. Dogs in these studies simultaneously received a constant background intravenous infusion of secretin.

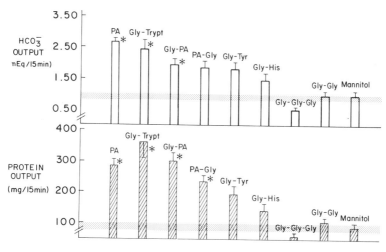

Figure 5. Pancreatic bicarbonate and protein responses to 30 mM perfused 1-peptides in dogs receiving a constant intravenous infusion of exogenous secretin (0.5 U/kg/hr). Perfusion rate was 25 ml/15 minutes. Control perfusions (300 mM mannitol or 30 mM 1-phenylalanine) were randomized with peptide perfusions.

481

Peptic digests of various proteins were prepared
in vitro and perfused at pH 7 into the gut of dogs
with pancreatic fistulas in which all endogenous pancreatic protease was diverted from the gut.   With
the exception of casein, undigested protein did not
stimulate; with the exception of gelatin, peptic digests of these proteins were potent stimuli of pancreatic protein secretion (Fig. 6).   Each digest
stimulated a juice with a ratio of bicarbonate-to-
protein output characteristic of exogenous purified
CCK.   None of the digests contained detectable
amounts of amino acids.

The effects of digests of bovine serum albumin (BSA)
were examined in detail.   Dialysis of peptic digests
of BSA removed about 20% of protein nitrogen, yet
did not alter the potency of the digest (Fig. 7).
Since dialysis removes oligopeptides, the dialyzed
BSA digests consisted of polypeptides which stimulated
pancreatic protein secretion.

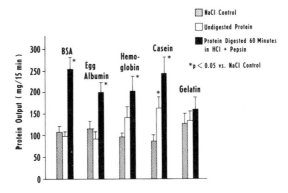

Figure 6.   Pancreatic protein outputs in
response to intestinally perfused proteins
or peptic digests of proteins.   Control
perfusions were 0.15 M NaCl instilled at
the same volume rate of flow as the protein
solutions.   In these experiments, endogenous
pancreatic protease was excluded from the
gut which was washed free of residual luminal protease before the experiments.[23]

   Peptic digests of BSA stimulated as much pancreatic
protein output as a mixture of all of the amino acids
in the BSA mixed in proportions that were the same as
in the protein (Fig. 8).

   It is clear from all these observations that many
types of protein hydrolytic products in the gut can
stimulate pancreatic protein secretion. These stimulants include some, but not all, 1-amino acids; some,
but not all, oligopeptides; and apparently some, but
not all, polypeptides, as peptic digests of gelatin
were without demonstrable effect.

   Although all of these various types of stimulants.
produce a CCK-like pancreatic response, it is not
known whether they act by independent receptor system
or ultimately through some common receptor pathway.
It is noteworthy that those peptic digests which were
effective stimulants contained N-terminal phenylalanine and leucine residues which were not found in the

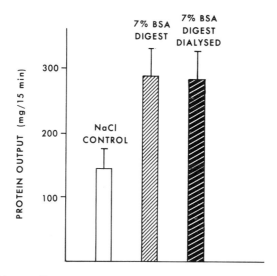

Figure 7. Pancreatic protein outputs in response to 0.15 M NaCl (control), peptic digests
of BSA dialyzed 48 hr against 0.15 M NaCl,
and the same peptic digests of BSA not dialyzed.[23]

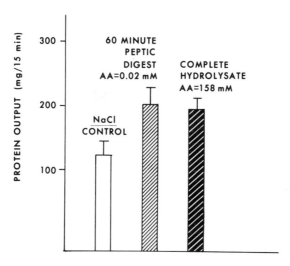

Figure 8.   Pancreatic protein responses to perfused peptic digest of 1.75% BSA and to amino acid mixture with a composition similar to a theoretically complete hydrolysate of the BSA. The peptic digest of BSA contained mostly polypeptides; free amino acids were not detectable in the peptic digest. Each perfusate was adjusted to an osmolarity of 320 mOsm.[23]

gelatin digests that were ineffective. Since the gut mucosa contains an N-terminal peptidase system,[15] it is possible that the activity of all proteolytic products ultimately derives from hydrolytic cleavage of a few potent amino acid residues such as phenylalanine (Table 1).

PRODUCTS OF FAT DIGESTION

When large amounts of triglyceride are instilled into the canine duodenum under conditions which preclude lipolysis, significant pancreatic stimulation is not observed.[20,26] Rather, stimulation of pancreatic secretion by luminal fat seems to depend on the presence of hydrolytic products of fat digestion. Monoglyceride appears to have a CCK-like effect.[20] Another potent stimulus of pancreatic secretion is the presence of fatty acids in the gut lumen.

Not all fatty acids stimulate; fatty acids of longer than eight carbons in chain length are potent stimuli of both pancreatic protein and bicarbonate secretion (Fig. 9). Even among medium and long chain fatty acids, pancreatic response varies. Medium chain fatty acids such as decanoate or dodecanoate stimulate more bicarbonate relative to protein output than long chain fatty acids.[20]

Moreover, even when responses to a single fatty acid such as oleate are examined over a range of concentrations of instilled oleate, bicarbonate output relative to protein output rises as the concentration of oleate is increased,[9,20] as shown in Figure 10, in which bicarbonate outputs are plotted against protein outputs. These responses to oleate are characteristic of neither exogenous secretin nor exogenous CCK. They could be explained by postulating that fatty acids release both hormones in proportions varying with chain length, or as here, with luminal concentrations of the infused fatty acid.[20] That fatty acids release CCK is corroborated by reports that medium or long chain fatty acids in the gut stimulate gallbladder contraction.[24] Whether the additional bicarbonate secretion is generated by the

Table 1. N-terminal amino acid analysis of peptic digests*

Peptic Digest	Pancreatic Stimulation	N-terminal Amino Acids
BSA	++	Phe, Leu, Val, Asp
Dialyzed BSA	++	Phe, Leu, Val, Asp
EGG Albumin	++	Phe, Leu, Val, Asp, Cys
Casein	++	Phe, Leu, Val, Asp, Ser, Thr
Hemoglobin	++	Phe, Leu, Val, Asp, Cys, Ser, Thr, Lys, Glu
Gelatin	0	Val, Asp

* N-terminal amino acids which cannot be identified by this system include Trp, His, Arg, Ile.[23]

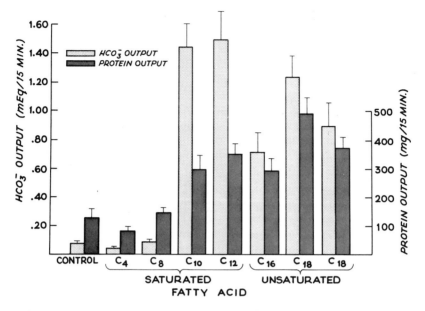

Figure 9. Pancreatic bicarbonate and protein outputs in response to various 80 mM fatty acid soaps (pH 9.2) perfused into the duodenum at 50 ml/15 min. Control = 0.15 M NaCl brought to pH 9.2 with NaOH.[20] (C$_{18}$, left = oleic acid; right = linoleic acid).

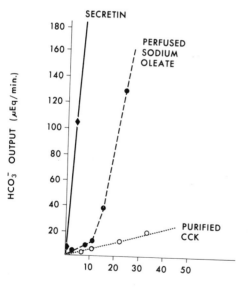

Figure 10. Pancreatic bicarbonate and protein responses to increasing doses of intravenous secretin, of intestinally perfused sodium oleate, or of intravenous purified CCK. Data modified from Debas and Grossman.[9]

release of secretin, remains moot. Because of strong
potentiation of bicarbonate output when secretin and
CCK circulate simultaneously, only small amounts of
endogenous secretin relative to large amounts of CCK
could account for this pattern of response to oleate.
As little as 0.125 U/kg/hr of secretin could produce
the largest bicarbonate response to oleate shown
here.[20] Immunoassays of portal vein blood obtained
during intestinal perfusion with oleate have failed
to demonstrate a rise in portal venous secretin.[6]
But the assay system used was not sensitive enough
to detect the small concentrations of secretin that
would be required to account for the pattern of
bicarbonate secretion shown here.

SUMMARY

In conclusion, several generalizations can be
made:
1)   Although bioassay is a powerful descriptive
tool that allows some characterization of the mode of
action of various luminal stimulants, it is incapable
of precisely defining which endogenous hormones or how
much hormone is released by any luminal stimulant.
2)   Despite the fallabilities of bioassay, it
is apparent that the gut has a limited capacity to
release either secretin or cholecystokinin.
3)   Both of these hormones appear to be distributed along, and releasable from, considerable lengths
of proximal gut, and it is likely that both hormones
are released by stimuli which are modified by diverse
processes along such lengths of gut.
4)   Acid in the gut lumen evokes responses
which can reasonably be explained by the release of
large amounts of secretin relative to small amounts
of CCK.
5)   Amino acids, oligopeptides, and polypeptides
stimulate a pancreatic secretion most like that stimulated by cholecystokinin.
6)   Fatty acids probably release CCK but produce pancreatic responses characteristic of neither
hormone; their actions could be explained by the release of large amounts of CCK relative to small
amounts of secretin.

Acknowledgments

This work was supported by research funds from the Veterans Administration.

References

1. Adibi SA, Mercer DW: Protein digestion in human intestine as reflected in luminal, mucosal, and plasma amino acid concentrations after meals. *J Clin Invest* 52: 1586–1594, 1973.
2. Barbezat GO, Grossman MI: Release of cholecystokinin by acid, submitted for publication.
3. Bloom SR, Bryant MG: Distribution of radioimmunoassayable gastrin, secretin, pancreozymin and enteroglucagon in rat, dog, and baboon gut, abstracted. *J Endocrinol* 59:xliv, 1973.
4. Bloom SR, Ogawa O: Radioimmunoassay of human peripheral plasma secretin, abstracted. *J Endocrinol* 58:24–25, 1973.
5. Bloom SR, Ward AS: Secretin release in man after intra-duodenal acid, abstracted. *Gut* 15:338, 1974.
6. Boden G, Noorjehan E, Owen OE: Effects of intraduodenal fatty acids, amino acids, and sugars on secretin levels, abstracted. *Clin Res* 22:354A, 1974.
7. Boden G, Essa N, Owen OE, Reichle FA: Effect of intra-duodenal administration of HCl and glucose on circulating immunoreactive secretin and insulin concentrations. *J Clin Invest* 53:1185–1193, 1974.
8. Brooks AM, Grossman MI: Postprandial pH and neutralizing capacity of the proximal duodenum in dogs. *Gastroenterology* 59:85–89, 1970.
9. Debas HT, Grossman MI: Pure cholecystokinin: Pancreatic protein and bicarbonate response. *Digestion* 9:469–481, 1973.
10. DiMagno EP, Go VLW, Summerskill WHJ: Location and regulation of pancreozymin secretion and action in man, abstracted. *J Lab Clin Med* 76:870–871, 1970.
11. Fara JW, Rubinstein EH, Sonnenschein RR: Intestinal hormones in mesenteric vasodilation after intraduodenal agents. *Am J Physiol* 223:1058–1067, 1972.
12. Go VLW, Hofmann AF, Summerskill WHJ: Pancreozymin bioassay in man based on pancreatic enzyme secretion: Potency of specific amino acids and other digestive products. *J Clin Invest* 49:1558–1564, 1968.

13. Grossman MI, Konturek SJ: Gastric acid does drive pancreatic bicarbonate secretion. *Scand J Gastroenterol* 9:299–302, 1974.
14. Ivy AC, Oldberg E: A hormone mechanism for gall-bladder contraction and evacuation. *Am J Physiol* 86:599–613, 1928.
15. Kim YS, Kim YW, Sleisenger MH: Studies on properties of peptide hydrolases in the brushborder and soluble fractions of small intestinal mucosa of rat and man. *Biochim Biophys Acta*
16. Konturek SJ, Dubiel J, Gabryś B: Effect of acid infusion into various levels of the intestine on gastric and pancreatic secretion in the cat. *Gut* 10:749–753, 1969.
17. Malagelada JR *et al*: Interactions of bile acid and digestive products on the release of cholecystokinin-pancreozymin in man, in preparation.
18. Meyer JH: Release of secretin and cholecystokinin, in Chey WY, Brooks FP (eds), *Endocrinology of the Gut*, Thorofare NJ: Charles B. Slack, Inc., 1974, pp 241–252.
19. Meyer JH, Grossman MI: Release of secretin and cholecystokinin, in Demling L (ed), *Gastrointestinal Hormones*, Stuttgart: Georg Thieme Verlag, 1972, pp 43–45.
20. Meyer JH, Jones RS: Canine pancreatic responses to intestinally perfused fat and products of fat digestion. *Am J Physiol* 226:1178–1187, 1974.
21. Meyer JH, Way LW, Grossman MI: Pancreatic bicarbonate response to various acids in duodenum of dog. *Am J Physiol* 219:964–970, 1970.
22. Meyer JH, Way LW, Grossman MI: Pancreatic response to acidification of various lengths of proximal intestine in the dog. *Am J Physiol* 219:971–977, 1970.
23. Meyer JH, Kelley GA, Jones RS, Spingola LJ: Effects of intestinally perfused products of protein digestion on canine pancreatic secretion, in preparation.
24. Snape WJ: Studies on the gall-bladder contraction in unanesthetized dogs before and after vagotomy. *Gastroenterology* 10:129–134, 1948.
25. Thomas JE, Crider J: A quantitative study of acid in the intestine as a stimulus for the pancreas. *Am J Physiol* 131:349–356, 1940.
26. Wang CC, Grossman MI: Physiological determination of release of secretin and pancreozymin from intestine of dogs with transplanted pancreas. *Am J Physiol* 164:527–545, 1951.
27. Wormsley KG: Response to duodenal acidification in man: III. Comparison with the effects of secretin and pancreozymin. *Scand J Gastroenterol* 5:353–360, 1970.

RELEASE OF GASTRIN FROM DOG ANTRAL MUCOSA
IN VITRO BY ACETYLCHOLINE

B. Schofield, Eva M. Kende,
B.L. Tepperman, Fern S. Tepperman

Division of Medical Physiology, University of Calgary,
Faculty of Medicine, Calgary, Alberta, Canada

Gastrin is known to be released from granules contained in the gastrin cells (G-cells) of the pyloric
antrum.[5] Currently, there are many gaps in knowledge
of this process. It is known that the release can
be effected by nerves and this aspect is thought to
be cholinergic.[1] Acetylcholine (Ach), applied topi-
cally to the antral mucosa, is the most effective
physiologic agent producing gastrin release, but the
concentrations used are pharmacologic. The mode of
action of physiologic secretagogues, such as polypeptides, is at present obscure since the original
concept that they operate by a local nervous reflex
is now thought doubtful. Most work has been done on
pouch dogs and there would seem to be considerable
value in studies done *in vitro*. The complex interactions of gastrointestinal hormones in the whole
animal are now well-known, and although it is not
reasonable to extrapolate directly from such a preparation to the whole animal, it provides considerable scope for the elucidation of fundamental mechanisms. The need for this is emphasized by the
recent suggestion[3] that releasing factors may exist
for the gastric hormones and that the polypeptide,
bombesin, or a related compound might fulfill this
role.
    When this study was begun, no previous reports of
gastrin release *in vitro* had been found. One study
in which rat tissue had been used, however, had been
submitted for presentation at the American Gastroen-
terological Association general meeting in May 1974.[4]

Our approach in these studies was to use tissue from the animal whose gastrin release mechanism had been most studied, that is, the dog. In view of the thickness of whole antral mucosa from dogs, attempts were made to achieve a thinner preparation. In 1959 Merritt and Kelly[6] described a procedure to obtain denervated antral mucosa for the preparation of grafted antral pouches. They used a dermatome to slice the mucosa superficial to the muscularis mucosae. Baugh (unpublished report) subsequently (in 1961) suggested but did not describe, a dissection procedure for the same purpose. We have developed this latter approach which in our hands has proved more satisfactory than the dermatome method.

METHODS

Mongrel dogs of both sexes and varying weight and age were used. The dogs were fasted for 24 hours before the experiment. They were anesthetized with intravenous thiopentone (15 mg/kg) and the gastric antrum was removed as rapidly as possible. The dog was then killed by intravenous chloroform. The antrum was rinsed with cold normal saline, pinned out on a parafilm-covered cork board, and the whole mucosa removed rapidly by splitting in the plane of submucosal cleavage. The muscularis externa was discarded. Portions of whole antral mucosa (WAM) containing mucosa, lamina propria, muscularis mucosae, and the submucosa were pinned out. The preparation was kept moist at all times with cold Krebs-Henseleit solution (NaCl 115.4 mM, NaHCO$_3$ 22.1 mM, KCl 7.4 mM, MgSO$_4$ 1.08 mM, CaCl$_2$ 2.23 mM and dextrose 8 mM in equilibrium with 95% O$_2$ containing 5% CO$_2$ pH 7.30). The muscularis mucosae and submucosa were dissected off leaving stripped antral mucosa (SAM).

Portions of SAM and WAM (about 0.5-cm square) from corresponding regions were prepared from each antrum. Each portion was cut into four to six small pieces. Pieces of each tissue (that is, SAM and WAM) were placed in 5 ml of Krebs-Henseleit solution previously aerated for one-half hour with 95% O$_2$ and 5% CO$_2$ in 25-ml Erlenmeyer flasks. Controls and flasks containing Ach chloride in the concentration range, 10^{-8} to 10^{-4} M, were prepared for both types of mucosa. The Ach was added immediately before the

tissue was placed in the flask. The incubation
flasks were placed in a Dubnoff metabolic shaker
bath under 95% O_2 at atmospheric pressure, and incubated at 37C for two hours. No change in pH was
produced by these additions and the pH remained unchanged during incubation.

The tissue was then removed by filtration (using
UniChem filter samplers, UniChem Corp., Fairburn,
Georgia) and dried in a 95C oven for dry weight
determination.   The incubation medium was then
assayed for gastrin content by a modification of the
Yalow and Berson[8] method for radioimmunoassay. The
antibody employed was raised in rabbits against
synthetic human gastrin (1-17) and has no cross-
reaction with cholecystokinin (CCK).

Gastrin was determined in duplicate in each of
three dilutions of each sample. In many assays one
of these dilutions did not fall within the limits
of the standard curve. Gastrin concentrations of
the experimental samples were determined by interpolation from the standard curve and the concentrations thus derived were then converted to picograms
of gastrin per milligram, dry weight, of tissue.
Unless otherwise stated, the output is expressed
for the whole two-hour incubation period. Most
previous work on gastrin content of tissue has been
expressed as picograms per wet weight of tissue.
Wet tissue weights are very approximate but a mean
ratio of wet/dry for dog antra in our experiments
is 7.4±0.2 to 1.

The incubation medium was shown in blank determinations not to interfere with the gastrin assay.
All reagents used in the incubation medium were
checked for possible interference with the assay,
and none were found to produce artifacts. High concentrations of tetracaine, however, may result in
precipitation with standard diluent used in the
assay. This precipitate can bind gastrin antibody,
which results in misleading gastrin concentrations.

RESULTS

Structural Features of Stripped and Whole Antral Mucosa

Figure 1A and B shows portions of stripped and
whole antral mucosa for comparison. It indicates
that complete removal of muscularis mucosae and

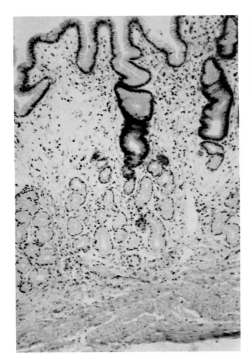 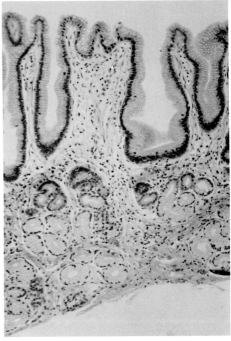

1A. Whole antral mucosa (WAM)   *1B.* Stripped antral mucosa
(×68)   (SAM) (×68)

Figure 1. The structural characteristics of whole and stripped antral mucosa. These figures indicate that complete separation of muscularis mucosae from mucosa is possible.

lamina propria can be obtained. In some specimens, discontinuous fragments of muscularis have remained adherent to the mucosa.

Resting Outputs of Gastrin

The mean resting output of gastrin from antral tissue slices was 1915±443 pg/mg dry weight of tissue/hr for WAM and 4993±885 pg/mg dry weight of tissue/hr for SAM. Considerable variation in resting output has occurred throughout the study so far. The reasons for this are being investigated. In most experiments, however, the above ratio of outputs between WAM and SAM has been maintained.

Ach Dose-Response of Whole Antral Mucosa

No evidence of stimulation of gastrin release by Ach in the concentration range 0 to 1×10^{-4} M was observed with this preparation (Figs. 2-4). In 12 experiments no significant peak was observed at any Ach concentration.

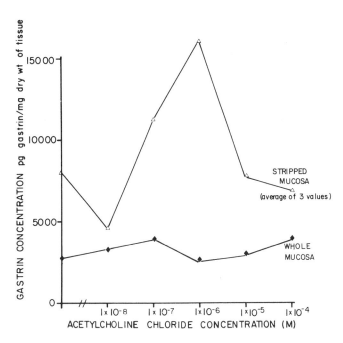

Figure 2. The dose response characteristics of a single experiment. A well-marked peak is evident at 1×10^{-6} M Ach chloride from SAM. No significant response is evident for WAM. In this experiment the SAM response to 1×10^{-7} M Ach is less than the resting output of gastrin. The reason for this is not at the moment apparent.

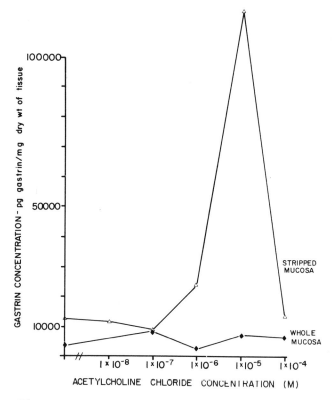

Figure 3. The Ach dose-response relationship in samples taken from a single vagotomized dog. A well-marked peak which is approximately nine times the control or resting level occurs at $1x10^{-6}$ M in SAM tissue. Once more, no response is evident from WAM. This is the greatest peak that has been obtained in any single experiment.

Ach Dose-Response of Stripped Antral Mucosa

Stripped dog antral mucosa incubated with Ach chloride in the concentration range 0 to 1×10^{-4} M produced a clear dose-response relationship with a peak at 1×10^{-5} M or 1×10^{-6} M Ach in most cases (nine out of 14 experiments peaked at 1×10^{-6} M and four peaked at 1×10^{-5} M and one experiment peaked at 1×10^{-4} M). Considerable variation occurred between individual experiments in absolute levels of gastrin released. Two experiments that peaked at 1×10^{-6} M and 1×10^{-5} M, respectively, are displayed with the corresponding gastrin output from WAM (Figs 2 & 3). The mean

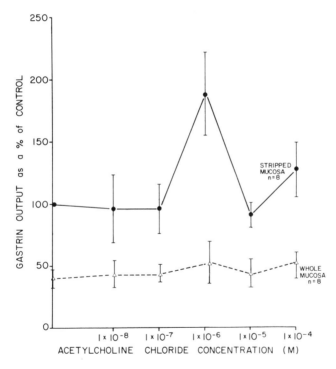

Figure 4. The mean response from eight experiments to doses of Ach chloride from 0 to 1×10^{-4} M. A significant ($p < 0.05$) peak occurs at 1×10^{-6} M Ach in the stripped tissue. No significant response occurs in WAM and all WAM values are significantly less ($p < 0.05$) than corresponding SAM values.

gastrin output expressed as a percent of resting or control levels at 1×10^{-6} M, is shown in Figure 4. All SAM values are significantly greater ($p < 0.05$) than the corresponding WAM response.

The single vagotomized dog displayed a greater capacity for release of gastrin into the bathing solution than did the intact dogs (Fig. 3). The peak increase in output (occurring at 1×10^{-5} M) is approximately nine times that of the control level.

Effect of Atropine

The addition of atropine sulfate (1.2 μg/ml) to the bathing solution, resulted in no significant alteration in the Ach dose response from WAM (Fig. 5). Atropine, however, resulted in a significant reduction ($p < 0.05$) in the gastrin response to 1×10^{-6} M Ach from SAM. The mean percent decrease at this dose of Ach is 73.2 ± 12.2. Atropine results in a slightly lower percent resting output of gastrin from SAM. This is not a significant decrease, however, from the nonatropinized state.

DISCUSSION

Histology and Improvement of Stripping Technique

Examination of histologic sections taken from experiments both before and after stripping of the submucosa and muscularis mucosae indicate that our dissection has not always been such as to ensure total removal of muscularis mucosae, although complete separation is possible (Fig. 1). Remnants of this tissue and portions of lamina propria have been found adhering to some portions from our tissue samples. There appears to be difficulty in some dogs in accurately defining the desired plane of separation during dissection, which has to be rapid. Small, noncontinuous adherent portions of muscularis mucosa and lamina propria seem unlikely to reduce diffusion of nutrients into the tissue very much, but a few ganglia might be capable of sustaining an effect of the whole plexus.

Ach Dose-Response Relationship

Our experiments so far show that gastrin release
from SAM is influenced in an appropriate fashion by
Ach, the most effective physiologic stimulant.   The
presence of a definite peak in the dose-response
curve appears analogous to the situation when Ach is
used to stimulate acid secretion by close arterial
injection into the fundic mucosa.   Pevsner and
Grossman[7] demonstrated that very low rates of intra-
arterial Ach infusion would produce acid secretion
and no acid secretion occurred above a definite rate.

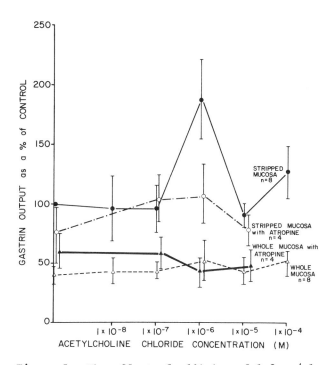

Figure 5. The effect of addition of 1.2 µg/ml
of atropine sulphate to the nutrient media for
both SAM and WAM.   Basal outputs are not significantly reduced but the peak at 10^{-6} M Ach has
been eliminated with addition of atropine.

One dose-response result has been on a dog vagotomized four months previously. In this dog the
peak Ach response was approximately nine times the
control, a ratio notably greater than those obtained
with intact dogs. This finding is in agreement with
the report of Becker, Reeder, and Thompson[2] who
found that the antra of vagotomized rats contained
considerably more gastrin than intact rats. This
point will be further investigated.

Effective gastrin release and a dose-response curve
to Ach have been obtained only from stripped antral
mucosa (SAM), that is, the material from which the
muscularis and Meissner plexus have been removed.
A fundamental point to be settled of course is whether
this difference depends on the thinness and consequent
increased permeability of the SAM preparation, or
whether it is related to the elimination of some inhibitory influence of the Meissner plexus. This
latter explanation seems unlikely but would require
elimination before a purely nutritional or respiratory
basis for the effect is assumed.

Effects of Atropine

Experiments show that the effects of Ach, at optimal
stimulation, are greatly reduced by atropine. So far,
however, it does not appear to affect the resting output significantly. Elucidation of this latter finding
seems important and will require further experimentation.

Possible Reasons for Confinement of Ach Responses to Stripped Antral Mucosa

The most likely possibility is the considerable reduction in thickness in the membrane after stripping
and the removal of an organized layer, which may be
difficult to permeate by nutrients and drugs.

A ganglionic layer has been eliminated, however,
and the possibility that it could exert an inhibitory
influence cannot be ignored until it has been excluded
by experiment.

If an inhibitory effect from the plexus were responsible, it might be removed by the use of a local
anesthetic in the nutrient fluid. So far, the one

preliminary experiment with tetracaine does not favor
this interpretation, since treatment with this agent
had no effect in increasing the gastrin output to a
range of Ach concentrations (Fig. 6). Anticholin-
esterase results are of interest to confirm the specificity of the dose-response effect and to permit ex-
trapolation of these data. They also allow investigation as to whether inherent Ach-producing mechanisms
with access to G-cells exist in both tissues. So far,
results with the drug eserine alone are available and
are at present incomplete.

Dose-Response Effects. On the SAM response, the few results we have are conflicting. The total output of
gastrin throughout the dose-response curve is not
raised by any level of eserine so far tested. This
was surprising initially, but would be compatible

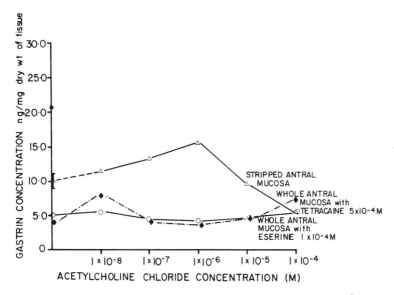

Figure 6. The effect of addition of tetracaine (5×10^{-4} M) and
eserine (1×10^{-4} M) to the WAM in a single experiment. The
dose-response curve from SAM in the one experiment is also expressed in the figure. Neither tetracaine nor eserine result
in a significant effect from WAM.

with a true Ach optimum at the G-cell receptors that
were obtained. If the concentration at the receptor
site depends on a balance between entry by diffusion
and cholinesterase destruction, then eserine would
raise the local concentration. One experiment so
far suggests a shift of the dose-response curve to
the left which also would be compatible with the
above concept and with a very narrow Ach optimum at
the receptor junctions. No effect at all was produced on the WAM curve which, at this stage, would
be compatible with the fact that this tissue is non-
functional because of inadequate nutrition. There
is no reason why eserine should improve this situation. Clearly, more work must be done before these
suggestions acquire true validity.

Possibility of Intrinsic Ach-Producing Mechanisms.   The
range of eserine concentrations that were tried did
not change the resting output of gastrin from either
tissue. For SAM the result obtained so far seems
reasonable, since the nerve terminations separated
from their ganglionic connections in the Meissner
plexus might not produce significant amounts of the
transmitter. The result with WAM, however, is again
compatible with the idea that this tissue is non-
functional, since it might have been expected that
nerves attached to their ganglia might have sufficient resting Ach production for eserine to have a
gastrin-releasing effect alone.

Our preliminary experiments, therefore, plus a
suggestion from the histology, do not favor an inhibitory effect from the Meissner plexus. This possibility cannot yet be regarded, however, as excluded
on the few experimental results so far available.

Final Comment

A procedure has been developed which permits the
study of gastrin release *in vitro* and which shows a
clear dose-response relationship for the most effective, generally recognized physiologic stimulant.
Supplies of bombesin did not reach us in time to be
included in this study. Our technique was originally
oriented toward dose-response effects, and we studied
Ach response against time. Clearly, this must be
done. A few preliminary results suggest that most of

the response to Ach occurs within the first half hour
Among our primary objectives, therefore, is the refinement of the procedure to one of long-term incubation
via short-term sampling to, it is hoped, a superfusion
of the portions of stripped antral tissue, both frag-
mented and in anatomic continuity and orientation.

SUMMARY

Portions of dog whole antral mucosa (WAM) dissected
from the muscularis externa and of mucosa stripped by
a further dissection of the muscularis mucosae (SAM)
were incubated at 37C in Krebs-Henreleit solution
under 95% O_2 and 5% CO_2 for two hours. Immunoreactive gastrin in the medium was assayed with an antigen
raised in rabbits to human synthetic G-17. Resting
outputs for WAM were 1915±443 and for SAM 4993±885
pg/mg dry tissue/hr. Ach chloride, 10^{-8} to 10^{-4} M,
increased gastrin output from SAM with a peak response at 10^{-6} M. Peak output ranged from 2 to 9
times control (range 3,000 to 5,800 pg/mg/hr). Output from WAM was not increased. Atropine, 1.2 pg/ml,
greatly reduced the peak response of SAM but not the
resting output of either tissue. Resting outputs
from either tissue were not increased by eserine 10^{-4}
or 10^{-5} M. The absence of an Ach response in WAM
persisted in the presence of 5×10^{-5} M tetracaine and
is probably due to inadequate nutrition of the thicker
tissue.

Acknowledgments

This work is supported by Canadian Medical Research Council
Grant MA-4322 and Medical Trust Fund of the University of Calgary.

References

1. Andersson S: Secretion of gastrointestinal hormones. *Ann
        Rev Physiol* 35:431-452, 1973.
2. Becker HD, Reeder DD, Thompson JC: Influence of vagotomy
        on tissue gastrin levels in stomach and pancreas in
        rats. *Surgery* 74:778-782, 1973.

3. Bertaccini G, Impicciatore M, Molina E, Zappie L: Action
     of some natural and synthetic peptides in the motility
     of human gastrointestinal tract "in vitro", in Daniel EE,
     Bowes K, Gilbert JAL, Schofield B, Schnitka TK, Scott G
     (eds), *Fourth International Symposium on Gastrointestinal
     Motility*, Vancouver: Mitchell Press, 1974, pp 287-292.
4. Dretler R, Wesdorp RIC, Fischer JE: Release of gastrin
     from isolated perfused gastric antra, abstracted.
     Gastroenterology 66:686, 1974.
5. McGuigan JE, Greider MH, Grawe L: Staining characteristics
     of the gastrin cell. *Gastroenterology* 62:959-969,
     1972.
6. Merritt JW, Kelly WD: Totally denervated pouches of gastric
     mucosa: Method and preliminary observations. *Surgery*
     46:486-495, 1959.
7. Pevsner L, Grossman MI: The mechanism of vagal stimulation
     of gastric acid secretion. *Gastroenterology* 28:493-499,
     1955.
8. Yalow RS, Berson SA: Radioimmunoassay of gastrin. *Gastro-
     enterology* 58:1-14, 1970.

NEW HORMONES

THE SECRETIN FAMILY AND EVOLUTION

Miklos Bodanszky

Department of Chemistry, Case Western
Reserve University, Cleveland, Ohio

Mere inspection of the sequences of the gastrointestinal hormones, secretin[13] and glucagon,[6] the vasoactive intestinal polypeptide (VIP),[5] and the gastric inhibitory polypeptide (GIP),[7] reveals conspicuous analogies. Even without statistical analysis, the existence of a "family" of hormones can be established beyond doubt (Table 1). The similarly obvious family of gastrin[12] will not be discussed here. The family concept is not restricted to peptide hormones; proteolytic enzymes,[19] steroid hormones and prostaglandins also form closely knit groups. Yet, peptide hormones lend themselves to a kind of analysis that was informative when applied to proteins; an investigation of homologies in the sequences of a given protein, for example, cytochrome C or hemoglobin from different species, can produce valuable data on evolution. Similar examination of the sequences of peptide hormones has been attempted repeatedly.[20,21]

In this report we try to demonstrate that the origin of hormone families cannot be treated in the same manner as the evolution of an enzyme or other functional protein. In the sequence of a peptide or protein from a series of different species, changes occur during evolution. These changes, usually due to single-base mutations, are mostly conservative and they do not significantly alter the functionality of the molecule; as examples, natural analogs of gastrin from the antral mucosa of different animals[12] are shown in Table 2. On the other hand, the two principal pituitary hormones, oxytocin and vasopressin, from the *same species* (that is, cattle) are compared in Table 3. A dramatic change can be observed in position 8: a neutral residue leucine in oxytocin and

507

arginine with basic side chain in vasopressin. The
difference between the two hormones is much more substantial than the differences found between the various natural analogs of the same hormone; leucine and
arginine are coded by triplets sufficiently different
to exclude single-base mutation that could transform
one hormone into the other. Moreover, the replacement
of leucine by arginine (or lysine in the hog) results
in major differences between the hormonal spectra of
the two peptides. The *nonconservative transformations*
that could lead from a potential common ancestor to
oxytocin and vasopressin are similar to the changes
that produced the individual members of the secretin
family (Table 1). As shown in Table 4, the differences

Table 1. The secretin family. The amino acid sequence of
secretin, the vasoactive intestinal peptide (VIP),
glucagon and the gastroinhibitory peptide (GIP)
(all from hog).

	1	2	3	4	5	6	7	8	9	10	11	12	13
Secretin	His	Ser	Asp	Gly	Thr	Phe	Thr	Ser	Glu	Leu	Ser	Arg	Leu-
VIP	His	Ser	Asp	Ala	Val	Phe	Thr	Asp	Asn	Tyr	Thr	Arg	Leu-
Glucagon	His	Ser	Gln	Gly	Thr	Phe	Thr	Ser	Asp	Tyr	Ser	Lys	Tyr-
GIP	Tyr	Ala	Glu	Gly	Thr	Phe	Ile	Ser	Asp	Tyr	Ser	Ile	Ala-

	14	15	16	17	18	19	20	21	22	23	24	25	26
Secretin	Arg	Asp	Ser	Ala	Arg	Leu	Gln	Arg	Leu	Leu	Gln	Gly	Leu-
VIP	Arg	Lys	Gln	Met	Ala	Val	Lys	Lys	Tyr	Leu	Asn	Ser	Ile-
Glucagon	Leu	Asp	Ser	Arg	Arg	Ala	Gln	Asp	Phe	Val	Gln	Trp	Leu-
GIP	Met	Asp	Lys	Ile	Arg	Gln	Gln	Asp	Phe	Val	Asn	Trp	Leu-

	27	28	29	30	31	32	33	34	35	36	37	38	39
Secretin	Val-NH$_2$												
VIP	Leu	Asn-NH$_2$											
Glucagon	Met	Asp	Thr										
GIP	Leu	Ala	Gln	Gln	Lys	Gly	Lys	Lys	Ser	Asp	Trp	Lys	His-

	40	41	42	43
GIP	Asn	Ile	Thr	Gln

Table 2. Gastrins from six different species. Variations in the sequence occur only in positions 5, 8, and 10 and can be rationalized by single-base mutations (Pyr = pyroglutamyl). The tyrosine in position 12 is present as sulfate ester in the gastrin II form.

	1	2	3	4	5	6	7	8	9
Pig	Pyr–Gly–Pro–Trp–**MET**–Glu–Glu–**GLU**–Glu–
Man	Pyr–Gly–Pro–Trp–**LEU**–Glu–Glu–**GLU**–Glu–
Cattle	Pyr–Gly–Pro–Trp–**VAL**–Glu–Glu–**GLU**–Glu–
Sheep	Pyr–Gly–Pro–Trp–**VAL**–Glu–Glu–**GLU**–Glu–
Cat	Pyr–Gly–Pro–Trp–**LEU**–Glu–Glu–**GLU**–Glu–
Dog	Pyr–Gly–Pro–Trp–**MET**–Glu–Glu–**ALA**–Glu–

	10	11	12	13	14	15	16	17
Pig	**GLU**–Ala–Tyr–Gly–Trp–Met–Asp–Phe–NH$_2$
Man	**GLU**–Ala–Tyr–Gly–Trp–Met–Asp–Phe–NH$_2$
Cattle	**ALA**–Ala–Tyr–Gly–Trp–Met–Asp–Phe–NH$_2$
Sheep	**ALA**–Ala–Tyr–Gly–Trp–Met–Asp–Phe–NH$_2$
Cat	**ALA**–Ala–Tyr–Gly–Trp–Met–Asp–Phe–NH$_2$
Dog	**GLU**–Ala–Tyr–Gly–Trp–Met–Asp–Phe–NH$_2$

Table 3. Oxytocin and vasopressin from the same species (cattle). The change in position 3 is due to single-base mutation; the difference in position 8 is nonconservative (a positively charged side chain in vasopressin) and cannot be explained by single-base mutation. The two peptides have different hormonal spectra.

	1	2	3	4	5	6	7	8	9
Oxytocin	Cys–Tyr–**ILE**–Gln–Asn–Cys–Pro–**LEU**–Gly–NH$_2$
Vasopressin	Cys–Tyr–**PHE**–Gln–Asn–Cys–Pro–**ARG**–Gly–NH$_2$

509

in the amino acid sequences of secretin, VIP and glucagon can be rationalized only in part by single-base mutations. Several positions (e.g., 14, 15, 21 and 28) provide examples for nonconservative transformations. For instance, in position 21 the change between VIP and secretin (lysine-arginine) is conservative. The same position in glucagon, however, is occupied by aspartic acid. This nonconservative transformation reverses the charge on the side chain

Table 4. Homology and binding sites in the secretin family*

Residue number	Secretin	VIP	Glu-cagon	Identical residues	Nonconservative changes	Potential binding functions
1	His	His	His	+ + +		+ + +
2	Ser	Ser	Ser	+ + +		H H H
3	Asp	Asp	Gln	+ +	+	- - H
4	Gly	Ala	Gly	+ +		
5	Thr	Val	Thr	+ +		0
6	Phe	Phe	Phe	+ + +		0 0 0
7	Thr	Thr	Thr	+ + +		
8	Ser	Asp	Ser	+ +	+	H - H
9	Glu	Asn	Asp		+	- H -
10	Leu	Tyr	Tyr	+ +		0 0 0
11	Ser	Thr	Ser	+ +		H H
12	Arg	Lys	Arg	+ +		+ + +
13	Leu	Leu	Tyr	+ +		0 0 0
14	Arg	Arg	Leu	+ +	+	+ + 0
15	Asp	Lys	Asp	+ +	+	- + -
16	Ser	Gln	Ser	+ +		H H H
17	Ala	Met	Arg		+	0 0 +
18	Arg	Ala	Arg	+ +	+	+ 0 +
19	Leu	Val	Ala			0 0 0
20	Gln	Lys	Gln	+ +	+	H + H
21	Arg	Lys	Asp		+	+ + -
22	Leu	Tyr	Phe			0 0 0
23	Leu	Leu	Val	+ +		0 0 0
24	Gln	Asn	Gln	+ +		H H H
25	Gly	Ser	Trp			H 0
26	Leu	Ile	Leu	+ +		0 0 0
27	Val	Leu	Met			0 0 0
28	---	Asn	Asp		+	H -

* H, hydrogen bonding; ±, ionic bonds; 0, hydrophobic interaction

from positive to negative. Of course, such major differences had to be expected: these peptides have different hormonal properties and they react with different receptors. Our inquiry aims at an understanding of the biologic significance and at the origin of the transformations.

THE CONDITIONS FOR HORMONAL ACTION

A minute amount of a hormone has to find its specific receptor in the relatively large volume and immense complexity of an organism and then to interact with it to trigger hormonal action. In this respect, it is irrelevant whether or not specific adenylate cyclases, phosphodiesterases or other molecules are the receptor. Still, for the present discussion, the not unreasonable assumption is made that the receptors are proteins. A specific interaction of the hormone with the receptor necessitates a very high binding constant, although the binding should be reversible to terminate the hormonal action. The presently conceivable models[1,18] require a) close molecular fit between hormone and receptor molecules, and b) complementarity of binding sites in two chains, that is, a negatively-charged group in the hormone opposite to a positively charged side chain in the receptor. Of course, other forces, such as hydrogen bonds or nonpolar interactions, can also participate in the binding. The multiple nature of the binding sites can produce very high binding constants, since physical separation of the two chains requires simultaneous dissociation of several pairs. There are indications for such molecular fit and some evidence for binding sites in the secretin family. The conspicuously high activity of the C-terminal pentadecapeptide part of VIP, as compared with the C-terminal tetradecapeptide, is most likely due to the presence of one more cationic binding site, since the only difference between the two peptides is an arginine residue.[3]

Close molecular fit of hormone with receptor assumes the presence of a well-defined architecture in both compounds, at least at the time of their interaction. The presence of an established geometry in the receptors, if these are indeed enzymes or more generally, proteins, is a modest postulate, since all the well-studied enzymes have such

structures. A preferred conformation in peptide hormones, especially in those with an open chain of
moderate length, is not so obvious. Our studies on
secretin, however, produced convincing evidence for
the existence of a preferred conformation,[4] for a
folded, partially helical molecule. The helical
stretch was tentatively proposed to be near the N-
terminal portion of the chain, starting beyond the
fourth amino acid.

Our recent investigations on the forces that stabilize the geometry of secretin demonstrated the influence of hydrophobic side chains in the area of
positions 5-7[11] and gave evidence of the role of the
carboxylic group containing side chains of residues
9 and 15.[10] No final proof for the exact location
of the helical stretch could be established so far.
In fact, the application of empiric rules[8,9,13,16,17]
suggests that the helix could well be in the C-terminal half of the chain. The same rules predict some
helicity in VIP and a low helix content in glucagon.
The ord spectra of the three peptides in water[2] vin-
dicate these expectations. On the other hand, the
three chains have some conformational freedom as
well and are able to assume similar shapes when relatively small amounts of organic solvents are added
to their aqueous solutions.

This is not unexpected: since VIP has both secretin
and glucagon-like activities, it should be able to
assume conformations that allow the postulated molecular fit with the secretin and glucagon receptors.
At this time, the conformational changes induced by
the contact with the specific receptors of these peptides are not known, but the solvent-induced changes
suggest that such changes can occur. The active conformations of secretin, VIP and glucagon might be
closely similar and the specificity of their hormonal
effects could rest on the differences in their respective binding sites.

Binding to the receptors could be synonymous with
hormonal action. Whether a differentiation between
binding sites and catalytic sites is justified or
not remains to be demonstrated. In the present examination of the secretin family, no such discrimination was made. A short scrutiny of Table 4 reveals
that the residues in positions 1, 2, 6 and 7 are
identical in secretin, VIP and glucagon. In position
3, nonconservative transformations produced acidic

side chains (Asp) in secretin and VIP, but a neutral
one (Gln) in glucagon. Position 4 shows only a conservative change (Gly, Ala). Similar comparisons
suggest additional single-base mutations, in positions 9, 10, 11, 12, 14, 15, 20, 22, 23, 24, 25, 26,
27 and 28. The number of positions where more than
a single mutation is needed to explain the variations
in the three sequences is still considerable. Thus,
although the three hormones are unquestionably members of a family, their individuality is not less
obvious. Positions 15 and 21 were mentioned earlier;
a reversal of charge suggests corresponding differences (with opposite signs) in the individual receptors. Charge differences are found in positions 9,
14, 17, 18, 20 and 28 as well. The specificity of
the hormonal action of the three chains probably
rests on more than just the distribution of charged
groups. These were pointed out only because the
differences are conspicuous. If other forces, for
example, hydrogen bonding or nonpolar interaction,
can bring about selective binding, then position 25
deserves consideration; we find serine with hydrogen
bonding ability in VIP, the potentially inert glycine in secretin and nonpolar tryptophan in glucagon.
Most of these contentions are speculative at this
time; only a very limited number of analogs of these
hormones were prepared[5] and the role of most of the
side chains remains to be explored. In general terms,
however, some of the differences in the sequences of
secretin, VIP, and glucagon allow the postulation of
corresponding differences in their respective
receptors.

EVOLUTION (?) OF FUNCTIONAL PROTEINS

The evolutionary changes in the amino acid sequence
of a protein, such as the extensively studied cytochrome C, might be substantial if the sequences of
the protein from two distant species are compared.
Yet in certain crucial positions the changes, if they
occur at all, are conservative. This could have been
anticipated; the function and hence the architecture
so closely related to function, can be maintained
only if the forces that stabilize the geometry of the
molecule remain intact. Therefore replacement of one
amino acid by an amino acid of different character

can be found only in relatively unimportant regions.
If a somewhat trivial analogy is permitted here, we
could compare these evolutionary changes to the alterations in subsequent models of an automobile.
Many details change, some may even improve the car,
others may deteriorate it, most of them contribute
only to new styling. The crucial features, however,
the motor, the wheels, the driving and steering
mechanisms, etc., remain essentially the same and
the car's *function* also remains unchanged. Therefore,
although the study of sequences can shed considerable
light on the evolutional order of different species,
it does not illuminate the origin of a given protein.
In fact, our ignorance is complete in this respect.

The "evolution" of a functional protein, such as
an enzyme, cannot be explained through a series that
starts with a simple molecule which then becomes
more complex and more perfect in its function through
random mutations and selection. Even the simplest
enzyme molecules are too sophisticated to allow such
speculations. The active sites reveal perfect en-
gineering; molecular steering requires orbital overlap,
which in turn is based on a highly defined geometric
arrangement of the functional groups.

It is very likely that possible alternative hypotheses of enzyme mechanisms are also unable to dis-
pense with the necessity of a well-determined conformation of the protein. Over and above the catalytic
effect, the specificity of enzyme action requires
organized, rigid areas near the catalytic site, for
example, a hole for aromatic side chains in chymo-
trypsin or for basic residues in trypsin. Furthermore,
these specific regions interact only with side chains
that are attached to residues of the L configuration.
On the other hand, the geometry of the catalytic and
specificity sites is determined by the architecture
of the entire molecule, which in turn is a function
of the amino acid sequence. The protein is held by
a series of strong and subtle intramolecular forces,
in a rigid conformation.

Without even entering the area of additional compli-
cations, such as allosteric regulation, it is obvious
that the formation of such functional molecules, as are
the enzymes, cannot be easily explained by a series of
random changes. A chain below a certain length cannot
be firmly held in a folded form; the long-range interactions on which most folds are based require a minimum chain length. Also, the side-chain interactions,

that stabilize a secondary-tertiary structure, are operative only when some contact can be established between the side chains of the participating amino acids. The involved residues might be far from each other if their distance is measured by position numbers in the sequence, but they will interact if brought into proximity by an appropriate folding of the chain.

On the other hand, this folding is stabilized by such "long-range" interactions. Thus, a short part of a sequence may not "make sense" in itself, but it becomes "reasonable" when regarded in the context of the entire molecule. Secretin provides a simple example: neither the N-terminal half nor the C-terminal half of its chain is helical when isolated; the entire molecule, however, has a preferred, folded, and partially helical geometry.[4] Because of such interdependence of separate parts of a peptide chain, it is easier to visualize the sudden appearance of a functional protein, like the birth of Pallas Athena from the head of Zeus, than to assume that its *functional complexity* is the result of gradual changes starting with something simple.

EVOLUTION (?) OF PEPTIDE HORMONES FROM A COMMON ANCESTOR

It is obviously intriguing to suggest that closely related hormones, such as the members of the secretin family, stem from a common ancestor, and are the products of evolutionary changes involving random mutation and selection. Yet, on closer examination such an assumption turns out to be probably untenable. The difficulties outlined in connection with the origin of functional proteins, for example, enzymes, appear further enhanced. In the secretin family (Table 1), we are looking at a series of homologous peptides, with *different functions*, but from the *same species* (hog). This alone seems to contradict evolutionary explanations. The functional specificity of these closely related compounds is based, at least in part, on certain differences in their sequences, that require corresponding differences in their counterparts, the specific receptors. Therefore, an evolutionary change in the hormone would necessitate a corresponding evolutionary alteration of the receptor.

For instance, the reversal of the positive charge
in position 21 in secretin to a negative charge in
the same position of glucagon (or vice versa) would
result in selective binding only if an opposite change
takes place in their individual receptors. For the
specific functions to be operative, it would also be
required that the changes in the hormone and in the
receptor occur simultaneously. This is hard to
accept. The argument that given enough time unlikely
events do occur cannot be used repeatedly in one
rationale and that *two* highly unlikely events should
by chance occur simultaneously at the same place has
to be considered fantastic.

As pointed out earlier, not all the differences
between the individual members of the secretin family
can be explained by single-base mutations. Also,
several of the differences correspond to nonconservative changes, and some of these differences seem to
account for the specificity in the hormonal spectrum.
Therefore an attempt to explain the existence of a
hormone family by evolution meets perhaps unsurmount-
able obstacles; random mutations followed by selection
should proceed both in the nucleotide sequence that
codes for the hormone and in the sequence that codes
for its receptor with the result of two peptide chains
that can interact with each other in a specific manner
through molecular fit and the correspondence of (the
newly formed) binding sites. It would not be more
arbitrary to propose that the changes leading from
one hormone to another in the same family first take
place in the peptide chains and next are transcribed--
contrary to the central dogma--into the coding nucleic
acids. In summary, a common-ancestor hypothesis for
the members of a hormone family lacks solid founda-
tions.

Unfortunately we cannot suggest, at least at this
time, a theory for the development of hormone families. The members of the secretin family are built
on common principles. They contain similar architectural features and can assume similar conformations,[8]
yet they also reveal differences in the distribution
of their binding sites (Table 4), differences that
are due to nonconservative changes, and that are often
consequences of more than single-base mutations.
These differences cannot be rationalized by simple
evolutionary schemes. Thus the secretin family and
the families of hormones in general present a major

challenge for an inquiry toward the understanding of their origin. The homology of certain regions in the gastrointestinal hormones with sequences of the seemingly unrelated peptides somatostatin and one of the Kazal-type pancreatic trypsin inhibitors (Asp-Gly-Thr-Phe-Thr-Ser-Glu-Leu-Ser in secretin, Thr-Phe-Thr-Ser in somatostatin, and Glu-Ala-Thr-Cys-Thr-Ser-Glu-Val-Ser in the trypsin inhibitor) supports the concept of architectural units in proteins.

SUMMARY

An examination of the sequences of secretin, the vasoactive intestinal polypeptide (VIP), and glucagon, all from porcine tissues, reveals extensive homologies, but also major differences, which account for their functional specificity. The origin of such hormone families cannot be explained by simple evolutionary schemes.

Acknowledgments

This study was supported by a grant from the U.S. Public Health Service (NIH AM-12473).

References

1. Bodanszky M: Gastrointestinal hormones, families of oligoelectrolytes, in Chey WY, Brooks FP (eds), *Endocrinology of the Gut*, Thorofare NJ: Charles B. Slack, Inc., 1974, pp 3-13.
2. Bodanszky M, Bodanszky A, Klausner YS, Said SI: A preferred conformation in the vasoactive intestinal peptide (VIP): Molecular architecture of gastrointestinal hormones. *Bioorg Chem* 3:133-140, 1974.
3. Bodanszky M, Klausner YS, Said SI: Biological activities of synthetic peptides corresponding to fragments of and to the entire sequence of vasoactive intestinal peptide. *Proc Natl Acad Sci USA* 70:382-384, 1973.
4. Bodanszky A, Ondetti MA, Mutt V, Bodanszky M: Synthesis of secretin: IV. Secondary structure in a miniature protein. *J Am Chem Soc* 91:944-949, 1969.

518   *M. Bodanszky*

5. Bodanszky M, Yang Lin C, Said SI: The vasoactive intestinal peptide (VIP): VI. The 17-norleucine analog of the sequence 14-28. *Bioorg Chem* 3:320-323.

6. Bromer WW, Sinn LG, Behrens OK: The amino acid sequence of glucagon: V. Location of amide groups, acid degradation studies and summary of sequential evidence. *J Am Chem Soc* 79:2807-2810, 1957.

7. Brown JC, Dryburgh JR: A gastric inhibitory polypeptide: II. The complete amino acid sequence. *Canad J Biochem* 49:867-872, 1971.

8. Chou PY, Fasman GD: Conformational parameters for amino acids in helical, β-sheet and random coil regions calculated from proteins. *Biochemistry* 13:211-222, 1974.

9. Chou PY, Fasman GD: Prediction of protein conformation. *Biochemistry* 13:222-245, 1974.

10. Fink MLT: *Side Chain Interactions in Synthetic Peptides,* dissertation, Case Western Reserve University, Cleveland, 1974, pp 108-148.

11. Funk KW: *Ortho-Nitrophenyl Esters in Peptide Synthesis,* dissertation, Case Western Reserve University, Cleveland, 1974, pp 70-91.

12. Grossman MI: Gastrin and its activities. *Nature* 228: 1147-1150, 1970.

13. Guzzo AV: The influence of amino acid sequence on protein structure. *Biophys J* 5:809-822, 1965.

14. Mutt V, Jorpes JE, Magnusson S: Structure of porcine secretin: The amino acid sequence. *Eur J Biochem* 15:513-519, 1970.

15. Mutt V, Said SI: Structure of the porcine vasoactive intestinal octacosapeptide. *Eur J Biochem* 42:581-589, 1974.

16. Prothero JW: Correlation between the distribution of amino acids and alpha helices. *Biophys J* 6:367-370, 1966.

17. Ptitsyn OB: Statistical analysis of the distribution of amino acid residues among helical and non-helical regions in globular proteins. *J Mol Biol* 42:501-510, 1969.

18. Schwyzer R: Molecular mechanism of polypeptide hormone action, in Hanson H, Jakubke HD (eds), *Peptides 1972,* Amsterdam: North-Holland Publishing, 1973, pp 424-430.

19. Stroud RM: A family of protein-cutting proteins. *Scientific American* 231:74-89, 1974.

20. Weinstein B: On the relationship between glucagon and secretin. *Experientia* 24:406-408, 1968.

21. Weinstein B: A generalized homology correlation for various hormones and proteins. *Experientia* 28:1517-1522, 1972.

GUT GLUCAGONOID (GLI) AND GUT GLUCAGON

Hideo Sasaki, B. Rubalcava,
C.B. Srikant, D. Baetens,
L. Orci, Roger H. Unger

Veterans Administration Hospital and the
University of Texas Southwestern Medical
School, Dallas, Texas and the Institute
of Histology and Embryology, Geneva,
Switzerland

In the quarter century since the discovery of
glucagon-like biologic activity in extracts of
canine gastrointestinal tissues by Sutherland and
DeDuve,[8] the status of glucagon-like polypeptides
of the gut has been uncertain, and their relationship, if any, to true pancreatic glucagon, confusing.
Recent collaborative studies from our laboratories
in Dallas (RHU) and Geneva (LO) suggest that much
of the confusion may result from the fact that at
least two independent species of glucagon-like
polypeptides coexist in the gut. One of these,
known as glucagon-like immunoreactivity or GLI, has
definite physicochemical, immunometric and biologic
differences from pancreatic glucagon, and may originate from cells resembling but, nevertheless,
distinguishable from so-called intestinal A-cells.[4]
The other has physicochemical, immunometric, and
biologic properties identical to pancreatic glucagon
and may well originate from cells, most prevalent
in the gastric fundus, which are morphologically
indistinguishable from pancreatic A-cells. Until
now there has been no effort to distinguish between
what may properly be referred to as "gut glucagon,"
"enteroglucagon," or "gastroglucagon" and "glucagon-
like immunoreactivity," "GLI," or "enteroglucagonoid."

MORPHOLOGY

In 1968 intestinal A-cells were first observed.[4]
These cells had predominantly round dense secretory
granules, but the significance of a halo between
the core and the enveloping membrane was not emphasized.   It was suggested that these cells might be
the site of GLI secretion.[4] Subsequent studies by
Polak and associates[5] have supported this prediction.
Indeed, they have observed immunofluorescent staining
of these cells by use of a nonspecific antiserum to
pancreatic glucagon, an antiserum which undoubtedly
cross-reacted with GLI.   Although the studies of Polak
do not differentiate between GLI-producing cells and
glucagon-producing cells, they do establish that at
least one of these two polypeptides is present in the
intestinal A-cells.
More recently, however, we have re-examined the
intestinal A-cells in the dog. A closer scrutiny
of the ultrastructural features of the secretory
granules allowed us to recognize two types of intestinal A-cells. One type (Fig. 1a), that we consider
to represent a true A-cell, is mainly concentrated
in the fundic mucosa and contains granules which fully
match those of pancreatic A-cells (presence of a distinct halo between the dense core and the enveloping
membrane) (Fig. 1b). The other type, more frequently
found in the postduodenal intestine, is characterized
by the presence of granules that have in general a
round shape and a limiting membrane closely applied
to the homogenous dense core (Fig. 2).
Although discriminatory immunohistologic studies
with pancreatoglucagon-specific antisera and GLI
cross-reacting antisera have yet to be done, the
"true" intestinal A-cells, on the basis of ultrastructural features, might be predicted to be the
source of any "true glucagon" originating in the
gastrointestinal tract.

PHYSICOCHEMICAL STUDIES

We have studied the glucagon-like immunoreactivity
in extracts of porcine duodenum kindly furnished by
Professor Viktor Mutt of the Karolinska Institute,
Stockholm, Sweden, and purified 50-fold in his laboratory. Gel filtration of such extracts on P-10

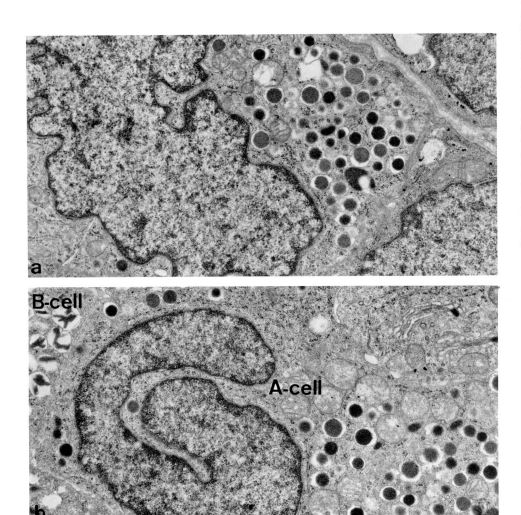

Figure 1. Comparison of a "true" gastrointestinal A-cell and a pancreatic A-cell. Note the complete morphologic resemblance between the secretory granules in each cell type.
(a) Dog fundic mucosa.   (b) Dog pancreatic islet.
(×10,500).

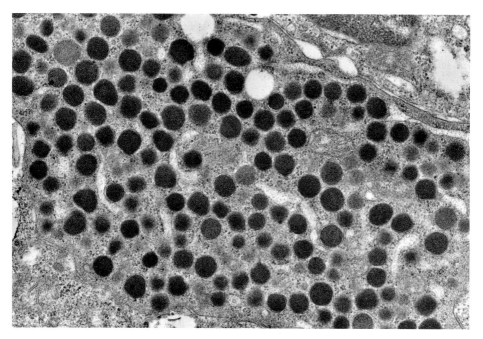

Figure 2. A-like cell in the dog duodenum. Most of the secretory granules appear round. The limiting membrane is closely
applied to the granule-core (×18,500).

Biogel columns reveal that most of the glucagon-like
immunoreactivity measured with the highly cross-
reactive antiglucagon serum, antiserum 78J, elutes
after the glucagon ^{125}I marker (Fig. 3). This peak
is estimated to have a molecular weight of 2900 compared to the 3485 molecular weight of pancreatic
glucagon. In almost all such chromatograms, however,
a "shoulder" or smaller peak, approximately 20% of
the total immunoreactivity, is also observed, preceding the 2900 molecular weight peak. This peak was
present in the eluates containing glucagon ^{125}I and
was estimated to have a molecular weight similar to
that of glucagon.
  Disc-gel electrophoresis at pH 8.3 and 4.7 revealed
that the electrophoretic properties of the 2900 molecular weight and 3500 molecular weight immunoreactivities differed strikingly. At pH 8.3 the 2900 molecular
weight material did not migrate from the origin,
whereas the 3500 molecular weight material moved into
the midportion of the gel; at pH 4.7, however, whereas
the 3500 molecular weight fraction, like pancreatic
glucagon, moved only slightly away from the origin,

522

the 2900 molecular weight moiety migrated into the midportion of the gel. These findings suggest that the 2900 molecular weight material is a strongly basic protein and could not, therefore, be derived from either pancreatic glucagon or from the 3500 molecular weight gut polypeptide which resembles it.

To determine the isoelectric point of these two duodenal immunoreactive fractions, they were subjected to isoelectric focusing by techniques described in detail elsewhere. The isoelectric point of the 2900 molecular weight moiety was found to be over 10, whereas the 3500 molecular weight material had an isoelectric point of 6.2, identical to that of pancreatic glucagon in the present system.

IMMUNOMETRIC COMPARISON OF 2900 AND 3500 MOLECULAR WEIGHT FRACTIONS

Antibodies formed against pancreatic glucagon vary in their ability to cross-react with gastrointestinal polypeptides such as the 2900 molecular weight material observed here. Antiserum 78J is the most cross-reactive antiserum available to us, whereas antisera 30K and G-58 are highly specific for pancreatic

Figure 3. Elution pattern of porcine duodenal extract chromatographed on Biogel P-10 column. Immunoactivity of eluted fraction measured using a specific GLI radio-immunoassay (antibody 78J) and a specific pancreatic glucagon radioimmunoassay (antibody 30K). Protein content estimated by measurement at OD_{280}. V_o=void volume, V_t=total elution volume.

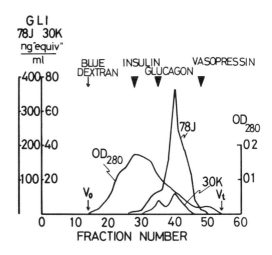

glucagon and cross-react with gastrointestinal extracts only very weakly. A given solution of pancreatic glucagon gives identical answers whether
assayed with a specific or with a cross-reacting
antiglucagon serum, whereas a solution containing
glucagon-like immunoreactivity from the gut, gives
much higher values with the cross-reacting antiserum
than with the pancreatoglucagon specific antisera.
Thus, the ratio of 78J immunoreactivity to 30K or
G-58 immunoreactivity provides an immunometric index
of resemblance to pancreatic glucagon, a ratio of 1
suggesting immunometric identity, and a higher ratio
suggesting immunometric dissimilarity.

As shown in Table 1, the 2900 molecular weight peak
gave a ratio of 61.1, whereas the 3500 molecular weight
peak gave a ratio of 0.9. Clearly then, the latter
fraction is immunometrically indistinguishable from
pancreatic glucagon, whereas the 2900 molecular
weight fraction differs greatly.

Since there is a small peak of 30K immunoreactivity
in the 2900 molecular weight zone, the question arises
as to whether this represents cross-reactivity between
the highly pancreatoglucagon-specific 30K antiserum
and the 2900 molecular weight fraction of GLI, or
whether it indicates that a different polypeptide of
similar molecular weight, perhaps a derivative of
the pancreatoglucagon-like 3500 molecular weight
moiety, is present in the GLI-containing eluates.
Disc-gel electrophoresis suggests the former possibility, that is, that the 2900 molecular weight
immunoreactivity represents 78J immunoactivity which
cross-reacts with 30K.

Table 1. Comparison of radioimmunoassay values for the 3500-
and 2900-molecular weight components of partially
purified porcine duodenal extract measured with cross-
reactive (78J) and relatively specific (30K) antisera

	Mean 78J Value (± SD)	Mean 30K Value (± SD)	Mean 78J/ 30K Ratio (± SD)
3500 MW immunoreactivity (ng equivalents/ml) (N=6)	6.1±0.4	7.0±0.3	0.9±0.13
2900 MW immunoreactivity (ng equivalents/ml) (N=6)	4450±106	72.8±26.9	61.1±22.6

BIOLOGIC ACTIVITIES

In the isolated perfused rat liver preparation of Mortimore,[9] used to detect glycogenolytic activity, the 2900 molecular weight fraction, when quantitated immunometrically by the 78J assay, was found to have approximately one-half the biologic activity of pancreatic glucagon; twenty 78J ng equivalents had the same glycogenolytic activity as 10 ng of glucagon. Twenty 78J ng of the 2900 molecular weight fraction contained only 1.2 30K ng equivalents of glucagon, which is not enough immunometric glucagon to cause a glycogenolytic response. Therefore, it is concluded that either the 2900 molecular weight material has intrinsic glycogenolytic activity, or that some other material in the GLI-containing eluates, not detectable by radioimmunoassay, is responsible for the glycogenolytic effect. Since VIP is known to have glycogenolytic activity, a VIP radioimmunoassay and bioassay, kindly performed by Dr. Said's laboratory, was employed to determine if sufficient VIP was present to account for the glycogenolytic activity; the values obtained by both assays were far below the minimal glycogenolytic dose. GLI itself is, therefore, the likely cause of the glycogenolysis.

This is supported further by experiments in which fractions containing varying amounts of 2900 molecular weight immunoreactivity were tested for ability to stimulate adenylate cyclase activity in the isolated rat liver cell membrane preparation of Neville.[3] Adenylate cyclase was measured by the method of Solomon and associates.[7] Excellent correspondence between the curve of adenylate cyclase activation and the curve of 78J immunoreactivity, was observed.

Similar experiments conducted with the 3500 molecular weight moiety also revealed that its glycogenolytic activity and its ability to stimulate adenylate cyclase activity are indistinguishable from the same dose of pancreatic glucagon. Moreover, adenylate cyclase activity and 30K immunoreactivity correspond to a remarkable degree, and the latter displaces glucagon ^{125}I from liver cell membranes at concentrations comparable to pancreatoglucagon.

DISTRIBUTION OF THE 2900 MOLECULAR WEIGHT GLI AND
3500 MOLECULAR WEIGHT PANCREATOGLUCAGON-LIKE MOIETIES

In preliminary studies it appears that the glucagon immunoreactivity of the fundus of the stomach
is largely in the 3500 molecular weight range and,
that like pancreatic glucagon, has a 78J to 30K ratio
of approximately 1. In the jejunum and ileum, however, the 78J to 30K ratio is much higher. This
suggests the presence of two different fractions of
immunoreactive material. The distribution of the
pancreatoglucagon-like material in the upper portions
of the gastrointestinal tract corresponds to the distribution of true A-cells, whereas the prevalence of
the GLI in the jejunum and ileum matches the distribution of the intestinal A-like cells[4] or EG-cells,[5]
which have been proposed as the source of GLI.

DISCUSSION

These studies reveal two clearly different polypeptides, one indistinguishable from pancreatic glucagon
in every respect tested; the other, although sharing
certain of the biologic and immunologic properties of
pancreatic glucagon, clearly distinguishable from it.
Moreover, two distinct intestinal A-cell types are
found, one mainly concentrated in the fundic mucosa,
which was indistinguishable from pancreatic A-cells,
and the other more prevalent in the postduodenal
intestine. To avoid compounding the already formi-
dable nomenclatural confusion, we propose, as indicated in Table 1, that the term gut "glucagon-like
immunoreactivity" or "GLI," or "glucagonoid,"be used
only for substances clearly distinguishable from
pancreatoglucagon, such as the 2900 molecular weight
material, obviously a different protein than pancreatic glucagon, and that the terms "gut glucagon" or
"enteroglucagon" (previously employed synonymously
with GLI) be used only to signify polypeptides which
can be differentiated from pancreatoglucagon only by
anatomic location.
These issues are of more than academic interest in
view of the fact that in dogs at least, the removal
of the pancreas causes only a modest and transient
reduction in the 30K immunoreactivity of plasma and
within 24 hours is followed by a remarkable increase

in immunoreactivity not indistinguishable immunometrically or by its molecular size from true pancreatoglucagon.[2,3,9] In view of recent studies indicating that the presence of glucagon, in addition
to insulin deficiency, may be a prerequisite for the
development of diabetic hyperglycemia,[1,6] the glucagon-
producing cells of the gastrointestinal tract may
prove to play a crucial role in diabetes mellitus as
well as in other diseases characterized by hyperglu-
cagonemia.

SUMMARY

Gastrointestinal extracts of hog duodenum contain
two distinct polypeptide families, both of which
react in certain of the radioimmunoassays in glucagon. One of these is a 2900 molecular weight moiety,
GLI, which cross-reacts to a variable degree with
antisera to pancreatic glucagon. GLI is a strongly
basic polypeptide with an isoelectric point over
10 and has considerably less glycogenolytic and
adenylate cyclase-stimulating activity than pancreatic glucagon, perhaps because of a lower affinity
for the glucagon-binding sites on isolated rat liver
membranes. The other polypeptide, like pancreatic
glucagon, has a molecular weight of 3500 and reacts
identically with all antisera to pancreatic glucagon.
It has an isoelectric point identical to that of
pancreatic glucagon and has the same affinity for
rat liver membranes as well as similar adenylate
cyclase-stimulating and glycogenolytic activity.
Cells indistinguishable from pancreatic A-cells have
been identified in the upper gastrointestinal tract
of dogs and may well be the source of this "true"
gut glucagon. It is suggested that the term "gut
glucagon" or "enteroglucagon" be restricted to this
polypeptide and that the term "GLI" or "enteroglucagonoid" be used to designate the 2900 molecular
weight polypeptide which originates primarily from
the A-like cells of postduodenal intestinal tract.

Acknowledgments

This work was supported by National Institutes of Health
grant 02700-15, Dallas, and the Fonds National Suisse de la
Recherche Scientifique (Grants 3.8080.72; 3.0310.73), Geneva.

REFERENCES

1. Dobbs R, Sakurai H, Unger RH: The essential role of glucagon in diabetic hyperglycemia and the effect of glucagon
   blockade in diabetes mellitus, abstracted. *Clin Res*
   22:648A, 1974.
2. Mashiter K, Harding PE, Chou M, Mashiter GD, Stout J,
   Diamond D, Field JB: Persistent pancreatic glucagon
   but not insulin response to arginine in depancreatized
   dogs, submitted.
3. Matsuyama T, Foa PP: Effects of pancreatectomy (PX) and
   of enteral administration of glucose (G) on plasma
   insulin (IRI), total (GLI) and pancreatic (IRG)
   glucagon, abstracted. *Diabetes* 23 (suppl 1):344, 1974.
4. Orci L, Pictet R, Forssmann WG, Renold AE, Rouiller C:
   Structural evidence for glucagon producing cells in
   the intestinal mucosa of the rat. *Diabetologia* 4:56-
   67, 1968.
5. Polak JM, Bloom S, Coulling I, Pearse AGE: Immunofluorescent localization of enteroglucagon cells in the
   gastrointestinal tract of the dog. *Gut* 12:311-318,
   1971.
6. Sakurai H, Blázquez E, Muñoz-Barragan L, Dobbs R, Unger RH:
   Prevention of hyperglycemia during insulin deficiency
   by glucagon blockade, abstracted. *Clin Res* 23:44A,
   1975.
7. Solomon Y, Londos C, Rodbell M: A highly sensitive adenylate
   cyclase assay. *Anal Biochem* 58:541-551, 1973.
8. Sutherland EW, DeDuve C: Origin and distribution of the
   hyperglycemic-glycogenolytic factor of the pancreas.
   J Biol Chem 175:663-674, 1948.
9. Vranic M, Pek S, Kawamori R: Increased "glucagon immunoreactivity" in plasma of totally depancreatized dogs.
   Diabetes 23:905-912, 1974.

HUMAN CIRCULATING GUT GLUCAGON: BINDING TO LIVER CELL PLASMA MEMBRANES

J.J. Holst, J.F. Rehfeld

Departments of Gastroenterology (A) and
Clinical Chemistry, Bispebjerg Hospital,
Copenhagen, Denmark

In 1973 we forwarded the hypothesis that increased release of gut glucagon might be the pathogenic factor in reactive hypoglycemia. It was postulated that gut glucagon might competitively inhibit the glycogenolytic action of pancreatic glucagon, which would otherwise counteract hypoglycemia.[7]

Evidence to support the hypothesis, however, must include demonstration of binding of gut glucagon to the hepatic glucagon receptor. Experiments with this objective are reported here.

MATERIAL AND METHODS

A 70-year-old female patient, who four years earlier had undergone truncal vagotomy and pyloroplasty for uncomplicated duodenal ulcer, showed symptoms of neuroglucopenia one to three hours after carbohydrate-rich meals.

A 100-g oral glucose tolerance test was performed, which showed reactive hypoglycemia and 20-fold increase in peripheral total glucagon concentration at the nadir of hypoglycemia (Fig. 1). Later another glucose tolerance test was performed and at the nadir of hypoglycemia, 300 ml of blood were drawn from an antecubital vein into chilled heparin-tubes containing aprotinin (Trasylol, Bayer), 500 KIU/ml blood.

The plasma was incubated with 10 ml of an antiglucagon immunosorbent (see below) for two hours at 4C under slow rotation.[1] The immunosorbent was then

529

packed in a column, and washed thoroughly with 0.05 M
sodium phosphate buffer, pH 7.5 containing in addition 0.15 M NaCl, and subsequently eluted with 10%
formic acid. All fractions were freeze-dried and
assayed for glucagon immunoreactivity. Glucose concentrations were determined on a Technicon Auto-
Analyzer by means of the hexokinase method. Glucagon radioimmunoassay was performed by an ethanol
precipitation technique. Plasma samples were extracted with ethanol before analysis.

Two different antisera were used, one (k 814, kindly
donated by LG Heding, the Novo Research Institute,
Copenhagen, Denmark) that is highly specific for pancreatic glucagon[2] and one (4304, X) that measures the
sum of glucagon immunoreactivity. This antiserum
yields completely superimposable dilution curves of
pancreatic glucagon and extracts of porcine intestinal
mucosa. The same antiserum was used for the preparation of the antiglucagon immunosorbent, which consists
of the gamma-globulin fraction of the antiserum covalently linked to CNBr-activated Sepharose 4B
(Pharmacia Fine Chemicals, Uppsala, Sweden) according
to the manufacturer's instruction.[3]

Binding of gut glucagon to hepatic glucagon receptors was studied by means of a glucagon radioreceptor-
assay, recently developed in this laboratory.[3] Standards or unknown samples and purified porcine liver
plasma membranes (200 µg protein) were incubated in
2 ml Krebs-Ringer-Bicarbonate buffer, containing in
addition 1% gelatine, for 30 minutes at room temper-
ature. Then 100 pg ^{125}I-labeled MonoComponent glucagon (Novo Research Institute, Copenhagen, Denmark)
were added to the mixture. After a total of 45 minutes, incubation separation is performed with centrifugation. Radioactivity in the precipitate is counted in an automatic gamma-scintillator (Selektronik,
Denmark). Sensitivity of the assay is 40 pg/ml.

RESULTS AND DISCUSSION

The changes in blood glucose, gut glucagon, and
pancreatic glucagon during an oral glucose tolerance
test in a patient with reactive hypoglycemia are
shown in Figure 1. The results of affinity chromatography for glucagon immunoreactivity of a 300-ml
blood sample obtained at the nadir of hypoglycemia

at a second glucose challenge are shown in Figure 2.
The binding capacity of the column was previously
determined to be 2.5 mg of pancreatic glucagon.[3]
A standard curve from the glucagon radioreceptor-
assay described is shown in Figure 3. When purified
human gut glucagon was subjected to receptorassay, a
clear concentration-dependent inhibition of binding
of the labeled glucagon was found in each of four
separate experiments. Corresponding radioimmunoassay
and radio-receptorassay results are listed in Table 1.
It appears that concentrations of gut glucagon four
to five times higher than pancreatic glucagon are
needed to produce the same inhibition. These results
are similar to those obtained with acid-ethanol extracts of porcine intestinal mucosa, shown in Figure
4.[3]

It seems probable in view of the present results
that human gut glucagon may bind to the human hepatic
glucagon receptor also. At this stage, however, two
problems present themselves.

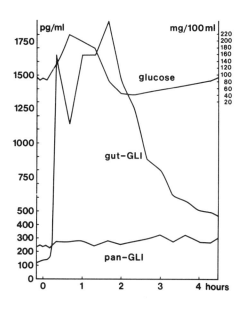

Figure 1. Gut glucagon
in reactive hypoglycemia.
Concentrations of glu-
cose, pancreatic gluca-
gon, and gut glucagon
during an oral glucose
tolerance test.

First, which are the consequences of gut glucagon binding to the hepatic receptor? A glycogenolytic activity of gut glucagon has been reported,[9] but coextracted vasoactive intestinal polypeptide[5] may be responsible for this. On the contrary, hypoglycemic activity was reported by Valverde and associates,[8] who injected a gut glucagon fraction into dogs, and by Marco and associates,[6] who investigated the metabolic consequences of endogenous gut glucagon release. Bataille and associates[1] reported stimulation of adenylate cyclase in rat liver plasma membranes when samples of these membranes were incubated

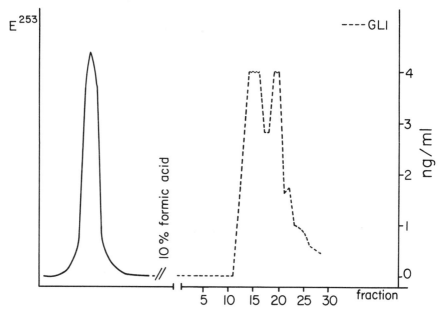

Figure 2. Affinity chromatography of human circulating gut glucagon; 300 ml plasma were incubated with 10 ml antiglucagon immunosorbent[3] for two hours, packed into a column and washed with sodium phosphate buffer. Glucagon immunoreactivity was eluted by means of 10% formic acid, and the eluted fractions assayed for immunoreactivity. Total yield was 50 µg. Content of pancreatic glucagon was less than 0.1%. Left column: readings in arbitrary units from an Uvicord (LKB), extinction coefficient (E) at 253 nm (vertical axis); collected fractions (horizontal axis).

with extracts of intestinal mucosa, but the activity was much lower than was expected from the results of binding studies - and again the results might be due to VIP-contamination.

Second, it is surprising that the secretion of pancreatic glucagon is not stimulated during hypoglycemia. We have found examples of such stimulation in other patients[7] but not in the present patient and a few others.

Clearly, this relative glucagon deficiency may be of importance in the pathogenesis of the hypoglycemia; the possibility then arises that gut glucagon may exert a kind of negative feedback control over the alpha cell.

Further experiments are necessary to clarify this problem.

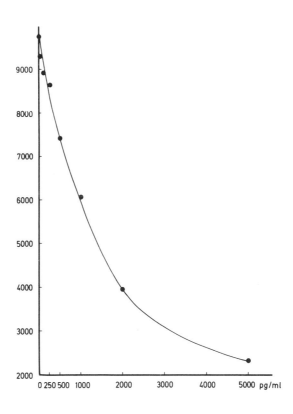

Figure 3. Standard curve from gut glucagon radioreceptorassay. Incubation conditions as described in text. Ordinate: counts in precipitate (bound fraction). Abscissa: concentration of glucagon in incubation mixture.

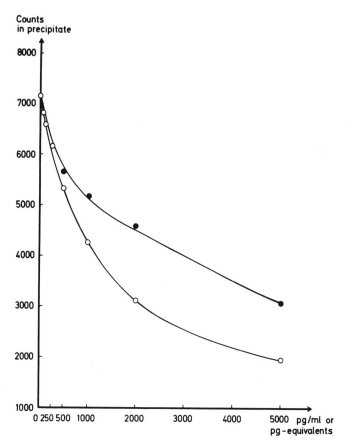

Figure 4. Binding of gut glucagon to porcine liver plasma membranes. Dilutions of pancreatic glucagon and gut glucagon are compared. Incubation conditions as described in the Methods section. Ordinate: counts in precipitate. Abscissa: concentrations of pancreatic glucagon (open circles) and concentrations of gut glucagon (closed circles), as measured by radioimmunoassay against standards of pancreatic glucagon.

Table 1. Binding of human circulating gut glucagon to porcine hepatic glucagon receptors

Concentration of gut glucagon in incubation mixture (ng/ml)*	Concentration of pancreatic glucagon that gives the same response (ng/ml)**
10	1.76
5	0.8
2	0.45

* Measured by means of specific radioimmunoassay.[4]
** Results of glucagon radioreceptorassay with standards of pancreatic glucagon.[3]

SUMMARY

In order to support the hypothesis that increased release of gut glucagon may be a pathogenic factor in reactive hypoglycemia, circulating human gut glucagon, obtained from a hypoglycemic patient, was purified by affinity chromatography and subjected to radioimmunoassay and radio-receptorassay, with pig liver plasma membranes used as the receptor. Human gut glucagon was found to compete with pancreatic glucagon for binding to receptor with an affinity similar to that observed with purified gut glucagon extracted from porcine intestinal mucosa. The results support the suggestion that gut glucagon may competitively inhibit the glycogenolytic activity of pancreatic glucagon *in vivo* under conditions with high levels of circulating gut glucagon.

References

1. Bataille DP, Freychet P, Kitabgi PE, Rosselin GE: Gut glucagon: A common receptor site with pancreatic glucagon in liver cell plasma membranes. *FEBS Lett* 30:215–218, 1973.
2. Heding LG: Radioimmunological determination of pancreatic and gut glucagon in plasma. *Diabetologia* 7:10–19, 1971.

3. Holst JJ: Development of a radioreceptor-assay for gluca-
      gon: Binding of enteroglucagon to liver plasma mem-
      branes, submitted.
4. Holst JJ, Aasted B: Production anu evaluation of glucagon
      antibodies for radioimmunoassay. *Acta Endocrinol (Kbh)*,
      in press.
5. Kerins C, Said SI: Hyperglycemic and glycogenolytic effects
      of vasoactive intestinal polypeptide. *Proc Soc Exp
      Biol Med* 142:1014-1017, 1973.
6. Marco J, Faloona GR, Unger R: Effect of endogenous intes-
      tinal glucagon-like immunoreactivity (GLI) on insulin
      secretion and glucose concentration in dogs. *J Clin
      Endocrinol Metab* 33:318-325, 1971.
7. Rehfeld JF, Heding LG, Holst JJ: Increased gut glucagon
      release as pathogenetic factor in reactive hypoglycaemia?
      Lancet 1:116-118, 1973.
8. Valverde I, Rigopoulou D, Exton J, Ohneda A, Eisentraut A,
      Unger RH: Demonstration and characterization of a
      second fraction of glucagon-like immunoreactivity in
      jejunal extracts. *Am J Med Sci* 255:415-420, 1968.
9. Valverde I, Rigopoulou D, Marco J, Faloona GR, Unger RH:
      Characterization of glucagon-like immunoreactivity.
      Diabetes 19:614-623, 1970.
10. Widdowson GM, Penton JR: Determination of serum or plasma
      glucose on the "Auto-Analyzer II" by use of the
      hexokinase reaction. *Clin Chem* 18:299-300, 1972.

THE CURRENT STATUS OF GIP

J.C. Brown, J.R. Dryburgh,
P. Moccia, R.A. Pederson

Department of Physiology, University of
British Columbia, Vancouver, British
Columbia, Canada

Gastric inhibitory polypeptide (GIP) obtained from porcine duodenal and jejunal mucosal extracts has been isolated and purified and the amino acid sequence determined.[3-7] The physiologic activities of this peptide have been described as follows: it was inhibitory for acid secretion from denervated pouches of the stomach of dogs, when the stimulus for acid secretion was pentagastrin, synthetic human gastrin I (SHG I), and histamine dihydrochloride. The stimulants for acid secretion were given in doses that produced 60% to 70% of maximum acid secretion. The degree of inhibition of pentagastrin-stimulated acid secretion was dose-dependent; maximum inhibition was obtained with GIP at an infusion rate of 1.0 µg/kg/hr.[12] Exogenous GIP also inhibited acid and pepsin secretion from innervated gastric remnants in dogs that were stimulated by insulin hypoglycemia. In these experiments, the isolated antral pouches were being perfused continuously with 0.1 M HCl.

GIP was also inhibitory for spontaneous motor activity in denervated pouches of the fundic gland area and pentagastrin-stimulated motor activity in antral pouches.[11] Two further actions of exogenously administered GIP have been described. These are stimulation of jejunal and ileal secretion[2] and release of insulin.[13] The enterogastrone-like effect (Cleator and Brown, unpublished observations) and the insulin-releasing effect, have been demonstrated in man.[9]

Development of a radioimmunoassay (RIA) for GIP has been described.[10] The antiserum used in the assay was

shown to have no cross-reactivity with glucagon, porcine secretin, porcine cholecystokinin-pancreozymin
(CCK-PZ), motilin, SHG I, vasoactive intestinal polypeptide (VIP), nor with insulin. This same antiserum
has been used in immunofluorescent studies to identify
the duodenojejunal cell that contains GIP,[14] which has
been identified as an endocrine polypeptide cell of
the APUD series and, provisionally, as the already
recognized D_1 cell.

In man immunoreactive GIP (IR-GIP) has been shown
to be released after ingestion of a meal. Mean fasting levels of IR-GIP, approximately 250 pg/ml of
serum, have been shown to rise almost immediately
after eating, to reach a peak in excess of 1000 pg/ml
within 45 minutes of the beginning of the meal, and
then to fall slowly over the next four hours.
Examination of the pattern of release showed that
there was at least a biphasic release of IR-GIP.

When oral administration of glucose, fat, and protein were investigated separately, it was found that
the initial peak response could be reproduced by
glucose, and the late plateau response by a triglyceride suspension (Lipomul). Protein, as a 280-g filet
steak (with 200 ml water) or meat extract (30 g
Bovril) did not produce an increase in serum IR-GIP.
The latter two stimulants would be expected to stimulate gastric acid secretion by the release of
gastrin and activation of other intragastric mechanisms, and the acidic gastric content would then be
passed on into the duodenum. The lack of an increase in IR-GIP was suggestive that acid in the
duodenum was not a secretagogue for IR-GIP release.
Further indirect evidence for lack of stimulation
of IR-GIP release by acid has been supplied by
studies in normal human volunteers, in whom pentagastrin was administered intravenously and the gastric contents allowed to pass into the duodenum.

Dogs have been prepared with extrinsically denervated pouches of the body of the stomach and Mann-
Bollman fistulae constructed to allow the introduction of secretagogues directly into the duodenum,
about 2 cm distal to the pyloroduodenal junction.
In addition, acid gastric contents were prevented
from entering the proximal small bowel by inserting
a wide-bore gastric cannula into the gastric remnant
and also by the preparation of a low gastrojejunostomy,
30 cm below the ligament of Treitz. The pyloroduodenal junction was divided and a pouch constructed of

the distal stomach. Acid secretion from the body of
the stomach was stimulated by a continuous intravenous
infusion of pentagastrin (1.0 µg/kg/hr) or histamine
dihydrochloride (10 µg/kg/hr) and after establishment
of a plateau of acid secretion, the duodenum was perfused with a solution of 20% dextrose (1.0 g/kg) or
60 ml of corn oil or 60 ml of 0.15 M HCl, introduced
via the Mann-Bollman fistula.

Both corn oil and glucose produced significant inhibition of pentagastrin-stimulated acid secretion
from the denervated fundic gland area pouches, with
simultaneous increases in serum IR-GIP (Figs. 1 & 2).
Corn oil was also tested against histamine-dihydro-
chloride-stimulated acid secretion, and a similar
degree of inhibition of acid secretion with an

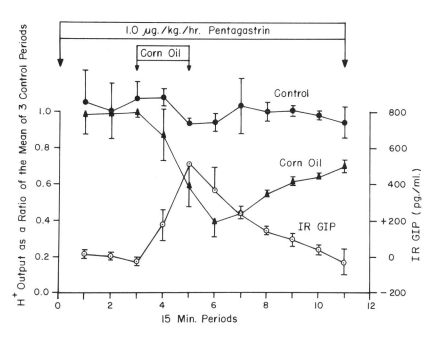

Figure 1. Effect of a 30-min duodenal perfusion of corn oil
(1.91 ml/min) on acid secretion from denervated fundic gland
area pouches stimulated by 1.0 µg/kg/hr pentagastrin and on
serum IR-GIP. Controls received only pentagastrin throughout
the experiment.

increase in circulating IR-GIP was observed (Fig. 3).
A similar inhibition of acid secretion was obtained
after duodenal perfusion with 0.15 M HCl.   In this
instance, however, there was no simultaneous increase
in circulating IR-GIP (Fig. 4).   It would appear then
that IR-GIP is not released when acid from the stomach
passes into the duodenum and therefore, perhaps, plays
no role in an autoregulatory mechanism.   The latter
observation lends support to the hypothesis of
Andersson and associates[1] that acid in the duodenal
bulb inhibited acid secretion from the stomach by a
humoral agent that was different from the characterized gastrointestinal peptides, which they named
bulbogastrone.
    Purification of GIP from EG stage I to EG stage II,[6]
began with a separation stage in which ion exchange
chromatography with carboxymethyl cellulose 11 (CM 11)
was used.   In this purification stage, three fractions

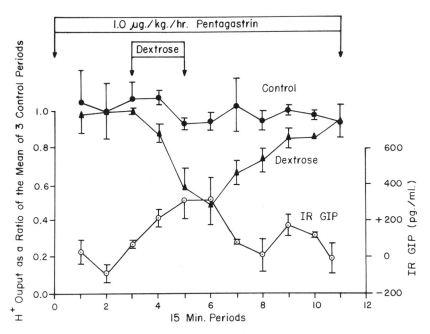

Figure 2.   Effect of a 30-min duodenal perfusion of 20% dextrose (1.0 g/kg) on acid secretion from denervated fundic gland
area pouches stimulated by 1.0 µg/kg/hr pentagastrin and on
serum IR-GIP.   Controls received only pentagastrin throughout
the experiment.

were separated and lettered A, B, and C. Fraction B contained almost pure GIP with little CCK-PZ activity, and fraction C contained the bulk of the CCK-PZ activity with little GIP. Fraction A, which because of the nature of the separatory procedure, would contain neutral or slightly acidic peptide material, was also inhibitory for acid secretion (Fig. 5).

Radioimmunoassay performed on this fraction showed very little IR-GIP, and polyacrylamide gel electrophoresis revealed it to contain several peptide bands. The material was quite impure and it is suggested that a potent inhibitor for acid secretion is present in this fraction.

The intravenous infusion of porcine GIP in man and dog produced inhibition of acid secretion by the stomach and release of insulin from the pancreas. These effects were observed when the dose of GIP administered raised the serum IR-GIP to levels that were less than could be obtained by feeding a mixed

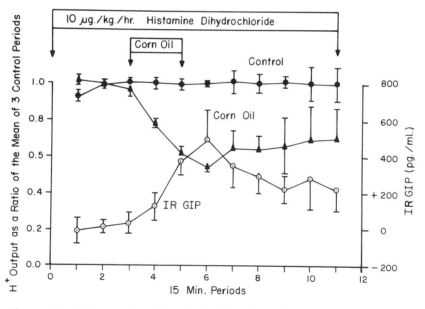

Figure 3. Effect of a 30-min duodenal perfusion of corn oil (1.91 ml/min) on acid secretion from denervated fundic gland area pouches stimulated by 10 µg/kg/hr histamine dihydrochloride and on serum IR-GIP. Controls received only histamine dihydrochloride throughout the experiment.

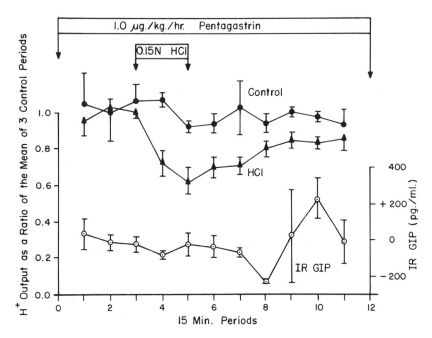

Figure 4. Effect of a 30-min duodenal perfusion of 0.15 N HCl
(1.91 ml/min) on acid secretion from denervated fundic gland
area pouches stimulated by 1.0 µg/kg/hr pentagastrin and on
IR-GIP. Controls received only pentagastrin throughout the
experiment.

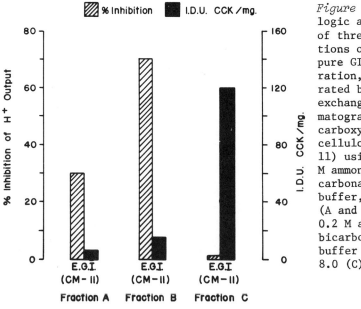

Figure 5. Bio-
logic activity
of three frac-
tions of an im-
pure GIP prepa-
ration, sepa-
rated by ion-
exchange chro-
matography on
carboxymethyl
cellulose (CM
11) using 0.01
M ammonium bi-
carbonate
buffer, pH 7.8
(A and B) and
0.2 M ammonium
bicarbonate
buffer pH
8.0 (C).

meal. When glucose was ingested, peak IR-GIP levels
in serum were reached within 45 minutes, the time
course of which correlated well with the increase in
serum glucose concentration and preceded the peak release of insulin. The time course of events was compatible with the suggestion that GIP is taking part
in the physiologic regulation of insulin secretion.
When the role of GIP as an enterogastrone is considered, however, the immediate release of GIP on feeding would produce inhibition of acid secretion at an
inappropriate time, when gastric digestion would be
far from complete. The time course of release of
IR-GIP when fat was ingested showed a peak response
between two and three hours, when gastric digestion
was more likely to be complete and when inhibition
of acid secretion would be appropriate. These observations suggest the possibility that at least
two immunoreactive components of GIP are being released, one by glucose and one by fat.

Serial dilutions of serum samples obtained 45 minutes after the ingestion of glucose and 150 minutes
after eating a mixed meal, were subjected to RIA for
GIP. Figure 6 shows that sera and fasting serum
samples (all from the same subject), obtained after
introduction of glucose or Lipomul, dilute out along
the standard curve, which demonstrates an appropriate
dose-response relationship between IR-GIP and antiserum under the RIA conditions. This does not necessarily mean that the IR-GIP is homogeneous. When
2.0 ml aliquots of the serum samples were subjected
to column chromatography on Sephadex G50, more than
one IR-GIP was observed (Fig. 7). The majority of
the immunoreactivity, however, eluted from the column at volumes corresponding to polypeptide with a
molecular weight of 5,000. There was also a larger
molecular weight component demonstrating immunoreactivity and a component eluting with the void volume.

SUMMARY

Porcine GIP administered intravenously to man, produced effects that were characteristic of both enterogastrone and insulin. The inability of duodenal
acidification to release IR-GIP suggests that yet
another peptide may be involved in the inhibition of
acid secretion, possibly bulbogastrone. The time-
course of release of IR-GIP after ingestion of oral

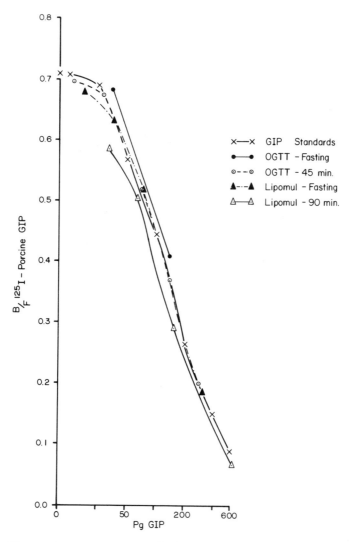

Figure 6. Comparison of the immunoreactivities of GIP and human sera obtained in the fasting situation and following oral ingestion of glucose (45 min) and Lipomul (150 min). The same subject was used in both experiments.

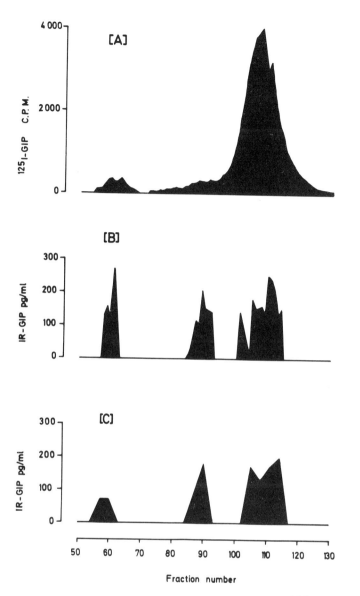

Figure 7. Sephadex G50 chromatography of ^{125}I–GIP (A) and human sera obtained 150 minutes after the ingestion of a mixed meal (B) and 45 minutes after ingestion of 75 g of dextrose (C).

glucose supports a possible role for GIP in a physiologic mechanism for insulin release. The time-course
of release of IR-GIP after ingestion of oral triglyceride supports a possible role for GIP in a physiologic mechanism for the inhibition of gastric acid
secretion. IR-GIP exists in more than one form but
the significance of this observation remains to be
elucidated.

Acknowledgments

This work was supported by a research grant from the Medical
Research Council of Canada.

References

1. Andersson S, Nilsson G, Sjodin L, Uvnäs B: Mechanism of
    duodenal inhibition of gastric acid secretion, in
    Andersson S (ed), *Nobel Symposium 16. Frontiers in
    Gastrointestinal Hormone Research,* Stockholm: Almquist
    and Wiksell, 1973, pp 223-238.
2. Barbezat GO, Grossman MI: Intestinal secretion: Stimula-
    tion by peptides. *Science* 174:422-424, 1971.
3. Brown JC: A gastric inhibitory polypeptide: I. The amino
    acid composition and the tryptic peptides. *Can J
    Biochem* 49:255-261, 1970.
4. Brown JC, Dryburgh JR: A gastric inhibitory polypeptide:
    II. The complete amino acid sequence. *Can J Biochem*
    49:867-872, 1971.
5. Brown JC, Mutt V, Pederson RA: Further purification of a
    polypeptide demonstrating enterogastrone activity.
    J Physiol 209:57-64, 1970.
6. Brown JC, Pederson RA: A multiparameter study on the
    action of preparations containing cholecystokinin-
    pancreozymin. *Scand J Gastroenterol* 5:537-541, 1970.
7. Brown JC, Pederson RA, Jorpes JE, Mutt V: Preparation of
    highly active enterogastrone. *Can J Physiol Pharmacol*
    47:113-114, 1969.
8. Cataland S, Crockett SE, Brown JC, Mazzaferri EL: Gastric
    inhibitory polypeptide (GIP) stimulation by oral glucose
    in man. *J Clin Endocrinol Metab* 39:223-228, 1974.
9. Dupre J, Ross SA, Watson D, Brown JC: Stimulation of in-
    sulin secretion by gastric inhibitory polypeptide in
    man. *J Clin Endocrinol Metab* 37:826-828, 1973.

10. Kuzio M, Dryburgh JR, Malloy KM, Brown JC: Radioimmuno-
    assay for gastric inhibitory polypeptide. *Gastroenter-
    ology* 66:357-364, 1974.
11. Pederson RA: *Physiological Studies on Gastric Inhibitory
    Polypeptide*, thesis. University of British Columbia,
    Vancouver, 1972.
12. Pederson RA, Brown JC: Inhibition of histamine-, penta-
    gastrin-, and insulin-stimulated canine gastric
    secretion by pure "gastric inhibitory polypeptide."
    Gastroenterology 62:393-400, 1972.
13. Pederson RA, Schubert HE, Brown JC: The insulinotropic
    action of gastric inhibitory polypeptide. *Can J
    Physiol Pharmacol*, in press.
14. Polak JM, Bloom SR, Kuzio M, Brown JC, Pearse AGE: Cellu-
    lar localization of gastric inhibitory polypeptide in
    the duodenum and jejunum. *Gut* 14:284-288, 1973.

CURRENT STATUS OF MOTILIN

J.C. Brown, J.R. Dryburgh

Department of Physiology, University of
British Columbia, Vancouver, British
Columbia, Canada

The intraduodenal instillation of alkaline buffer solutions or fresh porcine pancreatic juice increased the motor activity in transplanted pouches of the fundic gland area of the stomach of dogs.[5] A crude extract containing cholecystokinin-pancreozymin (CCK-PZ) (Boots Pancreozymin) was found to produce similar changes in motor activity, whereas purer CCK-PZ (GIH) did not.[1] A simple purification of Boots Pancreozymin, with Sephadex G75, separated a substance that was stimulatory for fundic pouch motor activity from material with pancreozymin activity.[2] Final purification of this substance[3] was achieved, with a side fraction obtained in the purification of secretin used as a starting material.[6]

The amino acid sequence has been reported as: Phe-Val-Pro-Ile-Phe-Thr-Tyr-Gly-Glu-Leu-Gln-Arg-Met-Glu-Glu-Lys-Glu-Arg-Asn-Lys-Gly-Gln, a 22-amino acid polypeptide with a molecular weight of 2700,[4] which was named motilin. Pure motilin, injected intravenously into dogs in doses as low as 50 ng/kg, induced increased motor activity in pouches of the body and of the antrum of the stomach, similar to those observed after alkalinization of the duodenum.

An analog of motilin has been synthesized, nor-leucine-13-motilin,[9] which has been shown to possess almost the complete biologic activity of natural porcine motilin (Fig. 1). A comparison of the electrophoretic mobilities of the tryptic peptides of the synthetic analog and natural porcine motilin, revealed the absence of the acidic peptide TR3 in the natural material.[8] Kinetic studies with leucine

aminopeptidase and dansyl-Edman degradations on this
peptide, revealed the presence of glutamine at position 14 and not glutamic acid as previously reported.
It was suggested that in the earlier preparation of
natural porcine motilin, deamidation of 14-glutamine
had occurred. From these studies it is apparent
that neither the 13-methionine nor the 14-amidated
glutamic acid contributes significantly to biologic
activity.

Antisera to porcine motilin have been raised in
guinea pigs by multiple injections of both conjugated
and unconjugated polypeptide and a radioimmunoassay
has been developed.[7] The antisera demonstrated no
cross-reactivity with glucagon, gastrin, secretin,
CCK-PZ, GIP, or VIP (Fig. 2). Cross-reactivity
studies with "Boots Pancreozymin" revealed the
preparation to contain 140±40 pg immunoreactive
motilin (IR-M) per microgram of "Pancreozymin" (Fig.
3). By bioassay, pure porcine motilin was found to
be 10,000 times purer than "Pancreozymin," a value
which compares well with the results obtained by
radioimmunoassay. It would appear then that natural
porcine motilin is the material that was present in
"Pancreozymin."

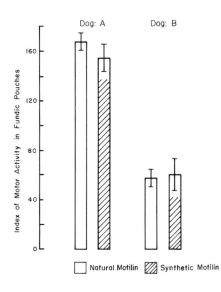

Figure 1. Comparison of the
biologic activity of synthetic norleucine-13-motilin
and natural porcine motilin
assayed by measuring in-
creases in motor activity
in denervated pouches of the
fundic gland area, after
single intravenous injections
of either peptide. Each pair
of results represents the
mean ± SEM of four experiments in two dogs.

The mean (± SEM) fasting serum levels for IR-M in eight dogs has been determined to be 294±44 pg/ml, whereas the motility index was 30.6±5.0. During duodenal perfusion with 50 ml 0.3 M Tris buffer, pH 10.2, the serum level rose to 498±100 pg/ml (2 min) and to a maximum of 916±92 pg/ml at 5 min (Fig. 4). We have begun studies on the distribution of IR-M in acid-alcohol extracts of various regions of the gastrointestinal tract of hogs. With a value of 100 assigned to the upper jejunal area, the following values have been obtained: fundus 0, antrum 0, duodenum 7, jejunum 100, ileum 0.06.

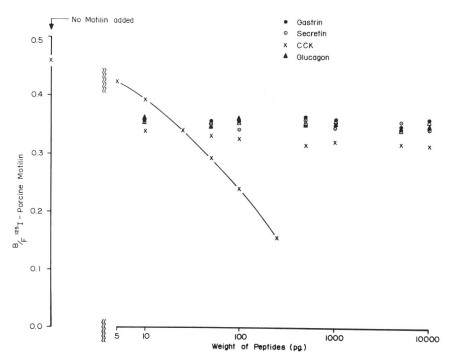

Figure 2. Comparative immunoreactivities of natural porcine motilin, synthetic human gastrin (SHG I), synthetic glucagon, natural porcine secretin, CCK-PZ (10% pure) (x——x = motilin).

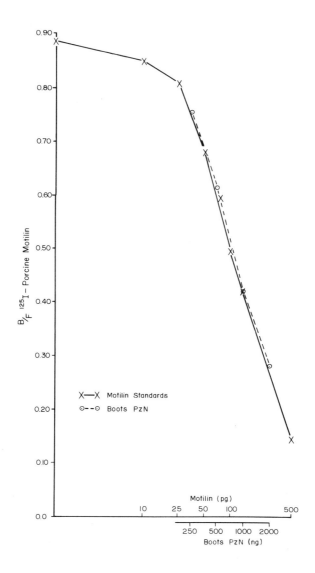

Figure 3. Comparative immunoreactivities of motilin and Boots' Pancreozymin. The 1.0 μg/ml dilution of pancreozymin was fitted to the motilin standard curve and other points plotted accordingly.

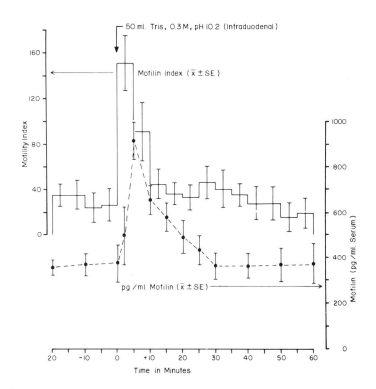

Figure 4. Fundic pouch motor activity expressed as an index of motility and circulating levels of IR-M in pg/ml serum after intraduodenal infusion of 0.3 M Tris buffer pH 10.2. Each motility index represents a five-minute period whilst the serum levels of motilin are measured at a specific time. Each result is the mean (± SEM) of five experiments in two dogs.

SUMMARY

   Comparison of the tryptic peptides of a synthetic motilin analog (nor-leucine-13-motilin) revealed the presence of glutamine in position 14. The synthetic peptide was immunologically indistinguishable from natural porcine motilin and possessed almost complete biologic activity. Radioimmunoassay revealed that "Boots Pancreozymin" contained IR-M at the concentration suggested by bioassay and that after alkalinization of the duodenojejunal region in dogs, there

553

was an increase in circulating IR-M that corresponded
to the increase in motor activity in the denervated
fundic gland area pouches.

Acknowledgments

This work was supported by a grant from the Medical Research
Council of Canada.

References

1. Brown JC: Presence of a gastric motor-stimulating property
    in duodenal extracts. *Gastroenterology* 52:225-229,
    1967.
2. Brown JC, Parkes CO: Effect on fundic pouch motor activity
    of stimulatory and inhibitory fractions separated from
    pancreozymin. *Gastroenterology* 53:731-736, 1967.
3. Brown JC, Cook MA, Dryburgh JR: Motilin, a gastric motor
    activity-stimulating polypeptide: Final purification,
    amino acid composition, and C-terminal residues.
    Gastroenterology 62:401-404, 1972.
4. Brown JC, Cook MA, Dryburgh JR: Motilin, a gastric motor
    activity stimulating polypeptide: The complete amino
    acid sequence. *Can J Biochem* 51:533-537, 1973.
5. Brown JC, Johnson LP, Magee DF: Effect of duodenal alkalin-
    ization on gastric motility. *Gastroenterology* 50:333-
    339, 1966.
6. Brown JC, Mutt V, Dryburgh JR: The further purification of
    motilin, a gastric motor activity stimulating polypep-
    tide from the mucosa of the small intestine of hogs.
    Can J Physiol Pharmacol 49:399-405, 1971.
7. Dryburgh JR, Brown JC: Radioimmunoassay for motilin,
    submitted.
8. Schubert H, Brown JC: Correction to the amino acid sequence
    of porcine motilin. *Can J Biochem* 52:7-8, 1974.
9. Wünsch E, Brown JC, Deimer KH, Drees F, Jaeger E, Musiol J,
    Scharf R, Stocker H, Thamm P, Wendelberger G: Zur
    Synthese von Norleucin-13-motilin. *Z Naturforsch* [C]
    28C:235-240, 1973.

BULBOGASTRONE

Sven Andersson

Department of Pharmacology,
Karolinska Institutet,
Stockholm, Sweden

The term bulbogastrone has been used to describe a humoral principle that is released from the duodenal bulb by acid and inhibits the gastric secretion of acid. The physiologic and biochemical evidence for the existence of this gastric inhibitory principle has recently been reviewed in detail[1] and therefore will not be further discussed in this presentation. Instead, the following questions will be considered:

Which gastric functions other than acid secretion will be affected when the duodenal bulb is acidified?

Can the duodenal bulb mechanism be stimulated by physiologic means, other than high acidity?

Is there any evidence for the existence of the duodenal pH-sensitive mechanism in species other than the dog?

Since the studies (for example, on the effects of various denervation procedures) that pertain to these questions are still not as extensive as those on the canine bulbar mechanism and its action on gastric secretion, it is better at the present state of knowledge not to use the word bulbogastrone but to speak about the duodenal bulb mechanism(s).

Figure 1 shows the profound inhibition of the acid secretory response of a Heidenhain pouch to gastrin after acidification of an isolated duodenal bulb. Similar acidification of the distal duodenum or the ileum was ineffective. What happens to the secretion of pepsin after acidification of the bulb? Recently, Nilsson[7] has shown that the pepsin output from Pavlov pouches in response to a meal was

significantly reduced upon acidification of the
duodenal bulb. In addition, the concentration of
pepsin in the gastric juice was reduced. Table 1
shows the mean values for the outputs of acid and
pepsin, as well as the pepsin concentration, with
and without acidification of the duodenal bulb.

In a recent series of experiments (Andersson and
Hjelmquist, unpublished data), we have attempted to
find out if acidification of the duodenal bulb influences the motor activity of the stomach. As yet,
we have only preliminary results but they suggest
that the bulbar mechanism can affect the motor activity in isolated fundic pouches. Figure 2 shows
a pressure recording from a Heidenhain pouch. In

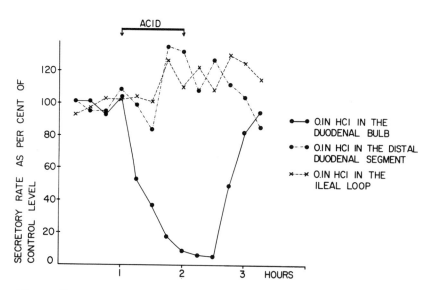

Figure 1. Acid output from Heidenhain pouch in response to
gastrin after perfusion of the duodenal bulb, the distal duodenal pouch, and an isolated ileal loop with 0.1 M HCl.
Each curve represents the mean value of three or four experiments. (Reproduced, with permission of *Acta Physiol Scand*
71:368–378, 1967.)

this instance we have studied the effect of bulbar
perfusion with either saline or acid on the spontaneous motor activity of the pouch. From the figure
it is evident that acidification of the duodenal bulb
more or less extinguishes the motor activity in the
pouch.

It is not yet possible to say anything definite
about the mechanism behind the observed effects on
pepsin secretion and motility. The findings may be
taken as preliminary evidence, however, that the
bulbar mechanism plays a physiologic role in controlling the pepsin secretion of the stomach as well
as its motility.

In a recent series of experiments, Nilsson[8] has
studied the effects of various hypertonic solutions
in the duodenal bulb on secretory responses from
Pavlov pouches (Table 2). As can be seen from this

Table 1. Acid output, pepsin output, and concentration in Pavlov pouch dogs in response to a test meal with and
without duodenal bulb acidification during the first
postprandial hour

		Hours after feeding			
	Basal hour	1	2	3	
ACID OUTPUT	0.07	4.73	4.61	3.40	Without acid*
mEq	0.05	1.98	2.47	3.23	With acid**
% inhibition	–	68	46	5	
PEPSIN OUTPUT	–	3204	1975	1465	Without acid*
units	–	1139	1140	1243	With acid**
% inhibition	–	64	42	15	
PEPSIN CONC.	–	215	141	150	Without acid*
units/ml	–	151	139	136	With acid**
% inhibition	–	30	2	9	

*   Mean of 25 experiments on five dogs

** Mean of 19 experiments on five dogs

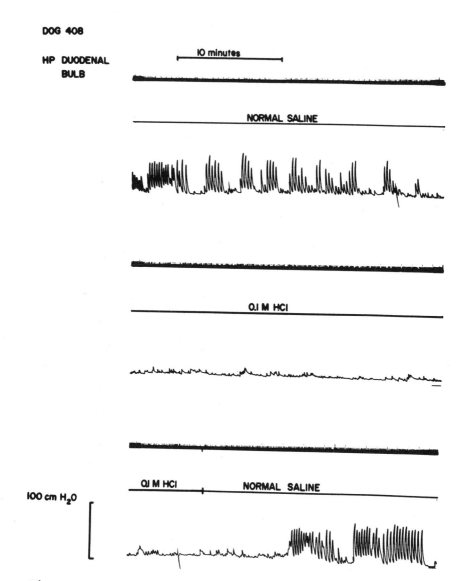

DOG 408

HP DUODENAL
BULB

10 minutes

NORMAL SALINE

0.1 M HCl

0.1 M HCl   NORMAL SALINE

100 cm H$_2$O

Figure 2. Inhibition of spontaneous motor activity in a Heidenhain pouch by perfusion of the isolated duodenal bulb with
hydrochloric acid.

table, acid produced its usual inhibition of gastric acid secretion, whereas none of the hypertonic solutions gave any inhibition. These studies suggest, therefore, that the duodenal inhibitory mechanism, which is sensitive to hypertonicity of the intestinal contents,[4] is located further down the small intestine. The finding that bulbar perfusion with acetylcholine produced gastric secretory inhibition, may indicate that the release mechanism for bulbogastrone is under cholinergic control.

In most studies on the inhibitory effects of duodenal acidification on gastric secretion, the dog has been the animal of choice. Several studies, however, have now been done on cats. Unfortunately, the results are divergent inasmuch as some authors[5] have found powerful gastric secretory inhibition and others[2,9] have been unsuccessful in this respect. Therefore, the question of whether or not a pH-sensitive mechanism inhibiting gastric acid secretion exists in the cat still seems to be open. In man, several studies[3,10] show that instillation of acid into the duodenum inhibits both acid and pepsin secretion. The localization of the inhibitory mechanism in the human duodenum is unknown.

Table 2. Mean gastric acid output (percent of control) in response to pentagastrin during duodenal bulb perfusion with acid, hypertonic solutions and acetylcholine

Bulbar perfusion with	Half-hour periods (duodenal perfusion during periods 1 and 2)				
	1	2	3	4	Mean of:
0.1 N HCl	40	14	24	78	9 experiments in 3 dogs
40% glucose	105	94	95	107	9 experiments in 3 dogs
40% peptone	113	110	114	126	7 experiments in 2 dogs
40% NaCl	102	103	101	99	9 experiments in 3 dogs
0.1% acetylcholine	60	85	95	90	6 experiments in 3 dogs

In a separate study,[6] we have tried to find evidence
for the existence of a duodenal inhibitory mechanism
in the rat in the following way. Gastric secretion in
groups of pylorus-ligated rats was compared with that
in groups of rats that had various duodenal ligations.
In one group, the duodenal ligation was placed immediately proximal to the entrance of the bile duct; in
another it was placed halfway between the pylorus and
the entrance of the bile duct. If we kept the rats
ligated for 10 to 16 hours, the acid output was progressively reduced, the further away from the pylorus
the ligature was placed (Fig. 3). The reduced acid
output was due exclusively to a reduction in acid
concentration. Since the acid gastric juice had free
access to the duodenum, and since it is known that
hydrogen ions are effectively eliminated by the duodenum, partly by absorption, it would be expected
that more hydrogen ions were absorbed with greater
length of the segment of the duodenum that was exposed to the gastric juice. With 10 and 16 hours of
ligation, therefore, it was impossible to determine

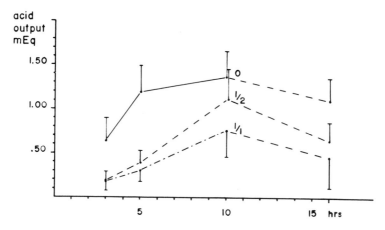

Figure 3. Gastric acid output in rats subjected to pyloric (0)
and duodenal (1/2, 1/1) ligation during 3, 5, 10 and 16 hours,
respectively.   0 = ligature at the pylorus;   1/1 = ligature
immediately proximal to the entrance of the bile duct;
1/2 = ligature halfway between pylorus and the entrance of
the bile duct.

whether the reduced acid output after the duodenal
ligations was due to inhibition of gastric secretion
or to a simple removal of hydrogen ions by absorption
through the duodenal mucosa.

By shortening the period of ligation to five or to
three hours, it was found that the volume as well as
acid output was decreased by the two duodenal ligations. In addition, it was shown that there was no
statistically significant difference in either volume
or acid output between duodenal ligations 1/1 and
1/2 in both the five-hour and three-hour groups.
Thus, it seems unlikely that absorption of hydrogen
ion is the major cause of gastric secretory inhibition. Instead, this observation indicates that the
upper duodenum of the rat contains a pH-sensitive
inhibitory mechanism similar to the one that has
been demonstrated in the duodenal bulb of dogs.

SUMMARY

In a series of experiments the importance of the
duodenal bulb for regulating gastric functions has
been investigated. Acidification of the isolated
duodenal bulb in dogs inhibits gastric acid and
pepsin secretion as well as spontaneous pressure
activity in gastric pouches. Possible mechanisms
behind these effects are discussed. A similar pH-
sensitive, gastric inhibitory mechanism has also
been shown to exist in the upper duodenum of the rat.
Perfusion of the canine bulb with various hypertonic
solutions had no effect on gastric secretion, whereas
acetylcholine produced a certain degree of secretory
inhibition.

References

1. Andersson S: Bulbogastrone, in Chey WY, Brooks FP (eds),
        Endocrinology of the Gut, Thorofare NJ: Charles B.
        Slack, Inc., 1974, pp 116-125.
2. Emås S, Svensson SO, Borg I: Effect of duodenal acidifi-
        cation or exogenous secretin on acid gastric secretion
        stimulated by histamine, pentagastrin or human gastrin
        I in conscious cats. *Digestion* 5:17-30, 1971.

3. Johnston D, Duthie HL: Inhibition of gastric secretion in
    the human stomach: Effect of acid in the duodenum.
    Lancet   2:1032-1036, 1965.
4. Konturek S, Grossman MI: Effect of perfusion of intestinal
    loops with acid, fat, or dextrose on gastric secretion.
    Gastroenterology   49:481-489, 1965.
5. Konturek S, Dubiel J, Gabrys B: Effect of acid infusion
    into various levels of the intestine on gastric and
    pancreatic secretion in the cat.   *Gut*   10:749-753, 1969.
6. Lundberg B, Andersson S: The role of the upper duodenum
    in controlling gastric acid secretion in the rat.   *Scand
    J Gastroenterol*   9:623-627, 1974.
7. Nilsson G: Effect of acid in the duodenal bulb on acid
    and pepsin responses to test meal in dogs, submitted.
8. Nilsson G: Effect of bulbar perfusion with acid, hyper-
    tonic solutions and acetylcholine on gastric acid
    secretion in dog, submitted.
9. Stening GF, Johnson LR, Grossman MI: Effect of secretin
    on acid and pepsin secretion in cat and dog.
    Gastroenterology   56:468-475, 1969.
10. Wormsley KG: Response to duodenal acidification in man:
    II. Effects on the gastric secretory response to
    pentagastrin.   *Scand J Gastroenterol*   5:207-215,
    1970.

CHYMODENIN: AN OVERVIEW

Joel W. Adelson

Department of Physiology, University of
California, San Francisco, California

This presentation is intended to be a general introduction to chymodenin, a peptide newly isolated
from porcine duodenum, which may well be a gastrointestinal hormone. First, I will briefly trace
the molecule's somewhat complicated early history,
then present the scheme finally developed for the
purification of the substance, focus upon the most
interesting aspect of its activity as we presently
understand it, and indicate how the action of the
molecule is likely to alter our view of the digestive
process. The reader who desires experimental details
is referred to the several publications subsequently
cited.

THE PEPTIDE'S EARLY HISTORY

The early history of the peptide is brief but complex. It is set forth here in the hope of clarifying
for the reader the flow of ideas and motivations,
both logical and serendipitous, which gave rise to
the final purification of the molecule. In 1967 I
began isolating various subcellular fractions of the
pancreas of the rat and incubating these subcellular
fractions in the presence of porcine duodenal extracts
which contained either secretin or CCK-PZ. These
studies were motivated by the hope that the interactions between the hormone-containing extracts and
the pancreatic organelles, would give clues to the
mechanisms of action of the hormones. The duodenal
extracts used in these studies were prepared commercially by the alcohol extraction method of Crick,
Harper and Raper;[8] in addition to the known hormones,

the extracts contained a variety of other uncharacterized substances including quite a number of peptides. The CCK-PZ-containing duodenal extract was
found to contain a material or materials which,
when incubated in low concentrations, *in vitro*,
with isolated rat pancreatic zymogen granules, led
to the rapid release of amylase and protease from
the granules.[3] The secretin-containing extract was
far less active in this regard.

In those days, before we had the present "dogmas"
that peptide hormones do not enter cells and that
peptide hormones require a "second messenger" to
reach the effector site of hormone action within the
cell, it was quite reasonable to imagine that the
action of the CCK-PZ-containing extract on the
zymogen granules mimicked, *in vitro*, what really
occurred in the cell; that is, that the mechanism
of action of CCK-PZ was directly to cause the zymogen granules to lyse and release their contents
into the pancreatic acini. We were quickly disappointed, however. Professor Viktor Mutt kindly
sent us some purer CCK-PZ with which we could run
the obvious control experiment intended to confirm
that it was, indeed, the CCK-PZ itself within the
Crick and associates extract, and not some other
substance, which released amylase from the granules.
In fact, no enzyme release was observed after the
incubation of the pure CCK-PZ with the granules,
even when extremely high doses of CCK-PZ were employed.[3,4] The negative result meant we had to
attribute the enzyme-releasing activity to another
substance and investigate further. The strategic
questions at this point were, if a biologically
active substance could be isolated from duodenal
extracts, what role it would play, if any, in pancreatic secretion, since CCK-PZ was thought to be
the unique duodenal hormone substance involved in
regulating the release of digestive enzymes from the
pancreas? Second, was there any real connection
between the enzyme-releasing activity and a yet-to-
be-found physiologic activity for the substance?

Our interest in the new substance was stimulated
further by several facets of its action. We were
satisfied that the activity was not due to secretin,
CCK-PZ, or a bile salt used in preparation of the
extract.[3,4] Thus it appeared to be a new or unique
activity. Enzymatic digestion revealed that the

molecule was proteinaceous in character; gel filtration chromatography indicated that it was likely a
peptide. We estimated from the apparent molecular
weight that the material was active *in vitro* at
10^{-6} M or lower.[4] These characteristics indicated
that there was some similarity to the other active
duodenal factors.

STARTING MATERIAL FOR PURIFICATION

The next problem was to find a more suitable source
of material for purification with respect to cost and
general availability; it would have to be obtainable
in the rather substantial quantities necessary to
attempt a purification. The late Professor J.E.
Jorpes and Professor Mutt were kind enough to let me
examine all the side-fractions produced during routine preparation of secretin and CCK-PZ in their
laboratory. The requisite enzyme-releasing activity
was found in a fraction produced at the stage of the
Mutt purification[11] where secretin was separated from
CCK-PZ. Secretin and the starting material were soluble in acidic methanol, which separated the material
from CCK-PZ. Neutralization of the methanol resulted
in precipitation of the starting material away from
the secretin. The starting material was thus an
*a*cidic *m*ethanol *s*oluble *n*eutral *i*nsoluble precipitate,
called by its acronym "AMESNI."

PURIFICATION OF THE PEPTIDE

The peptide was purified by chromatographic techniques. The development of the purification, however,
involved changes in the basic rationale which may be
confusing to the reader who tries to relate the
original enzyme-releasing activity *in vitro* to the
enzyme-specific secretion-stimulating activity described later. (I believe the occurrence of such
changes in rationale is not uncommon during hormone
purification, where the focus upon one activity
during purification may supplant the focus upon
another for a variety of reasons.) When AMESNI was
applied to SP-Sephadex, a rough separation of several peaks of basic peptides was obtained. When tested
for enzyme-releasing activity, several of these

peptidic peaks showed the ability to elicit enzyme
release from the zymogen granules, which raised the
question of the specificity of interaction of the
materials with the granules. In order to guide the
purification further, it was necessary to select a
more specific and biologic criterion of activity;
the ability of the material to alter the rate of
secretion of pancreatic fluid and protein by the rat
was therefore selected as a potential activity.
This choice of activity was rather arbitrary and
was based simply on the notion that if the peptides
interacted with pancreatic organelles, overall
effects on pancreatic secretion might also be predicted. If no such activity were observed, we would
have had to look elsewhere, but the problem of what
type of activity to seek would have been great, especially if we had to look beyond the pancreas.
Fortunately, one of the peaks obtained on SP-Sephadex
indeed showed both requisite activities; intravenous
injection in microgram doses in the rat stimulated
pancreatic fluid flow *in vivo,* and the material
caused enzyme release *in vitro,* so the purification
was continued on this material.[1,2]

Those persons familiar with the exigencies of hormone purification might well anticipate the next
problems: first, it is not possible to know before
purification how great the specific activity of the
final material will be, and therefore how little
active material may be obtained following any purification step from a large-appearing mass of starting
material. Second, as purification proceeds, the number of chromatographic fractions obtained multiplies
geometrically, and unless a convenient method is
available for quantitatively assaying the activity of
the materials obtained, the work becomes extraordinarily cumbersome. In our hands, it was next to impossible to assay the effect of all individual fractions upon pancreatic flow in the rat, so we pooled
fractions in large groups, suffering great loss of
resolution for the sake of convenience of assay.
This loss of resolution, combined with the high degree of variance obtained when observing pancreatic
flow in the rat, caused us to follow a false trail
on a number of occasions. We were finally able to
develop a satisfactory purification scheme[1,2] by
combining our two biologic assays with the counter-
migration-of-dye gel electrophoresis system of

Ahlroth and Mutt.[7] This electrophoresis system allowed us to visualize the peptides present in each major fraction clearly and to temper our choice of which active materials to include for further purification.

THE CHEMISTRY OF CHYMODENIN

The purification scheme shown in Table 1 summarizes the method finally developed to purify the peptide. The material obtained from Professor Mutt, "AMESNI," was sequentially subjected to two cation exchangers, both eluted by ammonium bicarbonate-containing gradients, followed by chromatography on a quarternary amine-containing anion exchanger at elevated pH under equilibrium conditions. Thus, the amphoteric nature of the substance was advantageous in purification. At times, we also found it useful to follow the ion exchangers with a single pass through a long gel filtration column to remove trace lower molecular weight contaminants.

Table 1. General purification scheme for chymodenin*

Step	Treatment	Conditions
1	Desalting by gel filtration on Sephadex G25, coarse	In ammonium bicarbonate
2	Cation exchange chromatography on SP-Sephadex C25	Ammonium bicarbonate,"steep" linear gradient
3	Cation exchange chromatography on CM-cellulose	Ammonium bicarbonate, "shallow" linear gradient
4	Anion exchange chromatography on QAE-Sephadex A25	Equilibrium conditions at pH 8.55 in low molarity sodium pyrophosphate
5	Desalting by gel filtration on Sephadex G25	In ammonium bicarbonate
6	Gel filtration on Sephadex G75	In acetic acid; optional step not always used

* Details are given in Adelson.[2]

The resultant peptide was found to be apparently homogeneous[1,2] by several of the usual criteria: gel electrophoresis at acid pH, SDS-gel electrophoresis, gel filtration, and the obtaining of near integral values upon amino acid analysis. The word "homogeneous" must, of course, be taken with caution; we have experienced some variation of the amino acid analysis of different batches, and we occasionally find trace impurities on electrophoresis gels. The material, in pure form, elicited (in nanogram doses) an increase in fluid output from the rat pancreas and (in microgram quantities) amylase release from zymogen granules.[2]

The chemical properties of the molecule may be briefly summarized[2] as follows: chymodenin is a basic polypeptide with a molecular weight just under 5000, well within the range found for other gastrointestinal hormones or putative hormones. The amino acid composition, as it is presently understood, is given in Table 2. This composition is distinct from other reported gastrointestinal materials and also appears not to allow chymodenin to act directly as a precursor or product of the other known substances. There is a possibility that the molecule contains a disulfide bridge; amino acid analyses have consistently shown the presence of between one and two cysteine residues. The N-terminus appears to be blocked to danzylation. The amino acid sequence has not yet been determined; this information will of course be of great interest for deciding whether or not chymodenin is a member of either of the two main gastrointestinal hormone families.

Table 2. Tentative amino acid composition of chymodenin*

Lysine	3	Serine	2	Valine	2
Histidine	1	Glutamic acid	4-5	Methionine	1?
Arginine	3	and glutamine		Isoleucine	2
Aspartic	5	Proline	2	Leucine	1
acid and		Glycine	2	Tyrosine	2
asparagine		Alanine	3	Phenylalanine	2
Threonine	2	Cysteine	2?	Tryptophan	1?

* Data from Adelson.[2]

THE ACTIVITY OF CHYMODENIN

Before generally describing the activity of chymodenin as we understand it at present, it should be
made clear to the reader that the molecule whose
purification was just described may very well not be
the one we set out to purify at the outset of the
work; although both the extract of Crick and associates[8] and pure chymodenin interact with zymogen
granules,[2,4] we have no evidence at present that
chymodenin, *per se,* is even present in the extracts
of Crick and associates.[8] Once a pure molecule
was obtained, however, it became reasonable to dis-
regard such issues and to describe the biologic
activity inherent within the molecule at hand without undue concern that the activities of a previously
known substance might be described, or a combination
of substances, known or unknown. The place to seek
such activity was clearly the pancreas. It had been
known for years, of course, that secretin's domain
of control was over electrolyte and water secretion;
that of CCK-PZ was over protein secretion. This left
at least theoretically, very little "room" for a new
substance to act upon exocrine secretion since a
hormone had been assigned to each of the two well
recognized exocrine functions of the pancreas.

In the few years immediately preceding and concomitant with the efforts described here, however,
Dr. S.S. Rothman and his collaborators had shown
that, in addition to indiscriminate, or massive overall protein secretion, the pancreas exhibited, under
a variety of conditions, the ability to secrete proteinaceous substances in a nonparallel, or enzyme-
selective fashion.[10,12-14,16] They showed further
that the pancreas called upon several distinct pools
and routes of protein secretion in order to accom-
plish such selective secretion.[10,15]

These exciting studies provided a potential role
for a substance such as chymodenin, and in collaboration with Dr. S.S. Rothman's laboratory, I have
studied, in the rabbit, the effects of chymodenin
on secretion by the pancreas. In studies employing
the rabbit pancreas *in situ,* we observed no major
effect of the peptide, in microgram doses, on fluid
output (Adelson and Rothman, unpublished data).
Using the same preparation, we surveyed a number of
pancreatic enzymes for peptide-elicited perturbances

in their outputs, and found that whereas gross protein output was stimulated only modestly by the peptide, a dramatic effect was seen specifically upon chymotrypsinogen output. A modest 40% rise in protein output was accompanied by a concomitant threefold rise in chymotrypsinogen output after injection of chymodenin (Table 3). Our "foil" enzyme, lipase, showed no change in output after administration of the new peptide.[5] In most mammals where it has been studied, chymotrypsinogen comprises about 10% to 20% of the protein in the total pancreatic enzyme constellation. Thus we have speculated[5] that if the rabbit falls into the same range, the effect of the peptide on protein secretion may be attributed to a major, or possibly exclusive, increase specifically in chymotrypsinogen secretion, in the relative absence of the increased secretion of other enzymes. Currently we are investigating this directly, with affinity chromatography methods used to separate out the secreted chymotrypsinogen from the other digestive hydrolases.

We have now studied in greater detail the effect of the molecule on the stimulation of chymotrypsinogen secretion *in vitro*,[6] and our earlier results have been confirmed. Both *in situ* and *in vitro*, the peptide elicited a rapid rise (within 15-20 minutes) in chymotrypsinogen secretion with no concomitant enhancement of lipase output, and the increase in protein output obtained after administration of chymodenin was so modest that the bulk of the increase can likely be attributed specifically

Table 3. Response to chymodenin in rabbit pancreas, *in situ*, in basal state*

	Control$_{(n)}$	Chymodenin$_{(n)}$	p
Chymotrypsinogen output	100±3 (9)	286±64 (16)	<0.01
Protein output	100±8 (10)	140±13 (15)	<0.025
Lipase output	100±20 (11)	107±16 (16)	NS

* Data from Adelson and Rothman.[5] The basal state of pancreatic secretion *in situ* employed in this comparison, was defined in reference 5. The data were normalized to allow the control output means to equal 100%. The number in parenthesis is n, the number of independent injections of chymodenin (10 µg in saline) or saline given to the series of nine control and nine treated rabbits as described in Adelson and Rothman.[5]

to chymotrypsinogen. Using the *in vitro* system, we have sequentially tested the effects of chymodenin and a cholinergic stimulus upon chymotrypsinogen total protein and lipase outputs. The results were unequivocal, the new peptide increased chymotrypsinogen output greatly relative to lipase; cholinergic stimulation (with methacholine chloride) increased the output of both enzymes, but we were surprised to find that lipase was increased far more than chymotrypsinogen (Table 4). The conclusion to be drawn is quite direct: the pancreas is capable, in the short term, of modifying its specific enzyme output in response to external, hormone-like stimuli.

The name "chymodenin" was of course chosen as a contraction of *chymo*trypsinogen, reflecting our present knowledge of the peptide's activity, and duo*de*num, the peptide's source. At this early stage certain conclusions should be avoided. First, it is not yet known that chymodenin *is* a hormone, and second, *if* chymodenin is in fact a hormone, it would be premature to conclude that its function was to stimulate chymotrypsinogen secretion, although this is our most attractive present possibility. What of chymodenin's ability to selectively stimulate the secretion of chymotrypsinogen? Chymodenin provides the first direct link between the duodenum and a highly enzyme-specific pancreatic response which does not elicit a massive protein release from the gland. The existence of chymodenin poses great problems for the exocytosis model[9] of pancreatic secretion, which demands parallel secretion of all enzymes in the constellation of hydrolases. Chymodenin is a putative regulator of enzyme-specific secretion.

Table 4. Effect of chymodenin and methacholine chloride on pancreatic secretion, *in vitro**

Treatment	Chymotrypsin-ogen output	Lipase Output	Total Protein Output	Ratio: Chymo-trypsinogen Lipase
Chymodenin	Increased	Unaffected	Modest increase	Increased
Methacholine chloride	Increased	Increased greatly	Increased greatly	Decreased

* Data from Adelson and Rothman[6] presented here as a qualitative summary of the original quantitative data.

At the functional level, what may chymodenin's existence mean? First, that pancreatic secretion of enzymes is potentially a highly specific process, giving rise to selective digestive hydrolyses, at least under certain circumstances. Perhaps diet immediately influences the pancreatic exocrine response in a fashion which has heretofore gone unappreciated. If there is a chymodenin, why not also for example a "lipodenin" or an "amylodenin," the release of which would follow from selective dietary input? Second, upon consideration one may readily ask if it is so surprising that the pancreas appears to be capable of what many other glands are, that is, responding to external stimuli with a response exactly and specifically matched with respect to both quantity (amount of enzyme output) as well as quality (type of enzyme output) for the maintenance of an organism's homeostasis? Such selective digestive ability would certainly be advantageous in preventing the undue expenditure of overall metabolic energy for digestive enzyme synthesis and secretion.

Chymodenin is at this stage a putative hormone, it resembles a hormone chemically, and it evokes in nanogram and microgram doses responses "at a distance," *in vitro* and *in vivo*. Future work including development of a radioimmunoassay, will determine if it is indeed released and by which specific stimuli into the blood stream. For now, we remain quite fascinated with the response chymodenin elicits from the pancreas.

SUMMARY

Chymodenin, a newly isolated hormone-like substance from porcine duodenum, is a basic peptide with a molecular weight just below 5000. It contains all the common amino acids, as well as a possible disulfide bridge. The molecule was isolated from an acidic methanol soluble, neutral pH insoluble "side-fraction" produced in the routine preparation of secretin and cholecystokinin-pancreozymin. The molecule was originally purified on the basis of its ability to elicit the release of enzymes from isolated pancreatic zymogen granules of the rat, *in vitro*. Later, partially purified extracts of the enzyme-releasing factors were found to cause stimulation of rat pancreatic fluid and protein secretion, *in situ*. After purification to apparent homogeneity, the peptide obtained was shown to exhibit, in addition to the aforementioned activities, the ability to elicit a dramatically increased enzyme-specific secretion of chymotrypsinogen by the pancreas of the rabbit. This secretion occurred accompanied by only a modest elevation in total protein, and no change in lipase output. Studies with chymodenin have shown the pancreas to be capable of enzyme-specific secretion; it is therefore possible that the digestive process itself is a process regulated at the molecular level.

Acknowledgments

Without the help, collaboration, advice, facilities, and funds of the following persons and agencies, this work would not have been possible: E.R. Blout, A. Ehrlich, the late J.E. Jorpes, V. Mutt, and S.S. Rothman; the National Cystic Fibrosis Research Foundation, the National Institutes of Health, and the Swedish Medical Research Council.

References

1. Adelson JW: Un nouveau polypeptide, extrait du duodénum porcin, possédant une activité biologique chez le rat, abstracted, *Biol Gastroenterol (Paris)* 4:355, 1971.
2. Adelson JW: Purification and characterization of chymodenin, a hormone-like peptide from porcine duodenum, in preparation.
3. Adelson JW, Ehrlich A: *In vitro* release of amylase from zymogen granules by factors from porcine duodenal mucosa, abstracted. *Fed Proc* 27:573, 1968.
4. Adelson JW, Ehrlich A: The effect of porcine duodenal mucosa extract upon enzyme release from pancreatic zymogen granules *in vitro*. *Endocrinology* 90:60-66, 1972.
5. Adelson JW, Rothman SS: Selective pancreatic enzyme secretion due to a new peptide called chymodenin. *Science* 183:1087-1089, 1974.
6. Adelson JW, Rothman SS: Chymodenin-induced selective secretion of chymotrypsinogen by the pancreas: Regulation and mechanistic implications, in preparation.

7. Ahlroth A, Mutt V: Polyacrylamide gel electrophoresis of polypeptides from the intestinal wall, with counter-migration of dye. *Anal Biochem* 37:125–128, 1970.

8. Crick J, Harper AA, Raper HS: On the preparation of secretin and pancreozymin. *J Physiol* 110:367–376, 1950.

9. Jamieson JD: The secretion process in the pancreatic exocrine cell: Morphological and biochemical aspects, in Jorpes JE, Mutt V (eds), *Secretin, Cholecystokinin, Pancreozymin, and Gastrin,* Berlin: Springer-Verlag, 1973, pp 195–217.

10. Liebow C, Rothman SS: Membrane transport of proteins. *Nature* 240:176–178, 1972.

11. Mutt V: Preparation of highly purified secretin. *Arkh Kemi* 15:69–74, 1959.

12. Rothman SS: "Non-parallel transport" of enzyme protein by the pancreas. *Nature* 213:460–462, 1967.

13. Rothman SS: Intracellular storage of exportable protein in functionally hypertrophied pancreas. *Am J Physiol* 219:1652–1657, 1970.

14. Rothman SS: Molecular regulation of digestion: Short term and bond specific. *Am J Physiol* 226:77–83, 1974.

15. Rothman SS, Isenman LD: Secretion of digestive enzyme derived from two parallel intracellular pools. *Am J Physiol* 226:1082–1087, 1974.

16. Rothman SS, Wells H: Selective effects of dietary egg white trypsin inhibitor on pancreatic enzyme secretion. *Am J Physiol* 216:504–507, 1969.

ACTIONS OF BOMBESIN ON SECRETIONS AND MOTILITY OF THE GASTROINTESTINAL TRACT

V. Erspamer, P. Melchiorri

Institute of Medical Pharmacology I,
University of Rome, Rome, Italy

In the course of a systematic screening carried out on extracts of the skin of 500 amphibian species collected throughout the world, a number of active peptides have been isolated, belonging to different families.[11] The family of bombesin-like peptides is so far represented by four members (Table 1).

In the present report the actions of bombesin on the gastrointestinal tract will be briefly described. It will be seen that the polypeptide displayed a complex spectrum of effects on gastric and pancreatic secretions, on gallbladder motility, and on gut electrical and mechanical activity.

Table 1. Amino acid sequences of bombesin and bombesin-like peptides

Bombesin	Glp*-Glu-Arg-Leu-Gly-Asn-Gln-Trp-		
Alytesin	Glp*-Gly-Arg-Leu-Gly-Thr-Gln-Trp-		
Ranatensin	Glp*		Val-Pro-Gln-Trp-
Litorin	Glp*		Gln-Trp-
Bombesin	Ala-Val-Gly-His-Leu-Met-NH_2		
Alytesin	Ala-Val-Gly-His-Leu-Met-NH_2		
Ranatensin	Ala-Val-Gly-His-Phe-Met-NH_2		
Litorin	Ala-Val-Gly-His-Phe-Met-NH_2		

* Glp = Pyroglutamyl

ACTION ON GASTRIC ACID SECRETION: RELEASE OF GASTRIN

Bombesin was found to be a potent stimulant of gastric acid secretion in gastric fistula dogs with Heidenhain pouches. The effect could be elicited not only by intravenous infusion of the polypeptide but also by subcutaneous injection. Rapid intravenous injection was considerably less effective.[2,3]

The following pieces of evidence unequivocally demonstrate that the gastric secretagogue activity of bombesin was due to release of gastrin from the G-cells of the antral mucosa:[1,3,16]

1) Gastric acid secretion was preceded and accompanied by an increase in plasma levels of

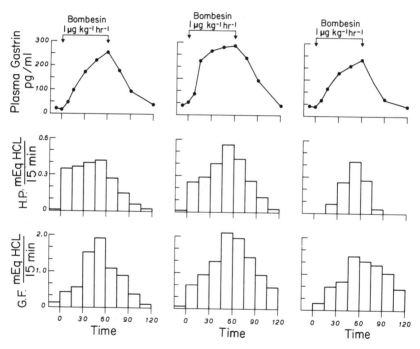

Figure 1. Gastric fistula dogs provided with Heidenhain pouches. Plasma gastrin levels and acid outputs, in the Heidenhain pouch (HP) and in the main stomach (GF), following intravenous infusion of 1 µg/kg/hr of bombesin for 60 minutes. Three single experiments in three different dogs.

immunoreactive gastrin. After intravenous infusion of bombesin, the increase in gastrin concentration was prompt, reached its maximum after approximately 30 minutes, and then, provided that the acid juice secreted in the main stomach was freely drained to the exterior, remained at a steady level throughout the duration of an experiment (Fig. 1). After cessation of the bombesin infusion, plasma gastrin returned to basal levels in less than one hour.

From threshold infusion rates (0.1 µg/kg/hr) up to the doses that produced optimum responses (1 µg/kg/hr), there was an evident dose-response relationship. Peak increases of gastrin concentrations above plasma basal levels were of the order of 150-220 pg/ml. No other known stimulus of gastrin release was more potent than bombesin. Peak acid responses to bombesin infusion were of the same magnitude as maximal responses to pentagastrin infusion.

2)   Antrectomy reduced the gastrin response to bombesin and the stimulation of acid gastric secretion by 85% to 90%. The same result was obtained after removal of the antral mucosa; regeneration of the mucosa gradually restored the response to bombesin.

3)   Blood collected from the gastroduodenal vein 30 minutes after start of an intravenous infusion of bombesin (0.6 µg/kg/hr) contained three times as much gastrin as that taken from a femoral artery (380 pg/ml versus 135 pg/ml).

Cholinergic mechanisms did not seem to play any important role in the release of gastrin by bombesin, as shown by the lack of effect of both antral denervation (Fig. 2) and premedication with atropine.

In dogs provided with antral pouches, acidification of the antrum caused a delay in gastrin release, or a temporary reduction of gastrin release stimulated by bombesin. Delay occurred when the acid was perfused throughout the period of bombesin infusion, temporary reduction occurred when the transition from neutral to acidified antrum was made during a bombesin infusion. The inhibitory effect of antral acidification, however, could be surmounted by increasing either the duration or rate of bombesin infusion. The effect of antral acidification on response to bombesin was the same for innervated and denervated antral pouches.

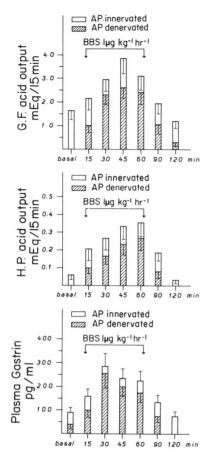

Figure 2. Gastric fistula dogs provided with Heidenhain pouches and antral pouches. Plasma gastrin levels and acid outputs, in the Heidenhain pouch (HP) and in the main stomach (GF), following intravenous infusion of 1 µg/kg/hr of bombesin for 45 minutes. Bombesin infusions were repeated in the same dogs before and after denervation of the antral pouches. Mean values ± SE of three measurements in each of four dogs.

Changes in gastrin release and gastric acid secretion similar to those produced by acidification of antral pouches, were caused by closing the gastric fistula during an infusion of bombesin (Fig. 3). In this situation, the gastric fistula dog behaved like the intact dog, presenting a reduced sensitiveness to the peptide.

Although atropine did not affect gastrin release by bombesin, it did strongly inhibit gastric acid secretion (as expected). A somewhat less intense inhibiting effect on acid output was exhibited also by metiamide, a blocking agent for histamine H_2-receptors. Secretin (1.5 U/kg/hr) only moderately reduced gastrin release (by 20%-30%) while sharply

decreasing gastric acid secretion (by 80%) stimulated
by bombesin.

In preliminary experiments, bombesin was infused
in gastric fistula dogs provided with Heidenhain
pouches at a rate of 0.6 µg/kg/hr for 12 to 15 hours.
As usual, plasma gastrin levels reached their maximum after 30 minutes (threefold increase), remained
at this level for approximately two hours, then gradually declined to attain basal values after 10 hours.
Food given at this time while continuing bombesin
infusion no longer produced any significant change
in plasma gastrin levels. It is conceivable that
this is due to exhaustion of depletable gastrin
stores in the G-cells.

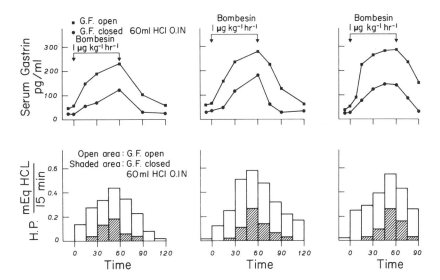

Figure 3. Gastric fistula dogs provided with Heidenhain
pouches. Plasma gastrin levels and acid output in the Heidenhain pouch (HP) following intravenous infusion of 1 µg/kg/hr
of bombesin for 60 minutes. During bombesin infusion the
gastric fistula was kept either open or closed, after 60 ml
of 0.1 N HCl had been introduced into the main stomach. Three
single experiments in three different dogs.

In a few experiments the form of gastrin released under the influence of bombesin was investigated. As shown in Figure 4, it appeared that at the beginning of the infusion (that is, during the first 10 to 15 minutes) increase in plasma gastrin levels was chiefly due to gastrin-17. Later on, this was gradually substituted by gastrin-34. Conclusions will be possible only after completion of our studies. It would seem, however, that gastrin-17, the gastrin form that appears to be predominant in the G-cells of the antral mucosa, is more promptly releasable than gastrin-34, which is mainly in extra-antral tissues.

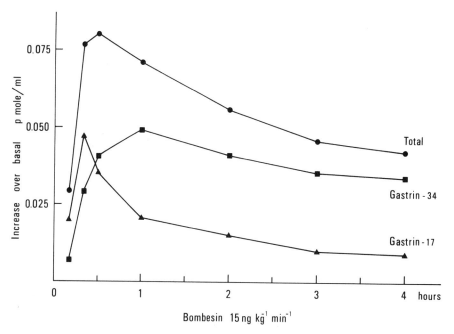

Figure 4. Gastric fistula dogs provided with Heidenhain pouches. Increase, above basal values, of plasma levels of total immunoreactive gastrin, as well as of levels of gastrin-17 and gastrin-34 produced by an intravenous infusion of 15 ng/kg/min of bombesin for four hours. Each point represents the mean of three experiments. Antibody used had the same affinity for gastrin-17 and gastrin-34.

The gastrin-releasing effect of bombesin was confirmed in man and cats. In man threshold infusion
rate of bombesin was of the order of 0.15 µg/kg/hr.
Optimum stimulation unaccompanied by untoward side
effects occurred with 0.6 µg/kg/hr. Peak increases
in plasma gastrin levels were significantly higher
in females than in males.

Cats were very sensitive to bombesin (threshold
0.02 µg/kg/hr; maximum response 0.5 µg/kg/hr), although increases in gastrin levels did not exceed
100 to 120 pg/ml. Secretin sharply reduced in this
species not only the secretagogue effect but also
the gastrin-releasing effect of bombesin.

Bombesin displayed a very poor stimulant action,
if any, on acid gastric secretion in the rat.[2] In
accordance with this observation, the gastrin-releasing effect of bombesin was also ambiguous, and
subcutaneous doses of the polypeptide as high as
500 µg/kg were required to raise plasma gastrin levels from 85 to 150 pg/ml. Subcutaneous doses of
50 to 200 µg/kg were ineffective.

ACTION ON GALLBLADDER MOTILITY AND PANCREATIC SECRETION:
RELEASE OF CHOLECYSTOKININ

Strong evidence suggests that bombesin releases
also cholecystokinin (CCK) from the duodenal mucosa.[13]
In fact, the intravenous infusion of bombesin elicited
the following events:

1) Contraction of the gallbladder in both
anesthetized and conscious dogs. Response appeared
after a latency period of 5-10 minutes and after
having gradually reached a maximum it persisted for
some time after the infusion was discontinued (Fig.5).
On the isolated dog gallbladder bombesin was virtually inactive (Fig. 6).

2) Relaxation of the choledochoduodenal junction.

3) Stimulation of flow of pancreatic juice,
again after a latency of approximately 10 minutes.
The juice was poor in bicarbonate but rich in protein
and enzymes. Amylase and trypsin concentrations rose
by 200% to 300%.

The pancreatic response was dose-related only between 0.1 and 1 µg/kg/hr. Increasing the infusion
rate above this level did not further increase protein output. Maximum output produced by infusion of

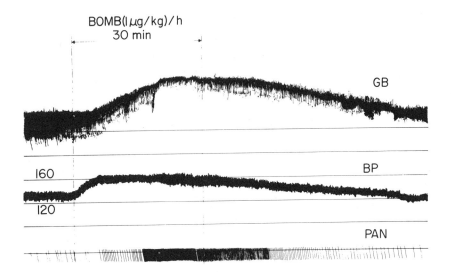

Figure 5. Dog anesthetized with sodium pentobarbital (30 mg/kg, intravenously). Responses elicited by the intravenous infusion of 1 μg/kg/hr of bombesin for 30 minutes. From top to bottom: gallbladder motility (GB), systemic blood pressure (BP), and flow of pancreatic juice, in drops (PAN).

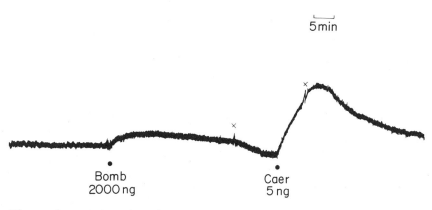

Figure 6. Isolated longitudinal strip of a dog gallbladder suspended in 10 ml of Krebs solution at 37C. Spasmogenic effect of 2000 ng bombesin and 5 ng caerulein.

porcine CCK or caerulein, however, was considerably higher than that caused by bombesin. One μg/kg/hr of bombesin produced approximately the same effect as 0.75 μg/kg/hr of CCK.

When the infusion of bombesin was continued for a sufficiently long time, protein output, after having reached a maximum, declined in spite of continuing the infusion. This result is similar to that obtained after intraduodenal infusion of L-tryptophan, capable of releasing endogenous CCK, but unlike that observed following infusion of exogenous CCK or caerulein, which produced a steady level of protein output throughout the infusion period. Similarly, a second bombesin infusion given shortly after the first one was much less effective.

Any intervention of antral gastrin in the production of the effects of bombesin on pancreatic secretion could be excluded because this polypeptide was equally effective before and after antrectomy.

Bombesin also caused contraction of the gallbladder in man and striking stimulation of pancreatic protein output. Maximum response, which was of the same magnitude as that obtainable with CCK, was elicited by infusion rates of 1.0-1.5 μg/kg/hr.

The chicken pancreas, too, was stimulated by bombesin to produce a scarce amount of juice, very rich in amylase and trypsin activity but poor in bicarbonate.

Measurements of CCK levels in plasma could not be performed as yet, owing to lack of reliable radioimmunoassay procedures.

ACTION ON MYOELECTRIC AND MECHANICAL ACTIVITY OF THE GUT

The effects of bombesin on the gastrointestinal musculature cannot be ascribed simply to release of peptides of the gastrin-CCK family. Whether we are dealing with direct effects of bombesin on the smooth muscle or with effects again mediated or with effects modulated by other agents, is a problem that remains to be solved.

In conscious dogs provided with electrodes chronically implanted on the serosal surface of different gastrointestinal segments, bombesin, infused for 30 minutes at a rate of 0.3 to 1.0 μg/kg/hr, produced the following events:

1)   significant increase in the frequency of
pacesetter potentials (PP) in antrum, duodenum,
jejunum and ileum. In the duodenum and jejunum,
the increase in frequency showed linear correlation
with the reduction of PP amplitude. The propagation
velocity of PP was approximately halved. Spikes
were not affected in the antrum and ileum, whereas
they were abolished in the duodenum and jejunum.
2)   disappearance of rhythmicity of contractions
of the duodenum and upper jejunum, with appearance
of an irregular sequence of slow and small potentials.
This could be interpreted as due to the failure of
coupling between relaxation oscillators over critical
maximal frequencies (Fig. 7).
During recovery, electrical activity gradually
returned towards preinfusion pattern.
3)   no consistent effect on the electrical activity of the colon.[5] The mechanical counterpart
was the disappearance of motility in the upper small
intestine which was observed also in man, by fluoroscopy and by balloon methods.[4],[7],[12]

EXTRAINTESTINAL ACTIONS OF BOMBESIN

The spectrum of biologic activity of bombesin is
not covered by the effects previously described. In
fact, the peptide was highly active on other target
organs and tissues outside the gastrointestinal
tract:
1)   *the vascular smooth muscle.* Generally
bombesin produced a moderate rise in systemic blood
pressure, but in the monkey it behaved like a potent
hypotensive agent. Tachyphylaxis was common.[9]
2)   *extravascular smooth muscles,* other than
the gut. In some cases, for example, in rat and
guinea-pig urinary bladder and guinea-pig bronchial
musculature, bombesin displayed a potent spasmogenic
action. [8],[15]
3)   *the kidney,* especially that of the dog. In
this species bombesin produced a pronounced antidiuretic effect, proceeding occasionally to complete
arrest of urine flow. Antidiuresis was the result
of a reduction in glomerular filtration rate caused
by a fall in intraglomerular hydrostatic pressure.
This, in its turn, was provoked by afferent vasocon-
striction, which represented the first cause of another series of events leading to a conspicuous

activation of the renin-angiotensin system and, if
sufficiently prolonged and kept within certain limits,
to a considerable release of erythropoietin.[10]
   It is possible that in the dog the renal effects
of bombesin may contribute to some extent in main-
taining high gastrin levels in plasma, because the
kidney is considered to be one of the chief inactivation sites of gastrin.

RELATIVE POTENCY OF BOMBESIN-LIKE PEPTIDES

   As already stated, three other bombesin-like peptides have been isolated so far, in addition to bombesin, from the amphibian skin: the tetradecapeptide

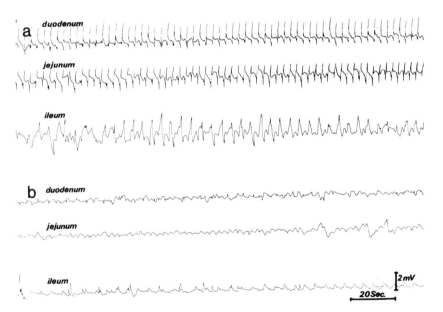

Figure 7. Conscious dog with electrodes chronically implanted
on the serosal surface of different intestinal segments.
Effects of an intravenous infusion of 1 μg/kg/hr of bombesin
on the electrical activity (pacesetter potentials) of duodenum,
jejunum, and ileum. Records were taken before (a) and 30
minutes after (b) starting bombesin infusion.

alytesin, the endecapeptide ranatensin, and finally
the nonapeptide litorin, the last arrival.

The pharmacologic effects of alytesin, as tested
so far, were exactly superimposable on those of
bombesin. For ranatensin the only available data
concern isolated smooth muscle preparations and
blood pressure.[6,14]

Litorin has been compared with bombesin and with
the C-terminal nonapeptide of bombesin, representing
the shortest amino acid sequence which possessed the
full spectrum of activity of bombesin, at a comparable
degree of intensity. Partial results are shown in
Table 2, in which only the intensity of response
has been taken into consideration.

Whereas the C-terminal nonapeptide closely mimicked
bombesin in its effects, the effects of litorin, also
from a qualitative point of view, did diverge from
those of bombesin in many respects. For example,
total acid output observed in the dog stomach at comparable gastrin levels was less for litorin than for
bombesin.

Table 2. The relative potency, on a weight basis, of litorin
and C-terminal nonapeptide of bombesin (Bombesin =
100)

Effects on:	Litorin	C-terminal nonapeptide of bombesin
Rat uterus	200–600	150–300
Rat urinary bladder	150–500	150–300
Guinea-pig colon	200–500	100–120
Guinea-pig urinary bladder	150–250	200–350
Kitten small intestine	100–350	100–150
Gastrin release in dog	50–100	40–60
Myoelectric activity of dog intestine	50	75

DOES MAMMALIAN GASTROINTESTINAL MUCOSA CONTAIN
BOMBESIN-LIKE PEPTIDES?

We have repeatedly insisted[3],[11] on the possibility that bombesin-like peptides may occur in the gastro-intestinal mucosa of mammals. To solve the problem, an antibody to a bombesin-like decapeptide conjugated with bovine albumin was prepared in the rabbit. It showed a moderate affinity to bombesin.

With the use of this antibody a substance has been traced in methanol extracts of the antral and duode-nal mucosa of pigs and dogs which behaved like bom-besin in the radioimmunoassay. Concentrations, ex-pressed as bombesin, ranged between 50 and 150 ng/g. The immunoreactive substance was scarce in the jeju-nal mucosa (10 ng/g) and below the limits of sensi-tivity of our method (1 ng/ml) in the mucosa of the gastric fundus and the distal ileum, as well as in antral and duodenal musculature and in pancreas.

Bioassay gave only partially reliable results, owing to the presence of disturbing contaminants.

It is evident that our study is continuing in different directions.

It is hoped that data herein reported will stimu-late further work on bombesin and related peptides, potent releasers of gastrointestinal hormones of the gastrin-cholecystokinin family as well as singu-lar modulators of electrical and mechanical activi-ties of the gut musculature. It may be that bombe-sin will help in elucidating problems concerning gastrointestinal secretions and motility and will disclose the way to the identification of bombesin-like hormonal peptides in the mammalian gut.

SUMMARY

Bombesin, a tetradecapeptide isolated from amphi-bian skin, caused in the dog stimulation of gastric acid secretion, contraction of gallbladder, relaxa-tion of the choledochoduodenal junction and stimu-lation of pancreatic secretion, with production of a juice rich in protein and poor in bicarbonate. These effects could be ascribed to release, by bom-besin, of gastrin from the antral mucosa and of cholecystokinin from the duodenal mucosa. Release

of gastrin was demonstrated also directly by radioimmunoassay, a procedure which permitted determination of plasma gastrin levels under different conditions, such as antrectomy, acidification of innervated and denervated antral pouches, premedication
with atropine and metiamide. During a bombesin infusion first gastrin-17 was released, and later
gastrin-34. Bombesin displayed complex effects on
myoelectric activity of the dog gastrointestinal
tract. These effects were particularly striking in
duodenum and upper jejunum and consisted essentially
in an increase in frequency and a decrease in amplitude of pacesetter potentials, abolition of spikes,
and final "electrical disorganization." The mechanical counterpart was extinction of mechanical activity.
The above effects could be elicited also in man and
other animal species. Natural and synthetic bombesin-
like peptides possessed a spectrum of activity similar
to that of bombesin. Bombesin-like peptides may occur
in the mammalian gastrointestinal tract.

Acknowledgments

Results reported in this communication are the outcome of the
common effort of several groups of research workers active in
Rome and Parma. Research was supported throughout by grants
from the Consiglio Nazionale delle Ricerche, Rome, Italy.
Synthetic bombesin, litorin and bombesin C-terminal nonapeptide
were set at our disposal, in generous amounts, by the Farmitalia
Research Laboratories, Milan.

References

1. Basso N, Improta G, Melchiorri P, Sopranzi N: Gastrin re-
        lease by bombesin in the antral pouch dog. *Rendic
        Gastroenterol* 6:95-98, 1974.
2. Bertaccini G, Erspamer V, Impicciatore M: The actions of
        bombesin on gastric secretion of the dog and the rat.
        Br J Pharmacol 49:437-444, 1973.
3. Bertaccini G, Erspamer V, Melchiorri P, Sopranzi N: Gastrin
        release by bombesin in the dog. *Br J Pharmacol* 52:219-
        225, 1974.
4. Bertaccini G, Impicciatore M, Molina E, Zappia L: The action
        of bombesin on the human gastrointestinal tract. *Rendic
        Gastroenterol* 6:45-51, 1974.

5. Caprilli R, Melchiorri P, Improta G, Vernia P, Frieri G: Effects of bombesin and bombesin-like peptides on gastrointestinal myo-electric activity in the dog. *Gastroenterology* 68:1228-1235, 1975.

6. Clineschmidt BV, Geller RG, Govier WC, Pisano JJ, Tanimura T: Effects of ranatensin, a polypeptide from frog skin, on isolated smooth muscle. *Br J Pharmacol* 41:622-628, 1971.

7. Corazziari E, Delle Fave FG, Melchiorri P, Torsoli A: Effects of a new peptide, bombesin, on gall bladder and duodeno-jejunal mechanical activity in man, in Daniel EE et al (eds), *Proceedings of the 4th International Symposium on Gastrointestinal Motility*, Vancouver: Mitchell Press, 1974, pp 293-304.

8. Erspamer V, Falconieri Erspamer G, Inselvini M, Negri L: Occurrence of bombesin and alytesin in extracts of the skin of three European discoglossid frogs and pharmacological actions of bombesin on extravascular smooth muscle. *Br J Pharmacol* 45:333-348, 1972.

9. Erspamer V, Melchiorri P, Sopranzi N: The action of bombesin on the systemic arterial blood pressure of some experimental animals. *Br J Pharmacol* 45:442-450, 1972.

10. Erspamer V, Melchiorri P, Sopranzi N: The action of bombesin on the kidney of the anaesthetized dog. *Br J Pharmacol* 48:438-455, 1973.

11. Erspamer V, Melchiorri P: Active polypeptides of the amphibian skin and their synthetic analogues. *Pure Appl Chem* 35:463-494, 1973.

12. Erspamer V, Melchiorri P, Sopranzi N, Torsoli A, Corazziari E, Improta G: Preliminary data on the action of bombesin on secretion and motility of the gastrointestinal tract in man, abstracted. *Rendic Gastroenterol* 5:68, 1973.

13. Erspamer V, Improta G, Melchiorri P, Sopranzi N: Evidence of cholecystokinin release by bombesin in the dog. *Br J Pharmacol* 52:227-232, 1974.

14. Geller RG, Govier WC, Pisano JJ, Tanimura T, van Clineschmidt B: The action of ranatensin, a new polypeptide from amphibian skin, on the blood pressure of experimental animals. *Br J Pharmacol* 40:605-616, 1970.

15. Impicciatore M, Bertaccini G: The bronchoconstrictor action of the tetradecapeptide bombesin in the guinea-pig. *J Pharm Pharmacol* 25:872-875, 1973.

16. Impicciatore M, Debas H, Walsh JH, Grossman MI, Bertaccini G: Release of gastrin and stimulation of acid secretion by bombesin in dog. *Rendic Gastroenterol* 6:99-101, 1974.

VASOACTIVE INTESTINAL POLYPEPTIDE (VIP): CURRENT STATUS

Sami I. Said

Departments of Internal Medicine and
Pharmacology, University of Texas
Southwestern Medical School and
Veterans Administration Hospital,
Dallas, Texas

Originally discovered and identified on the basis of its peripheral vasodilator effect,[20,21] vasoactive intestinal polypeptide (VIP) is now known to have a wide spectrum of biologic activity.[19] Although its normal physiologic role (if any) remains to be determined, VIP is already known to occur naturally in human subjects, is associated with, and perhaps causally related to, certain clinical syndromes,[4,15,17] and shows promise as a useful therapeutic agent.[18]

CHEMICAL FEATURES

VIP is closely related in its amino-acid composition and sequence to secretin, and somewhat less closely to glucagon and to the gastric inhibitory peptide (GIP).[5,13] In the course of synthesizing VIP, Bodanszky and associates[5,6] found that synthetic fragments of it exhibited characteristic biologic activity; in general, this activity increased with progressive lengthening of the fragment, with only the entire sequence showing full biologic potency.

Recently, Nilsson and associates (unpublished observations) isolated a peptide from small intestine of chicken, which possessed vasoactivity like that of porcine VIP, though differing in certain other biologic actions, as well as in five amino acid positions.

BIOLOGIC ACTIONS

Cardiovascular System

VIP received its name because of its potent vasodilator and hypotensive effects. These actions also
provided the basis for its bioassay during isolation.
It induces vasodilation in peripheral systemic (for
example, femoral) vessels, in splanchnic vessels,
particularly the hepatic and pancreaticoduodenal
arteries, and in pulmonary vessels.

VIP has a positive inotropic effect on cardiac
muscle, which is similar in magnitude to that of
pancreatic glucagon. This effect is detectable by
an increase in tension of isolated, isometrically
contracting papillary muscle of cat's right ven-
tricle, and by an increase in left ventricular dp/dt
in intact anesthetized dogs, when the heart rate,
"preload" and "afterload" are kept constant.[16]

Recently, we have also found that VIP is a potent
coronary vasodilator. This effect is *not* secondary
to an increase in cardiac metabolism, and is apparent
in doses that are too small to affect total blood
flow or blood pressure.[24]

Lungs and Respiration

VIP relaxes isolated guinea-pig trachea and dilates
pulmonary vessels. The bronchial-relaxant action of
VIP has been confirmed in preliminary experiments *in
vivo*. In both cases, VIP can reduce or abolish the
effect of bronchoconstrictor agents, such as histamine, kallikrein, and prostaglandin $F_{2\alpha}$.[18] Compared
with adrenergic stimulants, for example, isoproterenol
the direct inotropic and chronotropic actions of VIP
are negligible in relation to its tracheal-relaxant
actions.

VIP also augments minute and alveolar ventilation,
and this augmentation is at least in part attributable to chemoreceptor stimulation. The full mechanisms of this stimulation remain to be determined.

Metabolism

Like glucagon, VIP stimulates both lipolysis[8,9]
and glycogenolysis.[10] VIP stimulates adenylate cyclase

in the membranes of the rat liver and fat cells, in intact fat cells, and in rabbit intestinal (ileal) mucosa.[2,8,22] The maximal stimulation of adenylate cyclase by VIP is identical to that caused by secretin, but the affinity of VIP toward the enzyme is about 100 times greater.[7] VIP binding sites in liver membranes are distinct from those of secretin.[7]

Gastrointestinal System

These effects are discussed in detail by Makhlouf and Said.[12] Briefly, VIP inhibits both histamine and pentagastrin-stimulated *gastric acid secretion,* and relaxes isolated rat *gastric muscle.* This relaxation is elicited by low concentrations (about 10 ng/ml), and has been useful for bioassay (secretin causes similar gastric muscle relaxation, and is about twice as potent as VIP on this tissue). VIP stimulates electrolyte and water secretion by the *pancreas* of the cat, but it is considerably less potent than secretin in this respect, and it relaxes isolated, superfused guinea-pig *gallbladder* and antagonizes the contractile effect of cholecystokinin in intact cats.[14] In large doses, VIP increases *bile flow* in the dog.[23] It is a potent stimulant of *small intestine secretion* in dogs.[1] It *increases levels of cyclic AMP* in rabbit ileal mucosa and stimulates adenylate cyclase in concentrations ranging from a threshold of 0.1 to a maximum of 2 µg/ml. Transmural ileal flux measurements show that VIP added to the serosal side reverses the direction of net *Na flux* from absorption to secretion, and enhances the net secretory flux of anions.[22] This finding may explain the association of watery diarrhea with increased circulating levels of VIP (see section on VIP-secreting tumors, below, and report by Bloom and Polak[3]).

Platelets

Experiments in collaboration with Drs. Nils Bang and Marjorie Chang at the Lilly Research Laboratory, University of Indiana, have shown VIP to inhibit platelet aggregation (induced by collagen or ADP) *in vitro,* in concentrations of 4-8 µg/ml.

FATE AND METABOLISM

Evidence in dogs suggests that the liver is the major site of inactivation of VIP.[11] During passage through the lung, however, the hypotensive activity of VIP is enhanced, either because of further activation, or because of the release of additional vasodilator substances.[11]

BIOLOGIC ROLE

VIP in Hepatic Cirrhosis

Using a radioimmunoassay we have recently developed, together with bioassay on isolated smooth muscle organs, we have demonstrated increased plasma levels of VIP in patients with hepatic cirrhosis.[17] These patients often exhibit cardiovascular and respiratory manifestations (for example, high cardiac output, peripheral vasodilation, respiratory alkalosis) that mimic the effects of VIP in experimental animals.

VIP-Secreting Tumors

We have found increased plasma levels of VIP (or VIP-like immunoreactivity) in some patients with watery diarrhea, flushing, or both. Many of these patients had tumors originating in the pancreas, lung, or other organs. This finding establishes VIP as a peptide that can occur naturally in human subjects, and may explain some clinical syndromes (including diarrhea, hypotension, flushing) which complicate certain ectopic endocrine tumors (unpublished data; similar conclusions have been reported).[3,4]

VIP as a Normal Hormone

The inactivation of VIP in the liver suggests that the actions of this peptide may be limited normally to the gastrointestinal tract, the liver, and the portal circulation. Possible effects of VIP on these systems include: suppression of gastric secretion, stimulation of intestinal secretion and adenylate cyclase activity, relaxation of gastric and

gallbladder smooth muscle, glycogenolysis, increased
bile flow, and dilation of splanchnic vessels. To
what extent, if any, VIP exerts these or other actions
in the normal state remains to be determined. It
should be added that two related hormones, glucagon
and secretin, are also degraded to a significant
degree in the liver, and thus hepatic inactivation
of VIP does not rule out a possible physiologic role
for this peptide, even outside the portal region.

VIP AS A THERAPEUTIC AGENT

Several actions of VIP suggest its potential usefulness as a therapeutic agent, for example, its
ability to relax tracheobronchial smooth muscle and
to antagonize the bronchoconstrictor action of
several agents, along with its prolonged action and
its independence of adrenergic receptors, make it
promising as a bronchodilator. In addition, the
peripheral vasodilator action of the peptide, especially on the coronary circulation, also could
prove useful, and the inhibition of gastric acid
secretion and the relaxation of most gastrointestinal smooth muscle tissues, have obvious potential
applications.

Acknowledgments

This research was supported by a Center Award (HL-14187)
from the National Heart and Lung Institute, National Institutes of Health, U.S. Public Health Service.

References

1. Barbezat GO, Grossman MI: Intestinal secretion: Stimu-
    lation by peptides. *Science* 174:422-424, 1971.
2. Bataille DD, Freychet P, Kitabgi PE, Rosselin GE: Gut
    glucagon: A common receptor site with pancreatic
    glucagon in liver cell plasma membranes. *FEBS Lett*
    30:215-218, 1973.
3. Bloom SR, Polak JM: The role of VIP in pancreatic cholera,
    in Thompson JC (ed), *Gastrointestinal Hormones*, Austin:
    University of Texas Press, 1975, pp 635-649.

4. Bloom SR, Polak JM, Pearse AGE: Vasoactive intestinal peptide and watery-diarrhea syndrome. *Lancet* 2:14-16, 1973.

5. Bodanszky M, Klausner YS, Said SI: Biological activities of synthetic peptides corresponding to fragments of and to the entire sequence of the vasoactive intestinal peptide. *Proc Natl Acad Sci USA* 70:382-284, 1973.

6. Bodanszky M, Klausner YS, Yang Lin C, Mutt V, Said SI: Synthesis of the vasoactive intestinal peptide (VIP). *J Am Chem Soc* 96:4973-4978, 1974.

7. Desbuquois B: The interaction of vasoactive intestinal polypeptide and secretin with liver-cell membranes. *Eur J Biochem* 46:439-450, 1974.

8. Desbuquois B, Laudat MH, Laudat P: Vasoactive intestinal polypeptide and glucagon: Stimulation of adenylate cyclase activity via distinct receptors in liver and fat cell membranes. *Biochem Biophys Res Commun* 53:1187-1194, 1973.

9. Frandsen EK, Moody AJ: Lipolytic action of a newly isolated vasoactive intestinal polypeptide. *Horm Metab Res* 5:196-199, 1973.

10. Kerins C, Said SI: Hyperglycemic and glycogenolytic effects of vasoactive intestinal polypeptide. *Proc Soc Exp Biol Med* 142:1014-1017, 1973.

11. Kitamura S, Yoshida T, Said SI: Vasoactive intestinal polypeptide: Inactivation in liver and potentiation in lung of anesthetized dogs. *Proc Soc Exp Biol Med*, in press.

12. Makhlouf GM, Said SI: The effect of vasoactive intestinal peptide (VIP) on digestive and hormonal function, in Thompson JC (ed), *Gastrointestinal Hormones*, Austin: University of Texas Press, 1975, pp 599-610.

13. Mutt V, Said SI: Structure of the porcine vasoactive intestinal octacosapeptide: The amino-acid sequence. Use of kallikrein in its determination. *Eur J Biochem* 42:581-589, 1974.

14. Said SI: Smooth-muscle relaxant activity of vasoactive intestinal polypeptide, in *Proceedings International Endocrinology Symposium*, London: William Heinemann, 1973, in press.

15. Said SI: Vasoactive intestinal peptide (VIP), pp 735-737, in Grossman MI and others: Candidate Hormones of the Gut. *Gastroenterology* 67:730-755, 1974.

16. Said SI, Bosher LP, Spath JA, Kontos HA: Positive inotropic action of newly isolated vasoactive intestinal polypeptide (VIP), abstracted. *Clin Res* 20:29, 1972.

17. Said SI, Faloona GR, Deon H, Unger RH, Siegel SR: Vaso-active intestinal polypeptide: Elevated levels in patients with hepatic cirrhosis, abstracted. *Clin Res* 22:367, 1974.
18. Said SI, Kitamura S, Yoshida T, Preskitt J, Holden LD: Humoral control of airways. *Ann NY Acad Sci* 221:103-114, 1974.
19. Said SI, Makhlouf GM: Vasoactive intestinal polypeptide: Spectrum of biological activity, in Chey WY, Brooks FP (eds), *Endocrinology of the Gut*, Thorofare NJ: Charles B. Slack, Inc, 1974, pp 83-87.
20. Said SI, Mutt V: Polypeptide with broad biological activity: Isolation from small intestine. *Science* 169:1217-1218, 1970.
21. Said SI, Mutt V: Isolation from porcine intestinal wall of a vasoactive octacosapeptide related to secretin and to glucagon. *Eur J Biochem* 28:199-204, 1972.
22. Schwartz CJ, Kimberg DV, Sherrin HE, Field M, Said SI: Vasoactive intestinal peptide stimulation of adenylate cyclase and active electrolyte secretion in intestinal mucosa. *J Clin Invest* 54:536-544, 1974.
23. Thulin L: Effect of gastro-intestinal polypeptide on hepatic bile flow and splanchnic circulation. *Acta Chir Scand (suppl)* 441:5-31, 1973.
24. Yoshida T, Geumei AM, Schmitt RJ, Said SI: Vasoactive intestinal peptide: A potent coronary vasodilator, abstracted. *Fed Proc* 33:378, 1974.

THE EFFECT OF VASOACTIVE INTESTINAL PEPTIDE (VIP) ON DIGESTIVE AND HORMONAL FUNCTION

Gabriel M. Makhlouf, Sami I. Said

Department of Medicine, Medical College of
Virginia, Richmond, Virginia and Department
of Medicine, The University of Texas
Southwestern Medical School, Dallas, Texas

Phylogenetic evidence and the pattern of structural similarities suggest that VIP and secretin are early molecular ancestors from which other intestinal peptides such as gastric inhibitory peptide (GIP) and the enteroglucagons have diversified.[8] VIP shares a number of properties with secretin and pancreatic glucagon[3,12] but its physiologic status as a hormone in mammals has yet to be established.

GASTRIC SECRETION

The effect of synthetic porcine VIP on pentagastrin-stimulated acid and pepsin secretion was investigated in three dogs equipped with gastric fistulae.[16] At the height of the response to pentagastrin (0.25 to 4 µg/kg/hr), VIP was infused in a dose of 0.5 µg/kg/min for 7.5 minutes. Prompt inhibition of acid secretion occurred which ranged from 60% inhibition at the lowest dose to 22% at the highest dose of pentagastrin (Fig. 1). Kinetic analysis showed that inhibition was of the competitive type: maximal response was unchanged but the D_{50} pentagastrin was nearly doubled. Accordingly, K_i for VIP was 0.5 µg/kg/min, which corresponded to the actual dose employed in this study. A similar order of K_i was reported for inhibition of histamine-stimulated acid secretion in denervated canine pouches.[1] VIP has also been reported to inhibit food-stimulated acid secretion from these pouches; its molar potency in this regard was equivalent to that of GIP.[10]

VIP inhibited the maximal pepsin response by 75%
but had no effect on the reversed pepsin response
observed at high doses of pentagastrin (Fig. 1).

Comparative studies with secretin (0.05 µg/kg/min)
showed that the extent of inhibition (59% to 67%)
was independent of the degree of stimulation, an outcome compatible with inhibition of the noncompetitive
types.

Thus, the effect of VIP on gastric secretion differs
in three respects from that of secretin with which it
shares nine amino acid identities: 1) VIP inhibits

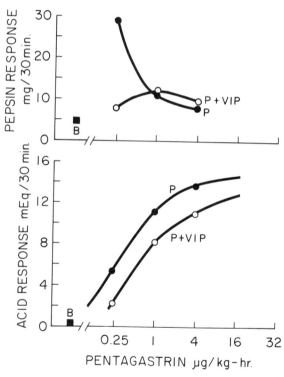

Figure 1. Dose-response curves to intravenous infusion of pentagastrin singly (P) and in combination
with VIP (P + VIP).

histamine as well as pentagastrin-stimulated acid
secretion, 2) inhibition of acid secretion by VIP is
of the competitive type, and 3) inhibition by VIP
extends to pepsin secretion. Inhibition by VIP is
more akin to that by GIP with which it shares few
(four) amino acid identities.[4]

INTESTINAL SECRETION

In contrast to its effect on gastric secretion,
VIP is an effective stimulant of small intestine
secretion, matched in this regard only by GIP and
glucagon.[1]
The comparative effects of VIP and glucagon, singly
and in combination, were studied in three dogs
equipped with Thiry-Vella loops of the proximal
jejunum.[14] VIP was infused in doses of 0.1 to 0.6
μg/kg/min for 15 minutes and glucagon in similar
doses for 30 minutes. The doses were given sequentially at one-hour intervals. VIP produced a dose-
dependent increase in intestinal secretion and blood
glucose levels (Fig. 2). Unlike secretion, blood
glucose did not return to control levels upon cessation of VIP infusion. A similar intestinal secretory
pattern was observed with glucagon; the rise in
blood glucose with the longer glucagon infusion was,
however, maximal from the start.
Dose-response analysis showed that while the D_{50}s
of VIP and glucagon were similar (0.2 μg/kg/min),
the maximal secretory responses were not (Fig. 3).
Correlative analysis of submaximal responses confirmed that glucagon was a partial agonist with an
efficacy of 0.55.
In separate experiments, a background dose of VIP
(0.1 μg/kg/min for 15 minutes) augmented the responses to increasing doses of glucagon (Fig. 4).
The augmentation was observed at all glucagon dose
levels; this outcome was expected kinetically
from the combination of a background dose of a full
agonist (VIP) with increasing doses of a partial
agonist (glucagon) (Fig. 5).
Schwartz and colleagues[17] have shown recently that
VIP increases the levels of cyclic AMP in human and
rabbit ileal mucosa *in vitro* and mimics the effects
of theophylline on ion flux and short circuit current. In these studies, neither GIP nor glucagon

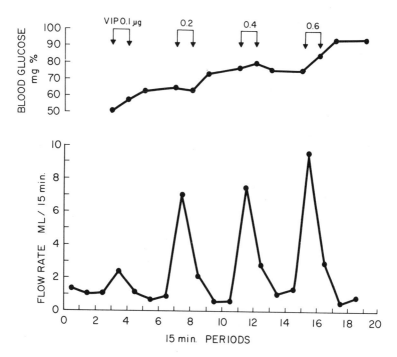

Figure 2. Effect of increasing doses of VIP on intestinal secretory rate and blood glucose levels. VIP was infused for
the first 15 minutes of every hour.

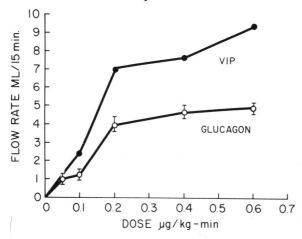

Figure 3. Arithmetic dose-response curves of the flow rate
of intestinal secretion in response to glucagon and VIP. The
maximal response to VIP is about twice the maximal response
to glucagon.

increased the levels of cyclic AMP in rabbit ileal mucosa. Glucagon was also tested on dog ileal mucosa and found ineffective. The differences between effects observed *in vivo* and *in vitro* deserve further study.

PANCREATIC AND BILIARY SECRETION

Acute studies in cats have shown that natural porcine VIP is a weak secretin-like stimulant of pancreatic flow and bicarbonate secretion.[13] A similar

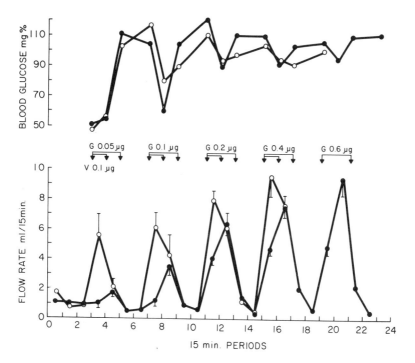

Figure 4. The effect of increasing doses of glucagon given for the first 30 minutes of every hour singly (closed circles) and in combination with a 15-minute infusion of VIP (open circles). A significant potentiatory effect on intestinal secretion is observed during the period of VIP infusion.

effect was observed with synthetic porcine VIP in
acute dogs with cannulated pancreatic and biliary
ducts.[9] Intravenous injection of VIP in doses of
1 to 4 µg/kg produced a prompt but short-lived pancreatic bicarbonate response which attained a peak
in the first five minutes after injection (Fig. 6).
The composition of secretion was similar to that
after injection of secretin, with high bicarbonate
and low protein concentration. Comparison of maximal bicarbonate responses to VIP and secretin showed
that VIP was a partial agonist with an efficacy of
0.27.

VIP given as a background to increasing intravenous doses of secretin (0.1 to 0.4 µg/kg) caused
an augmentation of submaximal responses but no
change in maximal response to secretin. VIP also
augmented the pancreatic flow response to the octapeptide of cholecystokinin by two- to fivefold. The
kinetic outcome in both instances was that expected

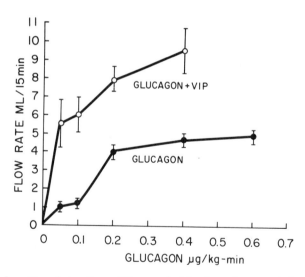

Figure 5. The data from Figure 4 displayed as arithmetic dose-
response curves. The augmentation elicited by VIP ranged from
sixfold at a glucagon dose of 0.05 µg/kg/min to twofold at a
dose of 0.4 µg/kg/min.

from the presence of a secretin-like partial agonist
of pancreatic secretion.

Both VIP and secretin doubled the flow of bile,
though the dose requirements for approximately equal
effects were about 10 times higher for VIP.

HORMONE RELEASE

In these experiments, blood glucose rose in parallel with insulin; the change in both indices was
first observed within two minutes of VIP injection
(Fig. 6). Total calcium levels also rose slightly
but significantly reaching a peak in the tenth
minute after VIP injection.

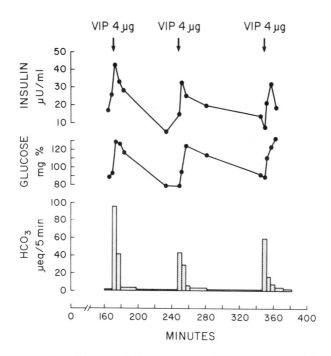

Figure 6. The effect of intravenous VIP on pancreatic bicarbonate secretion. A synchronous rise in blood glucose and
insulin levels occurs which reaches a peak in five minutes.

In view of the prompt hyperglycemia resulting from
hepatic glycogenolysis,[7] it could not be ascertained
whether VIP was directly insulinotropic *in vivo,*
that is, capable of releasing insulin independent
of the synchronous rise in blood glucose levels.   In
order to demonstrate this property of VIP, a preparation of saline-perfused cat pancreas was used *in
vitro.*   Prompt injection of 5 µg of VIP into the
perfusing fluid elicited a significant biphasic insulin response, as prompt as, but somewhat less than
the independent responses to injection of glucose
or octapeptide of cholecystokinin[15] (Fig. 7).   The
insulinotropic effect of VIP was also confirmed in
a preparation employing perfused slices of mouse
pancreas.

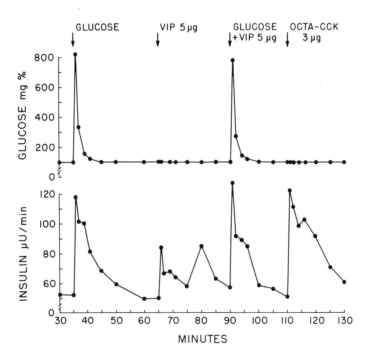

Figure 7.   The insulin response to pulse injections of glucose,
VIP and octapeptide of cholecystokinin into the medium perfusing the cat pancreas *in vitro.*

DIGESTIVE SMOOTH MUSCLE

VIP relaxes vascular and tracheal muscle as well as smooth muscle from the gallbladder, stomach, and colon.[11],[12] The only known exception is smooth muscle of the proximal (duodenal) and distal (ileal) small intestine.[6] The requirements of VIP for contracting small intestine muscle, however, are high with a mean C_{50} of 4×10^{-8} M (Fig. 8). By comparison with the octapeptide of cholecystokinin, VIP is only a partial agonist with an efficacy of 0.6. The effect of VIP, like that of the octapeptide of cholecystokinin, is reversibly blocked by tetrodotoxin which indicates that it too is neurally mediated.

STRUCTURE-ACTIVITY RELATIONSHIP

The effects of the N-terminal 1-3 and the C-terminal 18-28, 15-28 and 14-28 synthetic fragments were tested in all studies of secretory and motor function reported above. In no instance was a definite change observed. The requirements for activity are probably N-terminal and midzonal.

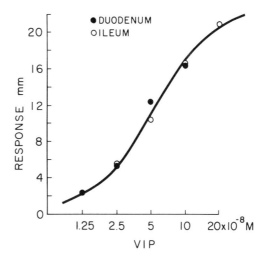

Figure 8. Contractile response of isolated duodenal and ileal longitudinal muscle to VIP.

PHYSIOLOGIC AND PATHOLOGIC STATUS

The physiologic status of VIP remains to be determined. It is possible that VIP is a vestigial peptide, released in small quantities during digestion
and promptly inactivated by the liver. It makes an
unwelcome appearance in tumors believed responsible
for the watery diarrhea syndrome (pancreatic cholera).[2,5] The spectrum of properties observed upon
intravenous injection of VIP, namely stimulation of
intestinal secretion, inhibition of gastric secretion, hyperglycemia, and slight hypercalcemia, conform well to the main components of the watery
diarrhea syndrome.

SUMMARY

The secretory, metabolic, and hormone-releasing
properties of synthetic porcine VIP were investigated
in dogs and cats. VIP inhibited pentagastrin-stimulated acid and pepsin secretion, but was a weak
stimulant of biliary and pancreatic bicarbonate
secretion with an efficacy relative to secretin of
0.25. In contrast, VIP was an effective stimulant
of small intestinal secretion capable of strongly
potentiating the effect of glucagon, a weaker intestinal secretory agonist. VIP raised the blood
glucose in a dose-dependent manner and simultaneously
blood insulin. Studies, in vitro, employing the perfused cat pancreas, showed that VIP was also directly
insulinotropic, independent of the simultaneous rise
in blood glucose. VIP contracted guinea pig intestinal longitudinal muscle, but otherwise relaxed all
other digestive smooth muscle. The spectrum of properties observed upon intravenous injection of VIP,
conform to the main components of the watery diarrhea
syndrome and support the immunochemical evidence
which implicates VIP in this disease.

Acknowledgments

These studies were performed in collaboration with Drs. J.T.
Farrar, A.M. Zfass, W.M. Yau, S.S. Jaffer and M. Schebalin.
The valuable technical assistance of Mrs. Susan Richey and Mr.
George Duckworth is gratefully aknowledged.

References

1. Barbezat GO, Grossman MI: Intestinal secretion: Stimulation by peptides. *Science* 174:422-424, 1971.
2. Bloom SR, Polak JM, Pearse AGE: Vasoactive intestinal peptide and watery diarrhea syndrome. *Lancet* 2:14-16 1973.
3. Bodanszky M, Klausner YS, Said SI: Biological activities of synthetic peptides corresponding to fragments of and to the entire sequence of the vasoactive intestinal peptide. *Proc Natl Acad Sci USA* 70:382-384, 1973.
4. Brown JC, Dryburgh JR, Pederson RA: Gastric inhibitory polypeptide and motilin, in Chey WY, Brooks FP (eds), *Endocrinology of the Gut*, Thorofare NJ: Charles B. Slack, Inc., 1974, pp 76-82.
5. Isenberg JI, Walsh JH, Grossman MI: Zollinger-Ellison syndrome. *Gastroenterology* 65:140-165, 1973.
6. Jaffer SS, Farrar JT, Yau WM, Makhlouf GM: Mode of action and interplay of vasoactive intestinal peptide (VIP), secretin, and octapeptide of cholecystokinin (Octa-CCK) on duodenal and ileal muscle in vitro, abstracted. *Gastroenterology* 66:716, 1974.
7. Kerins C, Said SI: Hyperglycemic and glycogenolytic effects of vasoactive intestinal polypeptide. *Proc Soc Exp Biol Med* 142:1014-1017, 1972.
8. Makhlouf GM: The neuroendocrine design of the gut. *Gastroenterology* 67:159-184, 1974.
9. Makhlouf GM, Said SI, Yau WM: Interplay of vasoactive intestinal peptide (VIP) and synthetic VIP fragments with secretin and octapeptide of cholecystokinin (Octa-CCK) on pancreatic and biliary secretion, abstracted. *Gastroenterology* 66:737, 1974.
10. Rayford PL, Villar HV, Reeder DD, Thompson JC: Effect of GIP and VIP on gastrin release and gastric secretion, abstracted. *Physiologist* 17:319, 1974.
11. Said SI, Makhlouf GM: Vasoactive intestinal polypeptide: Spectrum of biological activity, in Chey WY, Brooks FP (eds), *Endocrinology of the Gut*, Thorofare NJ: Charles B. Slack, Inc., 1974, pp 88-102.
12. Said SI and Mutt V: Polypeptide with broad biological activity: Isolation from small intestine. *Science* 169:1217-1218, 1970.
13. Said SI, Mutt V: Isolation from porcine-intestinal wall of a vasoactive octacosapeptide related to secretin and to glucagon. *Eur J Biochem* 28:199-204, 1972.

14. Schebalim R, Said SI, Makhlouf GM: Interplay of glucagon,
    vasoactive intestinal peptide (VIP) and synthetic
    fragments of VIP in intestinal secretin, abstracted.
    Clin Res 22:368A, 1974.

15. Schebalin M, Brooks AM, Said S, Makhlouf GM: The insulino-
    tropic effect of vasoactive intestinal peptide (VIP):
    Direct evidence from in vitro studies, abstracted.
    Gastroenterology 66:772, 1974.

16. Schorr BA, Said SI, Makhlouf GM: Inhibition of gastric
    secretion by synthetic vasointestinal peptide (VIP),
    abstracted. *Clin Res* 22:23A, 1974.

17. Schwartz CJ, Kimberg DV, Sheerin HE, Field M, Said SI:
    Vasoactive intestinal peptide stimulation of adenylate
    cyclase and active electrolyte secretion in intestinal
    mucosa. *J Clin Invest* 54:536-544, 1974.

VASOACTIVE INTESTINAL PEPTIDE: COMPARISON WITH SECRETIN FOR POTENCY AND SPECTRUM OF PHYSIOLOGIC ACTION

Stanisław J. Konturek, Piotr Thor, Artur Dembiński, Ryszard Król

Institute of Physiology, Medical Academy, Cracow, Poland

VIP isolated from extracts of the hog small intestine by Said and Mutt[25] and recently synthesized by Bodanszky and associates[2] resembles secretin, gastric inhibitory polypeptide (GIP) and glucagon in chemical structure and spectrum of biologic activity. It has been reported that VIP, like secretin, GIP, or glucagon, is capable of inhibiting gastric secretory activity and acts as a secretin-like partial agonist of pancreatic and biliary secretion.

This study was an attempt to compare VIP and secretin in regard to *inhibition* of gastric secretory and motor activities and *stimulation* of pancreatic and biliary secretions.

METHODS

Surgical Procedures

Three dogs weighing 15-18 kg were prepared surgically with gastric fistulas (GF) drained by a Thomas cannula[28] and a Heidenhain pouch (HP) drained by a Gregory cannula.[7] Three other dogs were provided with GF and denervated antral pouches for the studies on gastric secretion and motility.

Three dogs weighing 14-18 kg were prepared with GF and pancreatic fistulas (PF) made by a modification of the method of Herrera and associates[12] for the studies on pancreatic secretion.

Cholecystectomy was performed in two dogs weighing
12 kg. The minor pancreatic duct was ligated and a
biliary fistula (BF) was formed by the method described previously.[20]

Experimental Procedures

The tests were started at least four weeks after
the operations and were done on conscious dogs that
had been fasted about 18 hours. A continuous intravenous infusion of 0.15 M NaCl was given throughout
each test from a peristaltic pump (Unipan, Poland)
at a rate of 30 ml per hour.

Gastric Secretion. Throughout all tests the GF was open
and secretions from GF and HP were collected continuously and divided into 15-minute samples. The
volume of gastric juice was recorded and acid concentrations were determined by titration as described
previously.[18] Pepsin concentrations in the gastric
juice were determined by a modification[23] of the
Anson[1] hemoglobin method.

Aminopyrine clearance was used to measure mucosal
blood flow according to the procedure described by
Jacobson and associates.[13,14] By determining the
relationship of aminopyrine clearance (an estimate
of mucosal blood flow) to the rate of secretion
from GF or HP, a ratio (R) is obtained which provides information concerning the dynamics of secretion.

Basal secretion was collected for two 15-minute
periods and then the stimulant was given. In one
set of studies with pentagastrin-induced gastric
secretion, the exact comparison of the inhibitory
effectiveness of VIP and secretin was made. Three
different doses of VIP or secretin were given intravenously as single shots. The dose level differed
by a factor of three, so that the middle dose was
three times the lowest dose and the highest dose
was three times the middle dose. Two rapid intravenous injections of VIP or secretin were given
during each experiment, the first at 1½ hours and
the second at 3½ hours after the beginning of
pentagastrin infusion. VIP and synthetic secretin
were given alternately according to a randomized
block arrangement, so that each dose was given twice

as the first injection and twice as the second injection in each dog. In control tests in each dog,
the injection of VIP or secretin was replaced by
saline injection. These controls were done before,
during, and after the experiments with VIP or secretin. The inhibition of acid output, calculated for
the 30 minutes after the injection, was taken as
the difference between the control (saline) and the
test (VIP or secretin), expressed as a percentage
of the control. Since secretion had returned to
control level before the second injection, the data
obtained from both injections were pooled to calculate the mean inhibition.
    In another set of studies histamine was given in a
dose that has been shown to produce half-maximal
acid output. Ninety minutes after starting the infusion of histamine, when the secretory rate was
relatively stable, VIP or secretin was added to
intravenous infusion in a dose of 8 µg/kg/hr or
1 U/kg/hr, respectively. The doses of VIP and
secretin were selected as those that gave about 50%
inhibition of pentagastrin-induced gastric acid
secretion.

Gastric Motility. Motility records were made from the
intact stomach and from vagally denervated fundic
and antral pouches. The sensor consisted of a
water-filled polyvinyl tube with a side opening
1.5 mm in length, 2 cm from the closed end. The
tube was continuously perfused with 0.15 M NaCl
from an infusion pump at a constant rate of 7 ml/hr.
This rate did not cause any increase in pressure
when the tube was open to atmosphere. The tube was
connected to a transducer (Sanborn Co, Model 267 AC,
Waltham, Mass.), and pressure was recorded by a
Sanborn direct writer recorder. Atmospheric pressure was assigned 0 pressure. The pressure transducer was placed at the level of the open tip of the
tube. The sensor was introduced through the metal
cannula of GF into the stomach so that the opening
was about 3 cm distal to the internal opening of
the gastric cannula. The sensor was held in place
with a perforated rubber stopper which permitted
free drainage of secretion throughout the experiment.
The sensor used in the antral or fundic pouch was
the same as the one described above for use in the
intact stomach. The sensor was passed into the

innermost portion of the pouch and was maintained in
position by passing a piece of masking tape secured
to the tube around the abdomen. The sensor tube was
perfused with 0.15 M NaCl at a rate of 2.5 ml per
hour.

The motility tests were performed with graded-dose
injections of VIP or secretin. The motility pattern
was observed for a minimum of 30 minutes and then a
hormonal preparation was injected intravenously as
single shot. The recording was continued for an
additional 30 minutes or until motor activity returned to the control level. VIP and secretin were
injected in graded doses ranging from 2-16 µg/kg
and 0.25-2.0 U/kg, respectively. The doses of VIP
or secretin were given alternately as in the secretory tests. The interval between the injections was
long enough to allow motility to return to initial
level for at least 30 minutes.

Motility was analyzed by counting the number of
contractions per 15-minute period and measuring the
amplitude of each wave. To avoid inclusion of artifactual movements, only waves of greater pressure
than 3 cm H_2O were used in compiling the data reported here. In tests with graded-dose injections
of hormonal preparations, the average percentage
changes in motor activity occurring during 15 minutes
after injections were calculated at each dose level.

Pancreatic Secretion. Throughout all tests, the GF
was left open to allow drainage of gastric juice to
the outside and to prevent endogenous duodenal acidification.

Secretions from the PF were collected continuously
and divided into 10- or 15-minute samples. The
volume was recorded to the nearest 0.1 ml. Bicarbonate and protein concentrations were estimated as
described previously.[19] In some samples of pancreatic
juice the activities of amylase and trypsin were
measured. The activity of amylase was determined by
the method of Caraway.[4] Tryptic activity was measured by a modification of the method of Haverback
and associates.[11] Amylase and trypsin activities
were expressed in units and outputs were calculated
as volume times activity and expressed in units per
15 or 30 minutes.

For the comparison of secretory potencies, VIP or
secretin was infused intravenously in graded doses.

The dose level was changed every 60 minutes and differed by a factor of two.

The interaction of VIP or secretin with cholecysto-kinin was studied by intravenous infusion of graded doses of VIP or secretin in combination with a constant dose of synthetic caerulein. The dose level of VIP or secretin was changed every 60-minute period.

The interaction of VIP with secretin was determined by infusing VIP intravenously in various doses (1-8 µg/kg/hr) during an infusion of a constant dose of secretin (1 U/kg/hr). In control experiments the dogs received secretin alone for the duration of the test.

Biliary Secretion. Throughout all tests the BF was kept open as in tests with pancreatic secretion. Bile was collected every 15 minutes. The volume was recorded and bicarbonate concentration was determined in each sample by the technique used for analysis of bicar-bonate of pancreatic juice. A continuous intravenous infusion of 1% sodium taurocholate (Maybridge Chemi-cal Co, Tintagel, N. Cornwall, England) was given throughout each experiment at a rate of 1 ml/min.

For the comparison of secretory potencies, VIP or secretin was infused intravenously in graded doses. The dose level was changed every 60 minutes and differed by a factor of two.

RESULTS

Effect on Gastric Secretion

The injections of VIP or secretin against a background dose of pentagastrin (2 µg/kg/hr) producing half-maximal acid output, resulted in a dose-related inhibition of gastric acid secretion (Fig. 1). The dose-response curve for VIP and secretin showed no statistically significant difference. The potency of VIP inhibiting gastric acid secretion was 0.25 U/µg. A dose of 8 µg/kg/hr VIP or 1 U/kg/hr secretin caused about 50% inhibition (ED_{50}) of pentagastrin-induced half-maximal acid output.

With histamine stimulation (80 µg/kg/hr) the acid output from GF was as high as during pentagastrin infusion and remained fairly well sustained

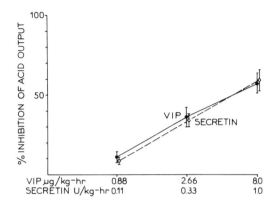

Figure 1. Relation between doses of VIP or secretin and the percent inhibition of acid output from GF stimulated by pentagastrin. In this and subsequent figures each line is the mean of three tests on each of three dogs. (Mean ± SEM).

Figure 2. Effect of VIP or secretin on histamine-induced gastric acid outputs from GF and HP.

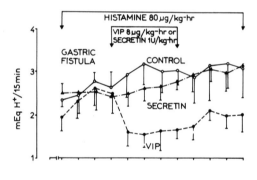

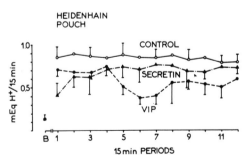

throughout the secretory test (Fig. 2). The acid
output from HP was about twice as high as in tests
with pentagastrin. VIP inhibited acid output, whereas secretin showed no difference in acid response to
histamine. Pepsin was secreted at low concentration
during histamine infusion. With VIP, pepsin output
was significantly decreased, whereas during secretin
infusion, pepsin output showed a tendency to increase
above the control level but this rise was not statistically significant (Fig. 3).

The clearance of aminopyrine in tests with histamine was significantly reduced by VIP (Fig. 4) but
unchanged by secretin. The R value with both VIP
and secretin remained unchanged throughout the
experiment.

Inhibition of Gastric Motility

In the intact stomach and in the denervated fundic
and antral pouches, regular contractions could easily

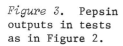

Figure 3. Pepsin
outputs in tests
as in Figure 2.

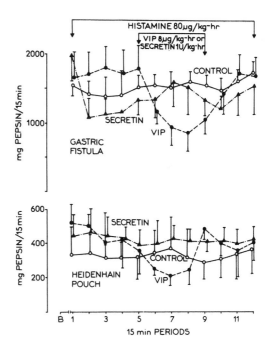

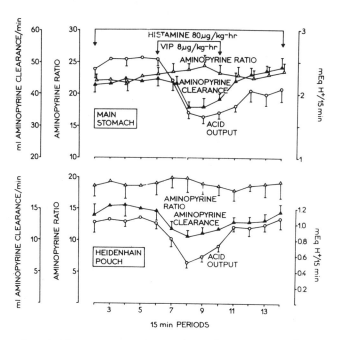

Figure 4. Acid output, aminopyrine clearance, and ratio values after histamine alone and histamine combined with VIP.

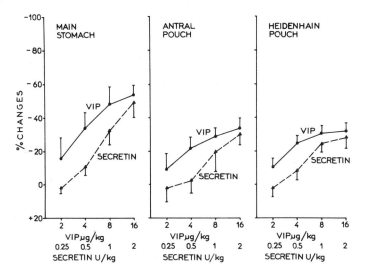

Figure 5. Percent changes in the number of contractions in the main stomach, denervated antral pouch, and HP in response to intravenous injections of graded doses of VIP or secretin.

be demonstrated in the fasting animal. The intravenous injection of either VIP or secretin resulted
in a prompt inhibition of this spontaneous motor
activity. Both VIP and secretin in all doses used
except the lowest, caused a significant inhibition
of motor activity. The inhibitory effect was most
pronounced during the first 15-minute period after
administration. As shown in Figure 5, increments
in the dosage of VIP or secretin were accompanied
by a corresponding increase in inhibition. The inhibitory effect was more pronounced in the main
stomach than in the denervated fundic or antral
pouches. The comparison of the dose-response curves
showed that 2 μg of VIP was not much more potent than
0.25 U of secretin. Parallel results were obtained
in the mean peak amplitude of gastric contraction
waves.

In the tests in which VIP or secretin was injected
intravenously in graded doses, pepsin output showed
a dose-related increase with both peptides (Fig. 6).

Effect on Pancreatic Secretion

The results on the comparison of pancreatic responses to VIP and secretin are shown in Figure 7.
Both VIP and secretin infused intravenously produced

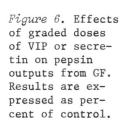

Figure 6. Effects
of graded doses
of VIP or secre-
tin on pepsin
outputs from GF.
Results are ex-
pressed as per-
cent of control.

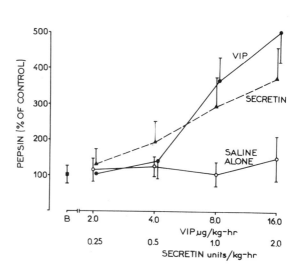

the peak response for volume and bicarbonate outputs
in the first or second 15-minute period and this
value was used to express the results. As shown in
Figure 7, graded doses of VIP and secretin evoked a
dose-related secretory response, achieving the highest
observed responses with VIP and secretin at the doses
of 8 µg/kg/hr and 4 U/kg/hr, respectively. The mean
(± SEM) maximal bicarbonate output that was observed
in response to VIP was 0.74±0.13 mEq/30 min and it was
about 17% of the response to secretin (4.16±0.73 mEq/
30 min). Dose-response analysis showed that mean
(± SEM) calculated maximal responses (CMR) for VIP and
secretin were 0.87±0.12 and 5.52±0.65 mEq/30 min, respectively (Fig. 8). Mean (± SEM) D_{50}s for VIP and
secretin were 1.81±0.14 µg/kg/hr and 1.31±0.12 U/kg/hr,
respectively. The efficacy of VIP was thus 0.17.

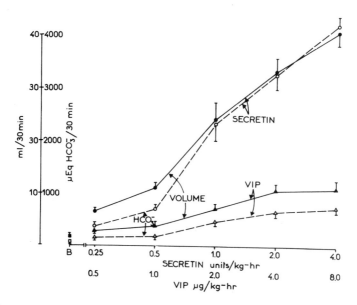

Figure 7. Effect of intravenous infusion of graded doses of
secretin or VIP on pancreatic volume flow and bicarbonate
outputs. In this and subsequent figures each line is a mean
of three tests on each of three dogs. Vertical bars are
standard errors of the mean.

Since the dose-response curves departed from parallel, the determination of the relative potency of VIP and secretin was possible only after additional secretory tests were performed in which secretin was infused intravenously in lower doses. The potency ratio of VIP to secretin was found to be about 8 µg/U (Fig. 9).

Both VIP and secretin infused intravenously in graded doses caused a sustained but dose-independent increase in protein and enzyme output (Figs. 10 & 11).

VIP in combination with a background dose of caerulein, produced a dose-related pancreatic volume flow and bicarbonate secretion that reached the highest observed output at a dose of 8 µg/kg/hr (Fig. 12). The bicarbonate response curve to VIP plus caerulein was significantly higher at all dose levels than to VIP alone. Similarly, the secretory response to secretin combined with caerulein background was significantly higher than to secretin alone at all dose

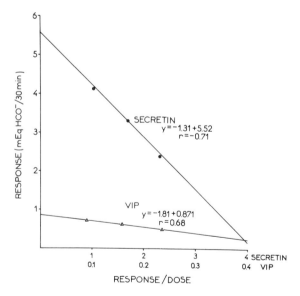

Figure 8. Linear plots of bicarbonate response against ratio of response/dose of secretin or VIP. Maximal responses (CMR) are given by the vertical intercepts and D_{50}s by the slopes.

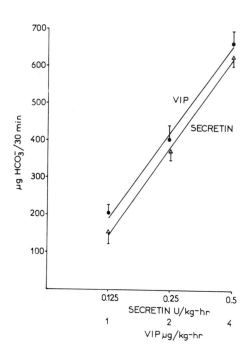

Figure 9. Pancreatic bicarbonate secretion after various doses of secretin or VIP infused intravenously.

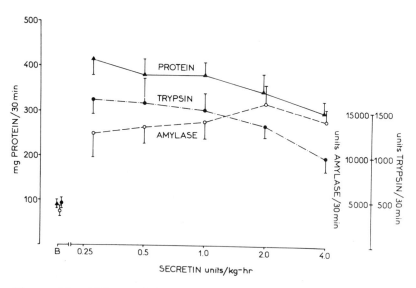

Figure 10. Effect of intravenous infusion of graded doses of secretin on pancreatic protein and enzyme secretion.

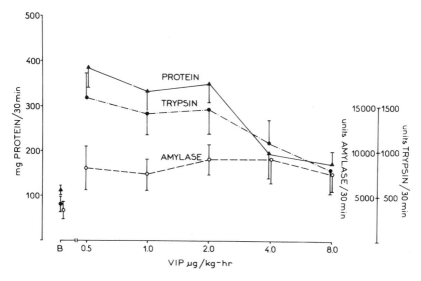

Figure 11. Effect of intravenous infusion of graded doses of VIP on pancreatic protein and enzyme secretion.

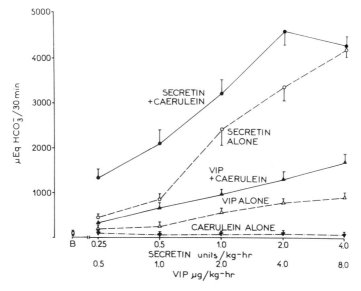

Figure 12. Pancreatic bicarbonate secretion in response to graded doses of secretin or VIP given alone or with a constant dose of caerulein.

levels except the highest (4 U/kg/hr). There was a
shift of the dose-response curve to VIP and secretin
to the left. The highest observed bicarbonate responses to the combined agents were supramaximal
compared with VIP or secretin alone and were greater
than a summed response. Caerulein alone evoked negligible pancreatic bicarbonate secretion.

The results on the interaction of VIP with secretin
are shown in Figures 13 to 15. The intravenous infusion of secretin in constant doses, produced a well
sustained plateau of pancreatic bicarbonate secretion.
The addition of VIP in a dose of 4 µg/kg/hr to intravenous infusion of secretin, caused a significant
inhibition of pancreatic volume and bicarbonate response to secretin. Over the wide range of doses
(0.5 to 4.0 U/kg/hr), doubling the dose of secretin
produced a corresponding increase in pancreatic
secretion both with and without VIP (Fig. 13). Although the percentage of inhibition decreased with
increasing doses of secretin, the absolute amounts

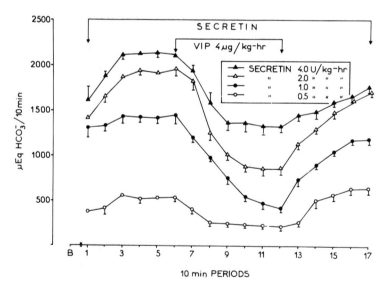

Figure 13. Effect of intravenous infusion of VIP upon pancreatic
bicarbonate outputs during infusion of varying doses of secretin.

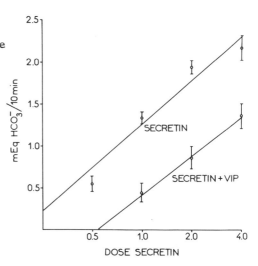

Figure 14. Dose-response curves to secretin and to secretin plus VIP. Points represent mean values obtained in last two 15-minute periods during VIP administration or comparable periods when secretin was infused alone.

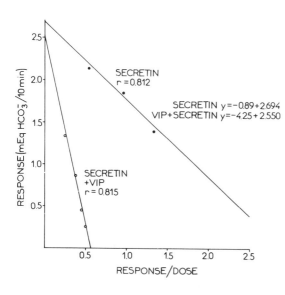

Figure 15. Data from Figure 10 plotted as the response against the response/dose. Equations for lines and coefficients of correlations are shown.

of inhibition remained essentially constant except
with the lowest dose of secretin (Fig. 14). When
the data from Figure 13 were plotted as response
against the response/dose in Figure 15, the plots
had widely different slopes and only slightly
differing intercepts with the Y axis. In this
particular transformation of Michaelis-Menten equation[5] the slope of the line is equal the D_{50} and
the intercept is equal the CMR. For secretin alone
the CMR equaled 2.55 mEq/30 min and the D_{50} equaled
0.98 U/kg/hr secretin, and for the combination of
VIP with various doses of secretin, D_{50} equaled
4 U/kg/hr secretin. The D_{50}s are significantly
different, whereas the difference in CMRs was statistically insignificant.

Doses of VIP doubling from and including 1 μg/kg/hr,
produced a prompt and significant inhibition of pancreatic secretion stimulated by near maximal dose of
secretin. The infusion of 1.0 μg/kg/hr VIP caused a
detectable and significant inhibition of secretin-
induced bicarbonate secretion. This dose may be
considered as the approximate threshold for VIP
inhibition. Maximal inhibition occurred with
8 μg/kg/hr (Fig. 16).

VIP infusion also resulted in an immediate reduction of the protein output due to a decrease in both
volume of the juice and protein concentration. Concurrently with the suppression of protein secretion,
there was also a decrease of amylase and trypsin
outputs (Fig. 17). The inhibition of protein and
enzyme outputs occurred at all doses of VIP but this
inhibition was not dose-related.

Effect on Bile Secretion

Secretin produced a dose-related increase of bile
flow and bicarbonate outputs from BF. VIP was also
an effective stimulant of bile secretion but the
increases in bile volume and bicarbonate outputs
were not dose-related.

DISCUSSION

VIP is a highly basic peptide which resembles
secretin, glucagon, and GIP in amino acid sequence

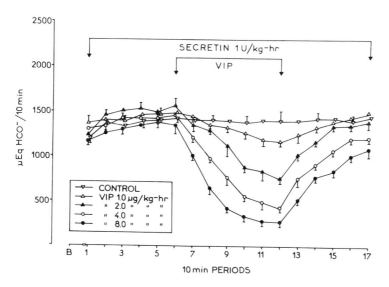

Figure 16. Effect of infusion of various doses of VIP on pancreatic bicarbonate secretion in response to secretin. Control received only secretin throughout the experiment.

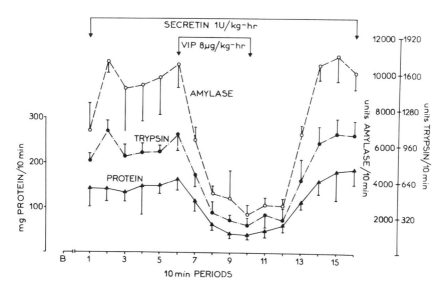

Figure 17. Effect of VIP on pancreatic protein and enzyme secretion in response to secretin.

and biologic actions.   It shares nine identities with
secretin, five with glucagon, and four with GIP, the
identities being widely dispersed in the molecule.
  The common feature of all four peptides is the
inhibitory action on gastric acid secretion.   This
study shows that VIP and secretin cause a dose-related
inhibition of pentagastrin-induced acid secretion.
VIP has a wider spectrum of inhibition than secretion,
for, unlike secretin, it is also able to inhibit
histamine-induced acid and pepsin secretion.   It is
of interest that the inhibition of gastric acid
secretion by VIP is accompanied by a parallel reduction in gastric mucosal blood flow as estimated by
the clearance of aminopyrine.   The ratio between
aminopyrine concentration in gastric juice and plasma
remained unchanged during the administration of VIP,
which indicates that it is unlikely that the reduction in blood flow is the primary factor of the inhibitory action.   The results would suggest that VIP
may have an as yet unknown direct inhibitory effect
on acid-producing cells.   A comparison of the inhibitory effect of VIP and secretin indicates that VIP
may differ from secretin by being a potent inhibitor
of histamine-induced gastric secretion.   Inhibition
of acid secretion by VIP is, therefore, more akin to
that by GIP.[9,27]
  The most striking difference in the action of these
two peptides is in the effect on pepsin secretion.
The pepsigogue effect of secretin has been recognized
since 1940 when Pratt[24] reported that crude secretin
increased pepsin secretion in response to histamine.
Johnson and Harrison,[16] using highly purified natural
secretin, demonstrated that this hormone stimulated
pepsin secretion in a dose-related manner and that
endogenous hormone released by duodenal acidification
can completely mimic the pepsigogue effect of exogenous hormone.   Among the intestinal hormonal peptides,
only secretin has so far been reported to stimulate
pepsin secretion.   Our study demonstrates that VIP
is capable of both stimulating pepsin secretion under
basal conditions and inhibiting pepsin output when
combined with a background stimulation by histamine.
The reason for the difference in the action of these
hormonal peptides on pepsin secretion is not apparent
from this report.
  Our study shows that VIP and secretin significantly
inhibit the spontaneous motor activity of the intact

stomach and vagally denervated portions of the fundic
and antral gland area. The degree of motor inhibition
is closely related to the dose of these peptides. The
motor responses of the vagally denervated portions
of the stomach are, however, less pronounced than
those of the intact stomach. It is of interest that
after vagal denervation of the stomach, secretin also
becomes a less potent inhibitor of gastric acid secretion, as reported previously.[3]

The contribution of VIP as well as secretin to the
regulation of gastric secretory and motor functions
under physiologic conditions remains to be assessed.
Johnson and Grossman[15] have suggested that secretin
is the only enterogastrone of physiologic significance
so far known to be released by acid from the duodenum.
The amount of secretin released by acid under normal
conditions, however, may be negligible and this hormone fails to inhibit histamine-induced gastric secretion. More recently Brown and associates[9] provided
evidence to support the notion that GIP accounts for
the action that has been called enterogastrone and
that it is released by a meal from the intestinal
mucosa. The mechanism and the site of release of
VIP are unknown. If released in amounts comparable
to those used in our present study, VIP may be also
considered as an enterogastrone, the idea of which
has been kept alive ever since Farrel and Ivy[6] found
that feeding fat inhibited the spontaneous motility
of a transplanted gastric pouch in the dog and then
Kosaka and Lim[21] extended this observation on acid
secretion induced by histamine from a HP.

Previous preliminary studies on the effect of VIP
on pancreatic secretion on anesthetized animals,[22,26]
showed that this peptide is a partial agonist of
pancreatic bicarbonate secretion and that, like
secretin, it augments the pancreatic response to CCK.
Our present study, performed on conscious dogs, confirmed this observation in part, and we also found
that VIP may competitively inhibit secretin-induced
pancreatic secretion.

Our data show that VIP given alone is a weak stimulant of pancreatic volume flow and bicarbonate
secretion and also causes negligible stimulation of
pancreatic protein and enzyme secretion. The maximal
observed rate of bicarbonate secretion attainable
with VIP is only about 17% of that obtained with
secretin, so VIP has a much lower efficacy as compared with secretin.

Caerulein clearly potentiates pancreatic bicarbonate response to VIP. Pancreatic bicarbonate response
to the combination of caerulein plus VIP is clearly
greater at each point on the dose-response curve than
to the sum of the effects of each agent alone. Thus,
by accepted criteria, caerulein potentiates the pancreatic bicarbonate response to various doses of VIP.
Similar considerations with regard to exogenous
secretin indicate that this hormone combined with
caerulein or a peptone meal also produces potentiated
pancreatic protein responses, as reported previously.[10]

The major finding of this study is the inhibition by
VIP of secretin-induced pancreatic secretion, which so
far as we know has not been previously reported. VIP
as a close homologue of secretin is assumed to act on
the same receptor sites of bicarbonate-producing cells.
Grossman[8] suggested that all digestive hormonal receptors possess a pair of interacting sites, one with
affinity for gastrin and related peptides and the other
with affinity for secretin and related peptides.
Receptor sites occupied by an agent with low efficacy
are blocked from reacting with homologue agents with
high efficacy. Since the efficacies of VIP and secretin differ greatly, as expected from the Grossman hypothesis, VIP with lower efficacy competitively inhibits secretin with higher efficacy. The characteristic features of competitive inhibition by VIP of
pancreatic secretion are an increased D_{50} and unchanged CMR.

It is of interest that VIP also causes inhibition of
pancreatic protein and enzyme secretion induced by
secretin. The inhibition can be attributed to the
reduction of pancreatic volume flow rather than to the
decrease in the protein and enzyme concentrations.
The possible mechanism of VIP-evoked inhibition of
pancreatic protein secretion was not studied, but
perhaps it was due to unspecific factors such as
hyperglycemia or interference with the splanchnic
circulation.[17,29]

The physiologic significance of VIP as a normal
hormone of pancreatic secretion has not been established. The pronounced inactivation of VIP in the
liver[9] suggests that the effect of this peptide may
be limited to the gastrointestinal system. The dual
effects of VIP on pancreatic secretion, stimulatory
when acting alone and inhibitory when combined with
secretin, suggest that this peptide may play a regulatory function in the control of pancreatic secretion.

SUMMARY

VIP and secretin were compared in regard to the inhibition of gastric secretory and motor activities, and to the stimulation of pancreatic and biliary secretion. Both VIP and secretin caused a dose-related inhibition of pentagastrin-induced gastric acid secretion. VIP in contrast to secretin, inhibited the acid and pepsin responses to histamine and reduced gastric mucosal blood flow. Both VIP and secretin resulted in a dose-related reduction in the rate and amplitude of the gastric contraction waves in the intact stomach and to a lesser degree in the denervated fundic and antral pouches. Comparison of pancreatic stimulatory potencies of both peptides showed that maximal bicarbonate response to VIP was about 17% of that to secretin. Caerulein clearly potentiated pancreatic bicarbonate response to VIP in a similar way to secretin. The interaction of these two peptides demonstrated that VIP is a competitive inhibitor of secretin-induced pancreatic bicarbonate secretion and is capable of suppressing secretin-induced pancreatic protein and enzyme secretion. These studies indicate that VIP has enterogastrone properties and shows biphasic stimulatory and inhibitory actions on pancreatic bicarbonate secretion as well as suppressive action on enzyme secretion.

References

1. Anson ML: The estimation of pepsin, trypsin, papain and cathepsin with hemoglobin. *J Gen Physiol* 22:79-89, 1948.
2. Bodanszky M, Klausner YS, Said SI: Biological activities of synthetic peptides corresponding to fragments of and to the entire sequence of the vasoactive intestinal peptide. *Proc Natl Acad Sci USA* 70:382-384, 1973.
3. Brooks AM, Stening GF, Grossman MI: Effect of gastric vagal denervation on inhibition of acid secretion by gastrin. *Am J Dig Dis* 16:193-202, 1971.
4. Caraway WT: A stable starch substrate for the determination of amylase in serum and other body fluids. *Am J Clin Path* 32:97-99, 1959.

5. Dowd JE, Riggs DS: A comparison of estimates of Michaelis-
    Menten kinetic constants from various linear transfor-
    mations. *J Biol Chem* 240:863–869, 1965.
6. Farrell JI, Ivy AC: Studies on the motility of the trans-
    planted gastric pouch, abstracted. *Am J Physiol* 76:
    227–228, 1926.
7. Gregory RA: Gastric secretory responses after portal venous
    ligation. *J Physiol* 144:123–127, 1958.
8. Grossman MI: Gastrin, cholecystokinin and secretin act on
    one receptor. *Lancet* 1:1088–1089, 1970.
9. Grossman MI and others: Candidate hormones of the gut.
    Gastroenterology 67:730–755, 1974.
10. Grossman MI, Konturek SJ: Gastric acid does drive pancreatic
    bicarbonate secretion. *Scand J Gastroenterol* 9:299–302,
    1974.
11. Haverback BJ, Dyce BJ, Gutentag PJ, Montgomery DW: Measure-
    ment of trypsin and chymotrypsin in stool: A diagnostic
    test for pancreatic exocrine insufficiency. *Gastro-
    enterology* 44:588–597, 1963.
12. Herrera F, Kemp DR, Tsukamoto M, Woodward ER, Dragstedt LR:
    A new cannula for the study of pancreatic function.
    J Appl Physiol 25:207–209, 1968.
13. Jacobson ED, Linford RH, Grossman MI: Gastric secretion in
    relation to mucosal blood flow studied by a clearance
    technique. *J Clin Invest* 45:1–13, 1966.
14. Jacobson ED, Swan KG, Grossman MI: Blood flow and secretion
    in the stomach. *Gastroenterology* 52:414–420, 1967.
15. Johnson LR, Grossman MI: Secretin: The enterogastrone
    released by acid in the duodenum. *Am J Physiol* 215:
    885–888, 1968.
16. Johnson LR, Harrison LA: Comparison of exogenous secretin
    and duodenal acidification on pepsin secretion in dogs.
    Am J Physiol 221:784–787, 1971.
17. Kerins C, Said SI: Hyperglycemic and glycogenolytic effects
    of vasoactive intestinal polypeptide. *Proc Soc Exp
    Biol Med* 142:1014–1017, 1973.
18. Konturek SJ, Tasler J, Obtułowicz W: Effect of metiamide,
    a histamine H_2-receptor antagonist, on mucosal blood
    flow and serum gastrin level. *Gastroenterology* 66:
    982–986, 1974.
19. Konturek SJ, Tasler J, Obtułowicz W: Characteristics of
    inhibition of pancreatic secretion by glucagon.
    Digestion 10:138–149, 1974.
20. Konturek SJ, Thor P: Effect of diversion and replacement
    of bile on pancreatic secretion. *Am J Dig Dis* 18:
    971–977, 1973.

21. Kosaka T, Lim RKS: On the mechanism of the inhibition of gastric secretion by fat: The role of bile and cystokinin. *Chin J Physiol* 4:213-220, 1930.
22. Makhlouf GM, Said SI, Yau WM: Interplay of vasoactive intestinal peptide (VIP) and synthetic VIP fragments with secretin and octapeptide of cholecystokinin (OCTA-CCK) on pancreatic and biliary secretion, abstracted. *Gastroenterology* 66:737, 1974.
23. Northrup JH, Kunitz M, Herriot RM: *Crystalline Enzymes,* ed 2, New York: Columbia University Press, 1948, pp 303-307.
24. Pratt CLG: The influence of secretin on gastric secretion, abstracted. *J Physiol* 98:1P-2P, 1940.
25. Said SI, Mutt V: Polypeptide with broad biological activity: Isolation from small intestine. *Science* 169:1217-1218, 1970.
26. Said SI, Mutt V: Isolation from porcine-intestinal wall of a vasoactive octacosapeptide related to secretin and to glucagon. *Eur J Biochem* 28:199-204, 1972.
27. Schorr BA, Said SI, Makhlouf GM: Inhibition of gastric secretion by synthetic vasointestinal peptide (VIP), abstracted. *Clin Res* 22:22a, 1974.
28. Thomas JE: An improved cannula for gastric and intestinal fistulas. *Proc Soc Exp Biol Med* 46:260-261, 1941.
29. Thulin L: Effect of gastrointestinal polypeptide on hepatic bile flow and splanchnic circulation. *Acta Chir Scand (suppl)* 441:5-31, 1973.

THE ROLE OF VIP IN PANCREATIC CHOLERA

S.R. Bloom, J.M. Polak

Department of Medicine and Department of
Histochemistry, The Royal Postgraduate
Medical School, The Hammersmith Hospital,
London, England

THE SYNDROME

In 1958 John Verner and Ashton Morrison drew atten-
tion to the association of severe refractory watery
diarrhoea with noninsulin-secreting islet cell adenomas
of the pancreas.[14] Other features of this syndrome
include hypokalaemia secondary to the diarrhoea, which
often requires large quantities of exogenous potassium
for correction, and hypo- or achlorhydria, which is
the main feature that distinguishes this syndrome from
the Zollinger-Ellison syndrome in which about a third
of the patients also have diarrhoea, albeit usually
less severe.[6] These main features have given rise to
the term WDHA syndrome (watery diarrhoea, hypokalaemia,
achlorhydria).[9] Because of the profuse and often
fatal diarrhoea, the more descriptive term "pancreatic
cholera" is also used.[10] Other frequent features of
the syndrome include diabetes mellitus, hypercalcaemia,
and skin flushing.[15] In a recent review of 55 cases,[15]
80% had a pancreatic tumour, whereas 20% did not, and
in the latter, diffuse nonbeta pancreatic islet hyperplasia was reported. Only 30% of the group were
completely cured by removal of a benign pancreatic
tumour, whereas in another 37%, metastases had already
occurred at the time of diagnosis. In the latter, a
good response to steroid therapy with considerable
reduction of diarrhoea was observed in many cases. The
mean time from onset of symptoms to diagnosis was
reported to be three years[8] and the diagnosis was
sometimes delayed by the occurrence of spontaneous

remissions. It has been pointed out that earlier
diagnosis of the syndrome would lead to much more
successful treatment.[15]

VIP

A vasoactive intestinal peptide (VIP) was isolated
from the upper small intestine of the pig by Said
and Mutt[11] in 1970. It was later found to have considerable amino acid homologies with secretin, glucagon, and gastric inhibitory peptide (GIP).[4] Like
secretin, it caused an alkaline juice flow from the
pancreas[12] and like glucagon it caused hyperglycaemia
by stimulating hepatic glycogenolysis.[7] Like GIP,
it inhibited even histamine-stimulated gastric acid
production.[1] In 1971 VIP was shown greatly to
stimulate flow of juices in the small intestine.[1]
Thus the actions of VIP fitted well with the abnor-
malities seen in the Verner-Morrison syndrome. Other
hormones have been suggested as possible causal
agents, of which the strongest candidate was secretin. This was based on the finding that tumour extracts caused a secretin-like stimulation of pancreatic juice flow in the dog.[13] In 1973, however,
high plasma and tumour levels of VIP were reported,
whereas secretin and GIP levels were found to be
within normal limits.[3] An earlier report that GIP
was involved[5] was proved incorrect. Several unanswered questions remained. First, as the VIP
assay was based on porcine VIP, was the immunoreactive material found in the Verner-Morrison syndrome
really of similar nature? Second, were all cases
of Verner-Morrison syndrome caused by a VIPoma?
Third, was VIP associated with those cases of pancreatic cholera where no pancreatic tumour was
found?

VIP RADIOIMMUNOASSAY

Pure porcine VIP was used to raise antibodies, and
after 12 to 18 months, about 10% of the rabbits
produced high affinity antisera. VIP was iodinated
with [125]Iodine using a modification of the Chloramine-
T technique.[2] Standard radioimmunoassay procedures
were employed, and a charcoal separation was used
after a five-day incubation at 4C. When the assay

mixture contained 20% plasma, differences between
adjacent samples of 12 pg/ml could be detected with
95% confidence. Two antisera giving this sensitivity
were employed, one giving full displacement with an
18-28 amino acid synthetic VIP fragment (C-terminal
binding), whereas the other showed virtually no
displacement with 18-28 or 15-28 amino acid fragments
(N-terminal binding). There was no cross-reaction,
even at high concentrations, with secretin, glucagon,
or GIP.

PLASMA VIP LEVELS IN THE VERNER-MORRISON SYNDROME

The initial plasma VIP level in 17 patients with
proven Verner-Morrison syndrome is shown in Figure 1.
The subjects included are all those who had severe
watery diarrhoea associated with a pancreatic tumour
(15 cases) or ganglioneuroma (2 cases) and from whom
we received a satisfactory plasma specimen. In only
three patients with proven Verner-Morrison syndrome
were the plasma specimens inadequate, and in these
patients, low VIP levels were found, probably because
of the rapid degradation of VIP by plasma proteolytic
enzymes. The unsatisfactory specimens included one
over four years old and one taken several hours after
death. Similar plasma levels were found in all cases
when the N-terminal and C-terminal assay results were

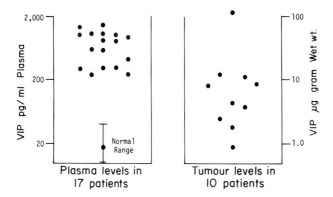

Figure 1. Plasma and tumour VIP levels in the Verner-Morrison
syndrome.

compared. Thus in answer to two of the questions
raised above, the human and porcine immunoreactivity
appears similar, and it seems that plasma VIP levels
are elevated to between 200 and 2000 pg/ml in all
cases of the classical Verner-Morrison syndrome.
Eight cases have been studied with a classical history of the Verner-Morrison syndrome but in whom no
pancreatic tumour was found, though in some cases
islet cell hypertrophy was observed. These patients
had VIP levels indistinguishable from normal and we
have termed these cases "pseudo-Verner-Morrison
syndrome." Many other plasma samples have been
received from colleagues since the first "VIP and
diarrhoea" report appeared. These came from patients
with diarrhoea of many aetiologies, including carcinoid syndrome, medullary carcinoma of the thyroid,
diarrhoea associated with bronchogenic carcinoma,
purgative addition, ulcerative colitis, and none of
these had VIP levels above 200 pg/ml.

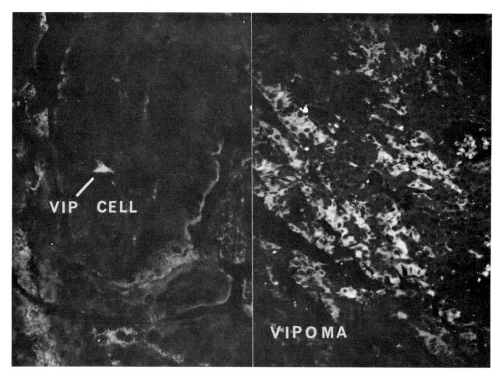

Figure 2. On the left is a section of human ileum and on the
right a section of a Verner-Morrison tumour. They have both
been stained by an immunohistochemical method employing an
antiserum against porcine VIP (×190).

GIP, secretin, and motilin plasma levels have been measured in both the Verner-Morrison and pseudo-Verner-Morrison syndromes and are entirely normal. Glucagon and gastrin, however, were slightly elevated in several cases and in one of these, the glucagon appeared to be coming from the tumour.

TUMOUR VIP CONTENT

Several tumours were obtained in a sufficient state of preservation for immunohistochemical staining and were positive for VIP, although negative for GIP and other hormones (Fig. 2). Electron microscopy demonstrated the presence of many cells with numerous electron-dense secretory granules of about 200 nm diameter and a limiting membrane leaving a wide halo (Fig. 3).

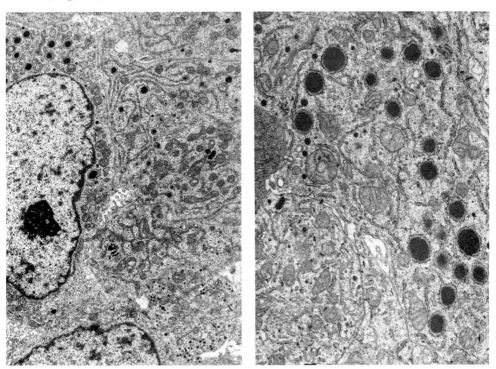

Figure 3. Electron micrographs of a Verner–Morrison tumour showing numerous electron–dense secretory granules with a limiting membrane leaving a wide halo (left, ×4400; right, ×9500).

Extraction of the tumours by acid alcohol gave
high VIP contents in every case studied (Fig. 1),
many times greater than the limit of detection
(0.5 ng/g). Figure 4 shows the elution pattern of
a fresh human ileal extract on a calibrated G50
Sephadex column. The VIP immunoreactivity elutes
as a single peak and leaves the column at exactly
the same position as did porcine VIP on a previous
occasion. Figure 5 shows human tumour VIP run on
the calibrated column. The immunoreactivity again
elutes as a single peak at the same position as the
porcine VIP. Three more tumours were also analysed
and gave identical patterns. Thus human ileal VIP,
tumour VIP and porcine VIP appear to be similar in
molecular size as well as in immunoreactivity.

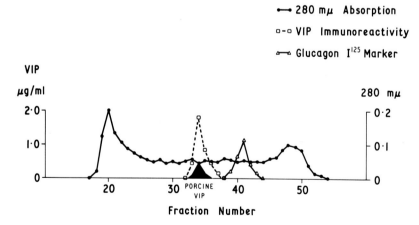

Figure 4. Elution pattern of immunoreactive VIP (dotted line)
from an extract of normal human ileum run on a 1-m G50
Sephadex column in 0.1 M formic acid. The expected position
of porcine VIP, obtained from previous runs, is marked.

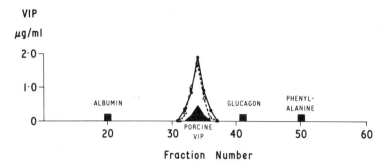

Figure 5. Elution pattern of human Verner-Morrison tumour extracts run on the same column as used for Figure 4. The tumour immunoreactivity is shown as solid and dotted lines, and the expected position of porcine VIP is marked.

SUMMARY

The diagnosis of a VIPoma producing the Verner-Morrison syndrome appears to require only the measurement of a single plasma VIP level. Current experience suggests false negatives and false positives must be rare.

A separate syndrome has been delineated, the "pseudo-Verner-Morrison syndrome" whose cause is unknown.

Acknowledgments

We wish to thank Mr. M.G. Bryant and Mrs. S.J. Mitchell for their considerable help with these studies and also Professor M. Bodanszky for very kindly supplying the VIP fragments. The pure porcine VIP was very generously supplied by Professor V. Mutt. Numerous colleagues donated plasma, tissue, and information on patients under their care, without which this study could not have been carried out.

References

1. Barbezat GO, Grossman MI: Intestinal secretion: Stimulation by peptides. *Science* 174:422-424, 1971.
2. Bloom SR: Hormones of the gastrointestinal tract. *Br Med Bull* 30:62-67, 1974.
3. Bloom SR, Polak JM, Pearse AGE: Vasoactive intestinal peptide and watery-diarrhoea syndrome. *Lancet* 2: 14-16, 1973.
4. Bodanszky M, Klausner YS, Said SI: Biological activities of synthetic peptides corresponding to fragments of and to the entire sequence of the vasoactive intestinal peptide. *Proc Natl Acad Sci USA* 70:382-384, 1973.
5. Elias E, Polak JM, Bloom SR, Pearse AGE, Welbourn RB, Booth CC, Kuzio M, Brown JC: Pancreatic cholera due to production of gastric inhibitory polypeptide. *Lancet* 2:791-793, 1972.
6. Isenberg JI, Walsh JH, Grossman MI: Zollinger-Ellison syndrome. *Gastroenterology* 65:140-165, 1973.
7. Kerins C, Said SI: Hyperglycemic and glycogenolytic effects of vasoactive intestinal polypeptide. *Proc Soc Exp Biol Med* 142:1014-1017, 1972.
8. Kraft AR, Tompkins RK, Zollinger RM: Recognition and management of the diarrheal syndrome caused by nonbeta islet cell tumors of the pancreas. *Am J Surg* 119: 163-170, 1970.
9. Marks IN, Bank S, Louw JH: Islet cell tumour of the pancreas with reversible watery diarrhea and achlorhydria. *Gastroenterology* 52:695-708, 1967.
10. Matsumoto KK, Peter JB, Schultz RG, Hakim AA, Franck PT: Watery diarrhea and hypokalemia associated with pancreatic islet cell adenoma. *Gastroenterology* 50:231-242, 1966.
11. Said SI, Mutt V: Polypeptide with broad biological activity: Isolation from small intestine. *Science* 169:1217-1218, 1970.
12. Said SI, Mutt V: Isolation from porcine intestinal wall of a vasoactive octacosapeptide related to secretin and to glucagon. *Eur J Biochem* 28:199-204, 1972.
13. Sanzenbacher LJ, Mekhjian HS, King DR, Zollinger RM: Studies on the potential role of secretin in the islet cell tumor diarrheogenic syndrome. *Ann Surg* 176:394-402, 1972.
14. Verner JV, Morrison AB: Islet cell tumour and a syndrome of refractory watery diarrhea and hypokalemia. *Am J Med* 25:374-380, 1958.
15. Verner JV, Morrison AB: Endocrine pancreatic islet disease with diarrhea. *Arch Intern Med* 133:492-500, 1974.

CHOLECYSTOKININ AND CENTRAL NERVOUS REGULATION OF APPETITE

Nachum Dafny, Eugene D. Jacobson

Programs in Neural Structure and Function
and Physiology, The University of Texas
Medical School, Houston, Texas

The neurohumoral basis for satiety after eating is unknown. There is some evidence that cholecysto-kinin (CCK), which is released postprandially, may induce satiety as a negative feedback. The effect of CCK and of other gastrointestinal hormones on the electrophysiologic properties of those portions of the central nervous system which regulate appetite is not known.

Beaumont[1] noted that St. Martin required instilla-tion of food into the upper gastrointestinal tract to assuage his hunger. Parenteral injection of in-testinal mucosal extracts, presumably containing soluble polypeptide hormones, caused depression of hunger and weight loss in rabbits.[5] Gibbs and associates[3,4] injected unfed rats with purified CCK or the synthetic octapeptide (CCK-OP), which possesses all the biologic activity of the entire CCK molecule, and evoked satiety. Pentagastrin and secretin did not stimulate the satiety response in the rats. Satiety was evoked by feeding, which is also known to produce release of gastrointestinal hormones, including CCK.

The aim of our study was to determine electro-physiologic changes in the polysynaptic output of various areas of the brain to gastrointestinal hor-mones. Central effects of CCK or other gastroin-testinal hormones can be expected to result from modulation of neuronal activities, and such actions may be localized in one or more brain structures. The present study represents an initial attempt to elucidate the postsynaptic effects of gastrointestinal hormones in several structures within the central nervous system which are presumably involved in controlling and regulating the appetite.

Responses evoked by click (acoustic) stimuli were recorded simultaneously from the ventromedial hypothalamus (VMH), lateral hypothalamus (LH), anterior hypothalamus (AH), septum pellucidum (SPT), dorsal hippocampus (H), amygdala complex (A), raphe nucleus (RN), and caudate nucleus (CN) in the conscious, freely moving rat.[2] The responses were recorded monopolarly with chronically implanted nichrome electrodes of 50 μ in diameter and a reference electrode implanted in the frontal sinuses. One week before experimentation, electrodes were placed in anesthetized rats using stereotaxic coordinates, and the placement was verified histologically in all rats. The evoked potentials were displayed on a storage oscilloscope, averaged on line with NIC 1070 computer and recorded with an X-Y plotter.

The experiments were carried out on 18 Holtzman male rats weighing 250-350 g, divided into two groups: those that received pentagastrin (100 μg/kg) followed by synthetic secretin (1 μg/kg), and those that were injected intraperitoneally with CCK-OP (1 μg/kg). Each experiment consisted of an initial period of four hours of adaptation of the rat to the experimental setting, one hour of control recording taken every 10 minutes, administration of the hormone (gastrin or CCK) followed by recording every three minutes, starting 15 minutes after injection, administration of the second hormone (secretin) or a second set of recordings after the first set, again with recordings obtained 15 minutes after injection. Each recording consisted of the average field potentials evoked by 32 consecutive click stimuli at intervals of 2.5 seconds.

The configuration of the averaged acoustic evoked response (AAER) was closely similar in all the eight recording sites, and consisted of an initial diphasic (positive-negative) low amplitude spike succeeded by a large triphasic (positive-negative-positive) wave. These components were labeled as P_1, N_1, P_2, N_2 and P_3, respectively, and are evident in Figure 1.

The findings of major interest in the present experiments (Fig. 1, Table 1) are that CCK caused an early transient increase in electrical activity in

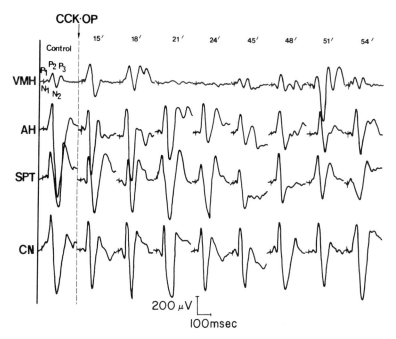

Figure 1. Average evoked responses to click stimuli recorded simultaneously from VMH, AH, SPT, and CN. Each
trace consists of the responses to 32 consecutive click
stimuli prior to drug injection (control) in the left side,
and the responses after intraperitoneal administration of
CCK-OP. Each amplitude response exhibits five components.
The first is the initial positive wave, P, followed by negative peak, N, the second positive, P_2, second negative,
N_2 and third positive wave, P_3. The numbers indicate time
in minutes after injection. In this particular rat CCK-OP
produced an initial increase (15' & 18') in the VMH, followed by a decrease in the responses and in the end, recovery. In AH the amplitude response decreased mainly from
24 minutes after injection and exhibited no recovery.
Similar results were recorded from the SPT. In CN, CCK-OP
did not alter the response.

the VMH followed by a prolonged decrease in the AAER which recovered after 50 minutes; in the LH, CCK caused an increase in the AAER at 21-24 minutes after injection; the AAER was attentuated in the AH from 45 to 60 minutes after injection of CCK; in the SPT, H and RN (all in the limbic system) mixed responses

Table 1. Summary of the general effects of CCK-OP in the various cerebral sites*

Structure	Number rats	Postinjection Time (minutes)			
		15-18	21-24	45-48	51-54
VMH	4	↑	↓	↓	–
LH	2	–	↑	–	–
RN	2	–	↑	↓	↓
AH	4	–	–	↓	↓
SPT	5	–	–	↓	↑
H	2	–	↑	–	↓
A	8	–	–	–	–
CN	2	–	–	–	–

* In ventromedial hypothalamus (VMH) we observed an initial increase followed by decreases and then recovery. In lateral hypothalamus (LH) there was no effect at the beginning, but at 21-24 minutes after injection, there was an increase in amplitudes and then recovery. In raphe nucleus (RN) no effect occurred at the beginning, but subsequently there were increases at 21-24 minutes after injection, and then the effect was reversed without recovery. In anterior hypothalamus (AH) the effect of CCK was late and was manifest as a decrease in the amplitude response without recovery. The septum pellucidum (SPT) responded late with a mixed effect -- decrease followed by increase. The dorsal hippocampus (H) also demonstrated mixed responses with only time and direction of the responses being different from the septum pellucidum. Both the amygdala complex (A) and the caudate nucleus (CN) failed to exhibit any changes in evoked responses after CCK-OP.

were recorded, and in the A (also limbic system) and CN (extrapyramidal system), no alteration in AAER was observed; and pentagastrin and secretin did not produce significant effects in any of these structures.

The specificity of these results is threefold, namely chemical, temporal, and spatial. CCK-OP, but not pentagastrin or synthetic secretin, initiated the changes in evoked responses; this specificity conforms to the observations of Gibbs and associates[3,4] that CCK-OP and CCK (but not the other two hormones) provoked satiety behavior in fasted rats. The onset of VMH depression and LH stimulation was about 20 minutes after injecting CCK-OP, and VMH changes persisted for about one-half hour; this time course is reasonable for a satiety factor. Finally, changes occurred in specific brain structures associated with regulation of appetite, namely those in the hypothalamus and limbic system, and not in the extrapyramidal system.

Our findings support the concept pictured in Figure 2. The "appetite center" interacts with upper centers, that is, the cortex, and with lower areas, which regulate vagal activity to initiate feeding and to stimulate gastrointestinal secretion and motility. The stomach empties food, containing lipid and protein, and acid into the upper gut. Contact by these dumped materials with the intestinal mucosa releases CCK into the blood. The hormone circulates to the

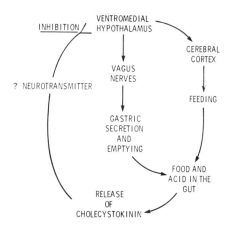

Figure 2. Our hypothesis describing the neurohumoral feedback regulation of appetite.

brain and probably interacts with at least one
neurotransmitter, that is, GABA, dopamine, norepi-
nephrine, cyclic AMP or GMP, serotonin, etc. This
leads to a change in electrophysiologic activity
of those brain areas that regulate the appetite,
namely hypothalamic and limbic structures, which
is interpreted as satiety. Some implications of
these findings in obesity and anorexia are apparent.

SUMMARY

   The onset of satiety after eating is delayed in
obesity. Satiety responses can be evoked in rats
by injection of the gastrointestinal hormone,
cholecystokinin or its biologically active synthetic
octapeptide (CCK-OP). An "appetite center" has
been postulated to exist in the ventromedial hypothalamus (VMH) and an anorectic center in the lateral
hypothalamus (LH). In conscious rats provided with
chronically implanted nichrome electrodes (50 μ
diameter) in the VMH and LH, the averaged acoustic
evoked response (AAER) from 32 repetitive click
stimuli was recorded simultaneously every three
minutes for hour-long periods of control and following injection of CCK-OP, pentagastrin or secretin.
Results were averaged on line with a computer.
Compared with control data, CCK-OP significantly
(p <0.01) decreased the AAER from the VMH at 21-48
minutes and increased AAER from the LH at 18-24
minutes after injection. Pentagastrin and synthetic
secretin were without effect. These findings are
consistent with the concept that a gastrointestinal
hormone released during feeding induces satiety by
altering central nervous electrical activity.
Obesity may be a hormone deficiency disease.

REFERENCES

1. Beaumont W: *Experiments and Observations on the Gastric
       Juice and Physiology of Digestion.* (facsimile of 1833
       edition). New York: Dover Publications, 1959, p 208.
2. Dafny N, Gilman S: L-DOPA and reserpine: Effects on
       evoked potentials in basal ganglia of freely moving
       rats. *Brain Res* 50:187-191, 1973.

3. Gibbs J, Young RC, Smith GP: Cholecystokinin decreases food intake in rats. *J Comp Physiol Psychol* 84: 488-495, 1973.

4. Gibbs J, Young RC, Smith GP: Cholecystokinin elicits satiety in rats with open gastric fistulas. *Nature* 245:323-325, 1973.

5. MacLagan NF: The role of appetite in the control of body weight. *J Physiol* 90:385-394, 1937.

APPENDIX

THE GASTRIN-CHOLECYSTOKININ FAMILY*

	Approximate molecular weight	
	I	II
Gastrin[a]		
Little gastrin (G-17)[14]		
Man	2096	2176
Hog	2114	2194
Dog	2038	2118
Cow and Sheep	2024	2104
Cat	2040	2120

Positions 1–17:

Man: Glp[b]-Gly-Pro-Trp-Leu-Glu-Glu-Glu-Glu-Glu-Ala-Tyr(SO$_3$H at 12)[c]-Gly-Trp-Met-Asp-Phe-NH$_2$

Hog: —Met— (6)
Dog: —Met— (6) —Ala— (8)
Cow and Sheep: —Met— (6) —Val— (5) —Ala— (8)
Cat: —Val— (5) —Ala— (8)

Minigastrin (G-13-I, 5-17)[12]		
Man	1647	

Leu-Glu-Glu-Glu-Glu-Ala-Tyr-Gly-Trp-Met-Asp-Phe-NH$_2$

Big gastrin (G-34-I)[11]		
Man	3839	

Glp[b]-Leu-Gly-Pro-Gln-Gly-His-Pro-Ser-Leu-Val-Ala-Asp-Pro-Ser-Lys-Lys[d]→
Gln-Gly-Pro-Trp-Leu-Glu-Glu-Glu-Glu-Ala-Tyr-Gly-Trp-Met-Asp-Phe-NH$_2$

Hog	3884	

Glp[b]-Leu-Gly-*Leu*-Gln-Gly-His-Pro-*Pro*-Leu-Val-Ala-Asp-*Leu-Ala*-Lys[d]→
Gln-Gly-Pro-Trp-*Met*-Glu-Glu-Glu-Glu-Ala-Tyr-Gly-Trp-Met-Asp-Phe-NH$_2$

Pentagastrin[15]	768	

N-t-butyloxycarbonyl-β-Ala-Trp-Met-Asp-Phe-NH$_2$

Cholecystokinin[13,16] (CCK-33)[e]	3919	

Lys-Ala-Pro-Ser-Gly-Arg-Val-Ser-Met-Ile-Lys-Asn-Leu-Gln-Ser-Leu-Asp-Pro-Ser-His-Arg-Ile-Ser-Asp-Arg-Asp-Tyr(SO$_3$H)-Met-Gly-Trp-Met-Asp-Phe-NH$_2$

Caerulein[2,3]	1352	

Glp[b]-Gln-Asp-Tyr(SO$_3$H)-Thr-Gly-Trp-Met-Asp-Phe-NH$_2$

Phyllocaerulein[1]	1206	

Glp[b]-Glu-Tyr(SO$_3$H)-Thr-Gly-Trp-Met-Asp-Phe-NH$_2$

* Modified from Thompson[18]

a Except where noted, the amino acid sequences for gastrins of different species are identical.

b Glp = Pyroglutamyl

c Gastrin of each species exists in form I and II; in form I, there is no SO$_3$H attached to Tyr in position 12.

d Points of cleavage by trypsin

e Another form of CCK with 39 amino acid residues [CCK-39] has been isolated; the two forms are equally potent.[8] The larger form is not yet chemically characterized.

THE SECRETIN-GLUCAGON FAMILY

(All sequences listed from porcine species)

Secretin[13] (mol wt 3055; 27 AA)

His-Ser-Asp-Gly-Thr-Phe-Thr-Ser-Glu-Leu-Ser-Arg-Leu-Arg-Asp-Ser-Ala-Arg-Leu-Gln-Arg-Leu-Leu-Gln-Gly-Leu-Val-NH$_2$

Glucagon[5] (mol wt 3485; 29 AA)

His-Ser-Gln-Gly-Thr-Phe-Thr-Ser-Asp-Tyr-Ser-Lys-Tyr-Leu-Asp-Ser-Arg-Arg-Ala-Gln-Asp-Phe-Val-Gln-Trp-Leu-Met-Asp-Thr

VIP[4] (mol wt 3381; 28 AA)

His-Ser-Asp-Ala-Val-Phe-Thr-Asp-Asn-Tyr-Thr-Arg-Leu-Arg-Lys-Gln-Met-Ala-Val-Lys-Lys-Tyr-Leu-Asn-Ser-Ile-Leu-Asn-NH$_2$

GIP[6] (mol wt 5105; 43 AA)

Tyr-Ala-Glu-Gly-Thr-Phe-Ile-Ser-Asp-Tyr-Ser-Ile-Ala-Met-Asp-Lys-Ile-Arg-Gln-Gln-Asp-Phe-Val-Asn-Trp-Leu-Leu-Ala-Gln-

Gln-Lys-Gly-Lys-Lys-Ser-Asp-Trp-Lys-His-Asn-Ile-Thr-Gln

RELATED COMPOUNDS

Motilin[7,17]   Phe-Val-Pro-Ile-Phe-Thr-Tyr-Gly-Glu-Leu-Gln-Arg-Met-Gln-Glu-Lys-Glu-Arg-Asn-Lys-Gly-Gln
(porcine)

Bombesin[9,10]   Glp^a-Glu-Arg-Leu-Gly-Asn-Gln-Trp-Ala-Val-Gly-His-Leu-Met-NH$_2$

a Glp = Pyroglutamyl

References

1. Anastasi A, Bertaccini G, Cei JM, DeCaro G, Erspamer V,
    Impicciatore M: Structure and pharmacological actions
    of phyllocaerulein, a caerulein-like nonapeptide: Its
    occurrence in extracts of the skin of *Phyllomedusa
    sauvagei* and related Phyllomedusa species. *Br J
    Pharmacol* 37:198-206, 1969.
2. Anastasi A, Erspamer V, Endean R: Isolation and structure
    of caerulein, an active decapeptide from the skin of
    Hyla caerulea. Experentia 23:699-700, 1967.
3. Anastasi A, Erspamer V, Endean R: Isolation and amino
    acid sequence of caerulein, the active decapeptide
    of the skin of *Hyla caerulea. Arch Biochem* 125:
    57-68, 1968.
4. Bodanszky M, Klausner YS, Said SI: Biological activities
    of synthetic peptides corresponding to fragments of
    and to the entire sequence of the vasoactive intestinal
    peptide. *Proc Natl Acad Sci USA* 70:382-383, 1973.
5. Bromer WW, Sinn LG, Behreno OK: The amino acid sequence of
    glucagon: V. Location of amide groups, acid degradation
    studies and summary of sequential evidence. *J Am Chem
    Soc* 79:2807-2810, 1957.
6. Brown JC, Dryburgh JR: A gastric inhibitory polypeptide II:
    The complete amino acid sequence. *Can J Biochem* 49:
    867-872, 1971.
7. Brown JC, Dryburgh JR: Current status of motilin, in
    Thompson JC (ed), *Gastrointestinal Hormones*, Austin:
    University of Texas Press, 1975, pp 549-554.
8. Debas HT, Grossman MI: Pure cholecystokinin: Pancreatic
    protein and bicarbonate response. *Digestion* 9:469-
    481, 1973.
9. Erspamer V, Melchiorri P: Active polypeptides of the
    amphibian skin and their synthetic analogues. *Pure
    Appl Chem* 35:463-494, 1973.
10. Erspamer V, Melchiorri P: Actions of bombesin on secretions
    and motility of the gastrointestinal tract, in Thompson
    JC (ed), *Gastrointestinal Hormones*, Austin: University
    of Texas Press, 1975, pp 575-589.
11. Gregory RA, Tracy HJ: The chemistry of the gastrins: Some
    recent advances, in Thompson JC (ed), *Gastrointestinal
    Hormones*, Austin: University of Texas Press, 1975,
    pp 13-24.
12. Grossman MI: Gastrointestinal Hormones, in Parsons JA (ed),
    Symposium on Peptide Hormones, London: Macmillan, 1974.
13. Jorpes JE: Memorial lecture: The isolation and chemistry
    of secretin and cholecystokinin. *Gastroenterology*
    55:157-164, 1968.

14. Kenner GW, Sheppard RC: Gastrins of various species, in Andersson S (ed), *Nobel Symposium 16. Frontiers in Gastrointestinal Hormone Research*, 1973, pp 137-142.
15. Morley JS, Tracy HJ, Gregory RA: Structure-function relationships in the active C-terminal tetrapeptide sequence of gastrin. *Nature* 207:1356-1359, 1965.
16. Mutt V, Jorpes JE: Isolation and primary structure of cholecystokinin-pancreozymin, in Andersson S (ed), *Nobel Symposium 16. Frontiers in Gastrointestinal Hormone Research*, 1973, pp 169-174.
17. Schubert H, Brown JC: Correction to the amino acid sequence of porcine motilin. *Can J Biochem* 52: 7-8, 1974.
18. Thompson JC: Chemical structure and biological actions of gastrin, cholecystokinin and related compounds, in Holton P (ed), *The International Encyclopedia of Pharmacology and Therapeutics*, Oxford: Pergamon Press, 1973, pp 261-286.

INDEXES